Pulmonary Medicine: A Case-Based Approach

Pulmonary Medicine: A Case-Based Approach

Editor: June Middleton

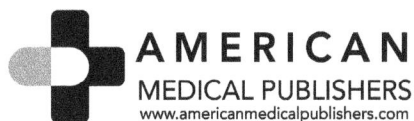

AMERICAN
MEDICAL PUBLISHERS
www.americanmedicalpublishers.com

AMERICAN
MEDICAL PUBLISHERS
www.americanmedicalpublishers.com

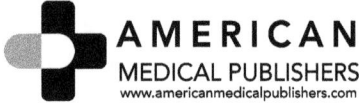

Cataloging-in-Publication Data

Pulmonary medicine : a case-based approach / edited by June Middleton.
    p. cm.
Includes bibliographical references and index.
ISBN 978-1-63927-464-2
1. Lungs--Diseases--Case studies. 2. Lungs--Diseases--Treatment--Case studies.
3. Respiratory organs--Diseases--Treatment--Case studies. I. Middleton, June.
RC756 .P85 2022
616.24--dc23

American Medical Publishers,
41 Flatbush Avenue,
1st Floor, New York,
NY 11217, USA

ISBN 978-1-63927-464-2 (Hardback)

Contents

Preface IX

Chapter 1   **Microbial yield from physiotherapy assisted sputum production in respiratory outpatients** 1
Philip J. Langridge, Reyenna L. Sheehan and David W. Denning

Chapter 2   **Observation management of pulmonary embolism and agreement with claims-based and clinical risk stratification criteria** 9
Elaine Nguyen, Craig I. Coleman, W. Frank Peacock, Philip S. Wells,
Erin R. Weeda, Veronica Ashton, Concetta Crivera, Peter Wildgoose,
Jeff R. Schein, Thomas J. Bunz and Gregory J. Fermann

Chapter 3   **Mechanical ventilation in idiopathic pulmonary fibrosis: a nationwide analysis of ventilator use, outcomes, and resource burden** 13
Joshua J. Mooney, Karina Raimundo, Eunice Chang and Michael S. Broder

Chapter 4   **Effect of sivelestat sodium in patients with acute lung injury or acute respiratory distress syndrome** 22
Shenglan Pu, Daoxin Wang, Daishun Liu, Yan Zhao, Di Qi,
Jing He and Guoqi Zhou

Chapter 5   **Impact of rapid investigation clinic on timeliness of lung cancer diagnosis and treatment** 31
Nicole Ezer, Asma Navasakulpong, Kevin Schwartzman,
Linda O iara and Anne V. Gonzalez

Chapter 6   **High-flow nasal cannula oxygen therapy versus conventional oxygen therapy in patients with acute respiratory failure** 39
Youfeng Zhu, Haiyan Yi, Rui Zhang and Jianrui Wei

Chapter 7   **Implication of species change of Nontuberculous Mycobacteria during or after treatment** 49
Jong Sik Lee, Jong Hyuk Lee, Soon Ho Yoon, Taek Soo Kim, Moon-Woo Seong,
Sung Koo Han and Jae-Joon Yim

Chapter 8   **The use of an alternate side lying positioning strategy during inhalation therapy does not prolong nebulisation time in adults with Cystic Fibrosis** 56
Ruth L. Dentice, Mark R. Elkins, Genevieve M. Dwyer and Peter T. P. Bye

Chapter 9   **The relationship between high-dose corticosteroid treatment and mortality in acute respiratory distress syndrome** 62
Takashi Kido, Keiji Muramatsu, Takeshi Asakawa, Hiroki Otsubo,
Takaaki Ogoshi, Keishi Oda, Tatsuhiko Kubo, Yoshihisa Fujino,
Shinya Matsuda, Toshihiko Mayumi, Hiroshi Mukae and Kazuhiro Yatera

Chapter 10   **Eplerenone attenuates pathological pulmonary vascular rather than right ventricular remodeling in pulmonary arterial hypertension** 69
Mario Boehm, Nadine Arnold, Adam Braithwaite, Josephine Pickworth,
Changwu Lu, Tatyana Novoyatleva, David G. Kiely, Friedrich Grimminger,
Hossein A. Ghofrani, Norbert Weissmann, Werner Seeger, Allan Lawrie,
Ralph T. Schermuly and Baktybek Kojonazarov

Chapter 11   **Comparative bench study evaluation of different infant interfaces for non-invasive ventilation** 77
Giorgio Conti, Giorgia Spinazzola, Cesare Gregoretti, Giuliano Ferrone,
Andrea Cortegiani, Olimpia Festa, Marco Piastra,
Luca Tortorolo and Roberta Costa

Chapter 12   **Anti-fibrotic effects of pirfenidone and rapamycin in primary IPF fibroblasts and human alveolar epithelial cells** 85
M. Molina-Molina, C. Machahua-Huamani, V. Vicens-Zygmunt,
R. Llatjós, I. Escobar, E. Sala-Llinas, P. Luburich-Hernaiz,
J. Dorca and A. Montes-Worboys

Chapter 13   **Management of acute respiratory failure in interstitial lung diseases: overview and clinical insights** 98
Paola Faverio, Federica De Giacomi, Luca Sardella, Giuseppe Fiorentino,
Mauro Carone, Francesco Salerno, Jousel Ora, Paola Rogliani, Giulia Pellegrino,
Giuseppe Francesco Sferrazza Papa, Francesco Bini, Bruno Dino Bodini,
Grazia Messinesi, Alberto Pesci and Antonio Esquinas

Chapter 14   **Balloon pulmonary angioplasty – efficient therapy of chronic thromboembolic pulmonary hypertension in the patient with advanced sarcoidosis** 111
Andrzej Labyk, Dominik Wretowski, Sabina Zybińska-Oksiutowicz,
Aleksandra Furdyna, Katarzyna Ciesielska, Dorota Piotrowska-Kownacka,
Olga Dzikowska –Diduch, Barbara Lichodziejewska, Andrzej Biederman,
Piotr Pruszczyk and Marek Roik

Chapter 15   **Lower mortality after early supervised pulmonary rehabilitation following COPD exacerbations** 116
Camilla Koch Ryrsø, Nina Skavlan Godtfredsen, Linette Marie Kofod,
Marie Lavesen, Line Mogensen, Randi Tobberup, Ingeborg Farver-Vestergaard,
Henriette Edemann Callesen, Britta Tendal,
Peter Lange and Ulrik Winning Iepsen

Chapter 16   **Role of medical Thoracoscopy in the Management of Multiloculated Empyema** 134
Kamran Khan Sumalani, Nadeem Ahmed Rizvi and Asif Asghar

Chapter 17   **Degree of control of patients with chronic obstructive pulmonary disease** 140
Adolfo Baloira, José Miguel Rodriguez Gonzalez-Moro, Estefanía Sanjuán,
Juan Antonio Trigueros and Ricard Casamor

Chapter 18   **National survey: current prevalence and characteristics of home mechanical ventilation** 148
Luca Valko, Szabolcs Baglyas, Janos Gal and Andras Lorx

Chapter 19   **Efficacy of 1, 5, and 20 mg oral sildenafil in the treatment of adults with pulmonary arterial hypertension**... 155
Carmine Dario Vizza, B. K. S. Sastry, Zeenat Safdar, Lutz Harnisch, Xiang Gao, Min Zhang, Manisha Lamba and Zhi-Cheng Jing

Chapter 20   **Effects of treadmill exercise versus Flutter® on respiratory flow and sputum properties in adults with cystic fibrosis**.. 167
Tiffany J. Dwyer, Rahizan Zainuldin, Evangelia Daviskas, Peter T. P. Bye, and Jennifer A. Alison

Chapter 21   **Successful treatment of severe *Pneumocystis* pneumonia in an immunosuppressed patient using caspofungin combined with clindamycin**............................. 175
Hongjuan Li, Haoming Huang and Hangyong He

Chapter 22   **Efficacy of concurrent treatments in idiopathic pulmonary fibrosis patients with a rapid progression of respiratory failure**... 181
Keishi Oda, Kazuhiro Yatera, Yoshihisa Fujino, Hiroshi Ishimoto, Hiroyuki Nakao, Tetsuya Hanaka, Takaaki Ogoshi, Takashi Kido, Kiyohide Fushimi, Shinya Matsuda and Hiroshi Mukae

Permissions

List of Contributors

Index

Preface

Over the recent decade, advancements and applications have progressed exponentially. This has led to the increased interest in this field and projects are being conducted to enhance knowledge. The main objective of this book is to present some of the critical challenges and provide insights into possible solutions. This book will answer the varied questions that arise in the field and also provide an increased scope for furthering studies.

Pulmonary medicine deals with the diseases that are associated with the respiratory tract. It manages patients needing advanced life support and mechanical ventilation. Pulmonary medicine is helpful in treating diseases like pneumonia, asthma, tuberculosis, emphysema, etc. Some of the clinical procedures that fall under its domain are spirometry, bronchoscopy, CT scanning, scintigraphy, etc. Inhalation of bronchodilators and steroids, and intake of oral antibiotics and leukotriene antagonists are important in the treatment of pulmonary diseases. Surgical procedures such as pleuroscopy and bronchoscopy are also performed in pulmonary medicine to treat severe diseases. This book studies, analyses and upholds the pillars of pulmonary medicine and its utmost significance in modern times. It is a compilation of chapters that discuss the most vital concepts and emerging trends in the field of pulmonary medicine. Those in search of information to further their knowledge will be greatly assisted by this book.

I hope that this book, with its visionary approach, will be a valuable addition and will promote interest among readers. Each of the authors has provided their extraordinary competence in their specific fields by providing different perspectives as they come from diverse nations and regions. I thank them for their contributions.

Editor

Microbial yield from physiotherapy assisted sputum production in respiratory outpatients

Philip J. Langridge[1], Reyenna L. Sheehan[1] and David W. Denning[1,2]*

Abstract

Background: Sputum is a key diagnostic sample for those with chronic chest conditions including chronic and allergic aspergillus-related disease, but often not obtained in clinic.
The objective of this study was to evaluate physiotherapeutic interventions to obtain sputum from those not able to spontaneously produce and the subsequent microbiological result.

Methods: Sputum samples were collected by physiotherapists from patients attending routine outpatient clinics managing their aspergillus-related diseases who were unable to spontaneously produce. Active Cycle of Breathing Techniques (ACBT) technique was applied first, for 10 min, followed by hypertonic saline induction using a Pari LC plus or Pari Sprint nebuliser, if necessary and deemed safe to do so. Samples processed in the laboratory using standard microbiological techniques for bacterial and fungal culture with the addition of *Aspergillus* real-time PCR.

Results: Samples were procured from 353 of 364 (97 %) patients, 231 (65 %) by ACBT and 119 (34 %) with administration of hypertonic saline. Three of 125 (2.4 %) patients had significant bronchospasm during sputum induction. Sixteen patients' sputum tested positive for *Aspergillus* culture, contrasting with 82 whose *Aspergillus* PCR was positive, 59 with a strong signal. PCR improved detection of *Aspergillus* by 350 %. Sputum from 124 (34 %) patients cultured other potentially pathogenic organisms which justified specific therapy.

Conclusions: Physiotherapeutic interventions safely and effectively procured sputum from patients unable to spontaneously produce. The method for sputum induction was well-tolerated and time-efficient, with important microbiological results.

Keywords: Sputum, Induced, Physiotherapy, Aspergillus, Hypertonic

Background

Induced sputum using nebulised saline to induce a productive cough has been studied for diagnosing *Pneumocystis* pneumonia (PCP) and pulmonary aspergillosis [1, 2]. Many patients attending clinics report they are not able to produce sputum spontaneously on request, having discarded their morning sputum. Yet a respiratory sample is critical for microbiological diagnosis of bacterial and fungal infections. Furthermore the yield of *Aspergillus* spp. from fungal cultures of sputum is poor and molecular diagnosis more sensitive, [3, 4], although improved means of processing specimens has been shown to improve culture yield [4, 5]. In patients with complex respiratory problems, multiple pathogens are common, the most common of which are *Streptococcus pneumoniae*, *Haemophilus influenzae*, *Pseudomonas aeruginosa* and *Aspergillus fumigatus*. Therapy of these different infections varies substantially and may be further influenced by resistance profiles. Hence accessing respiratory samples becomes an important part of clinical assessment and consequent improved outcomes, rather than relying on empirical choices, which are often unsuccessful.

The techniques for assisting sputum production include the Active Cycle of Breathing Techniques (ACBT) and sputum induction, prior to more invasive and costly

* Correspondence: ddenning@manchester.ac.uk
[1]The National Aspergillosis Centre, ERC, 2nd floor, University Hospital South Manchester, Southmoor Road, Manchester M23 9LT, UK
[2]The University of Manchester; Manchester Academic Health Science Centre, Manchester, UK

bronchoscopy. Induced sputum production with nebulised hypertonic saline was reported to carry a 14-27 % rate of significant bronchospasm, [6, 7].

Many of the patients attending the National Aspergillosis Centre have complex respiratory problems with an average of 2.5 underlying respiratory conditions [8]. The microbiological yield, adverse events and general challenges of regular use of sputum production using ACBT and nebulised hypertonic saline in the outpatient setting has not been studied previously. This became possible in our service because of the routine contribution made by experienced physiotherapists in our aspergillosis clinics, employed expressly to contribute to infection diagnosis, as well as providing patient advice and training and administering/ assessing safety of nebulised antibiotics and antifungals.

Here we review our experience of physiotherapist-directed efforts to acquire sputum samples, the sputum production rates, adverse events and the microbiological yield. Our service has an extremely low rate of pulmonary tuberculosis (PTB), so we infrequently requested mycobacterial culture, despite our clinical observation that the relative rate of non-tuberculous mycobacterial (NTM) infection in chronic pulmonary aspergillosis (CPA) is higher than in general respiratory practice. We therefore cannot comment on the performance of these techniques on mycobacterial smear or culture yield. The focus is on rapidly growing bacteria, fungal culture and *Aspergillus* PCR.

Methods

Patients and clinics

Three hundred and sixty four patients aged 22-90 years on treatment for, or thought to have *Aspergillus* disease, including chronic pulmonary aspergillosis (CPA), allergic bronchopulmonary aspergillosis (ABPA), severe asthma with fungal sensitization (SAFS) and/or *Aspergillus* bronchitis (Table 1) were referred for sputum induction. All were attending the National Aspergillosis Centre in Manchester and were unable to spontaneously produce a sputum sample. These samples were sent for microbiological testing as directed by the physician. This report is a retrospective service evaluation of all patients who underwent physiotherapy-assisted sputum production in the outpatient clinics between 25/04/2012 and 23/04/2014 to assess sample yield and safety, and as such is exempt from ethical review. These physiotherapeutic interventions were performed as part of their standard care in clinic and consent for each intervention was obtained accordingly.

Disease definitions

The diagnosis of CPA was based primarily on antibody and radiological data, [8, 9], ABPA primarily on clinical

Table 1 Working clinical diagnoses in 364 patients

Diagnosis	No of patients with provisional or confirmed diagnosis
Chronic pulmonary aspergillosis	183
ABPA	58
ABPA and CPA	9
Aspergillus bronchitis	41
Single aspergilloma	5
Severe Asthma with Fungal Sensitisation	8
Asthma with fungal sensitisation	3
Subacute invasive aspergillosis	7
Aspergillus airway colonisation	1
Aspergillus pericarditis	1
Aspergillus sinusitis	1
Candida bronchitis	2
Other	45

ABPA allergic bronchopulmonary aspergillosis, *CPA* chronic pulmonary aspergillosis

and serological data, [10], SAFS as described previously, [11, 12] and *Aspergillus* bronchitis as recently revisited [13].

Sputum production techniques

After gaining consent, patients were firstly instructed in ACBT which was performed for 10 min (see Fig 1). If this was unsuccessful, consideration was given to nebulised hypertonic saline (7 % NaCl) to induce sputum (Figs. 1, 2 and 3). Previous intolerance of nebulised hypertonic saline, lack of consent, and/or perceived exceptionally high clinical risk (e.g. FEV1 < 0.5 L) excluded patients from induction with hypertonic saline. Hypertonic saline was administered via the breath enhanced Pari LC plus or Pari Sprint nebulisers driven by Clement Clarke's Econoneb compressor. The patients excluded from sputum induction and unable to produce after 10 min of ACBT were offered alternative physiotherapeutic modalities including postural drainage, autogenic drainage and "bubble" positive expiratory pressure.

Microbiological methods

Generally 2 samples were provided, one for microscopy with gram stain and bacterial and fungal culture, the other for DNA extraction and *Aspergillus*-specific PCR. Sputum was digested with Sputasol® (ratio 1:1), vortexed, a slide prepared for gram stain and 10 μL-streaked on two Sabouraud dextrose agar plates [14] and incubated at 30 °C and 37 °C for 7 days. DNA extraction was performed from 0.5–3 mL of sample using the MycXtra kit

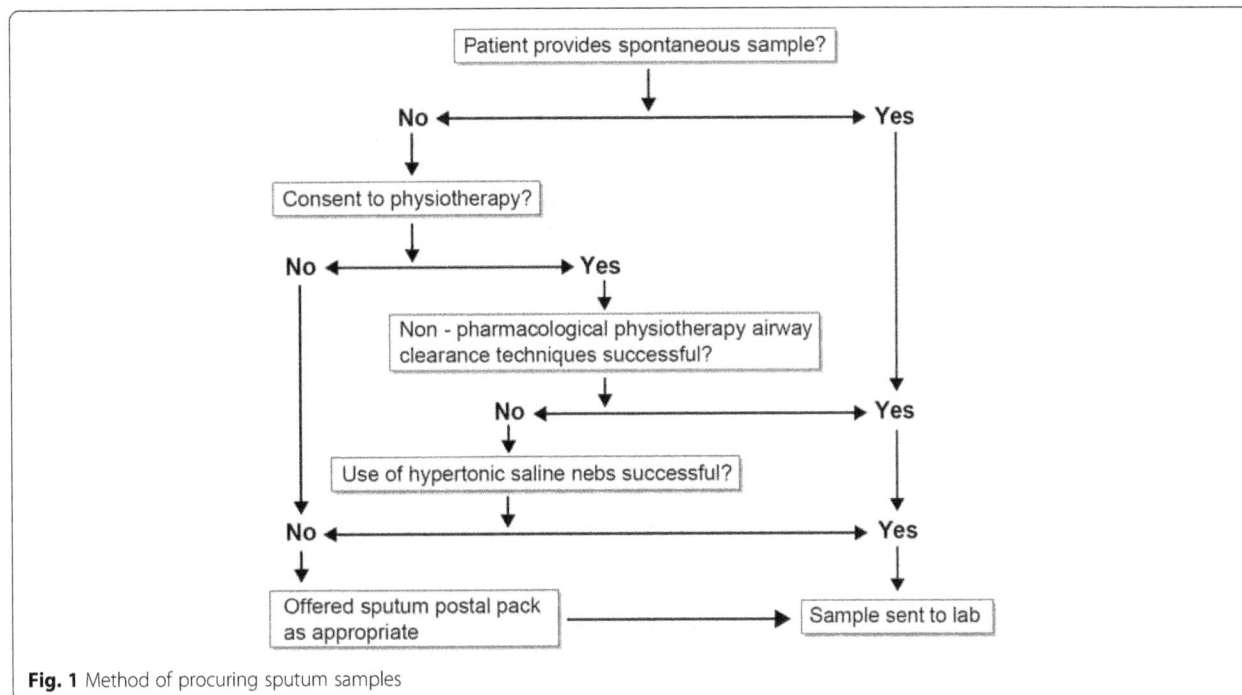

Fig. 1 Method of procuring sputum samples

(Myconostica, Cambridge, UK). DNA was eluted in 40 μL of buffer S5 and 10 μL was used for quantitative PCR (qPCR) with the MycAssay Aspergillus kit (Myconostica) [3]. As per the manufacturer instructions, a Ct of >38 is negative, a Ct from 36-38 is a weak positive and <36 is interpreted as a strong positive. Susceptibility testing of Aspergillus isolates was routinely done and reported, as previously described [15].

Results

Table 1 shows the working diagnoses of the patients on referral. Sputum was procured in 353 out of 364 patients (97 %) by ACBT (231 (65 %)) or hypertonic sputum induction 119 (34 %). Three of 125 (2.4 %) patients had significant bronchospasm during sputum induction. ACBT was unsuccessful in a further 8 patients who declined hypertonic sputum induction and sputum was not produced by 3 patients who underwent hypertonic sputum induction. Seven patients had sputa obtained from physiotherapists at multiple clinic dates. One patient, in the process of nebulised acetylcysteine challenge testing, produced sputum. Another patient required aseptic endotracheal suction via tracheostomy to gather sputum. ACBT took about 15 min per patient and if ACBT was followed by hypertonic saline induction, which took ~25 min per patient.

Several organisms were cultured from sputum samples (Table 2). One hundred and twenty three samples were culture positive - 56 probably significant bacteria, including one *Mycobacteria avium intracellulare*, 16 *Aspergillus* spp and 51 *Candida* spp., *Saccharomyces*

cerevisiae or other probably insignificant yeasts. Among the bacteria were two patients with MRSA, 19 with *Pseudomonas aeruginosa* and 2 with *Stenotrophomonas maltophilia*, classically organisms that do not respond to standard antibiotics for community acquired pneumonia.

Of the 3 methods used to detect *Aspergillus*, only 18 patients' sputum showed fungal elements on microscopy consistent with *Aspergillus* spp. and 16 grew *Aspergillus* in culture (Tables 2 and 3). Culture was slightly more often positive from ACBT samples (5 %) than hypertonic induced sputum (2 %), but this was not significant by Fisher Exact test ($p = 0.28$). Of the 18 microscopy positive samples, only 7 of these tested positive for *Aspergillus* PCR, consistent with other fungi being implicated in symptoms (one was *Scedosporium apiospermum*), *Candida* pseudohyphae being seen or contaminated microscopy materials. Eighty-two samples were *Aspergillus* PCR positive (Table 3), of which 59 (72 %) had strong signals; four had a technical failure. Twenty three samples were positive by PCR and culture and/or microscopy. Of the 74 samples negative for both fungal culture and microscopy, fungal PCR was strongly positive in 37 (50 %). There was a slightly higher frequency of strong signals from sputum obtained by ACBT than with induced sputum (76 % versus 64 %), but this was not significant by chi-square (p = 0.27).

Of the 16 *Aspergillus* isolates grown, 3 were not referred for susceptibility testing. The *A. terreus* isolate was resistant to amphotericin B (minimum inhibitory concentration (MIC) = >8 mg/L), and susceptble to itraconazole, voriconazole and posaconazole. Nine isolates

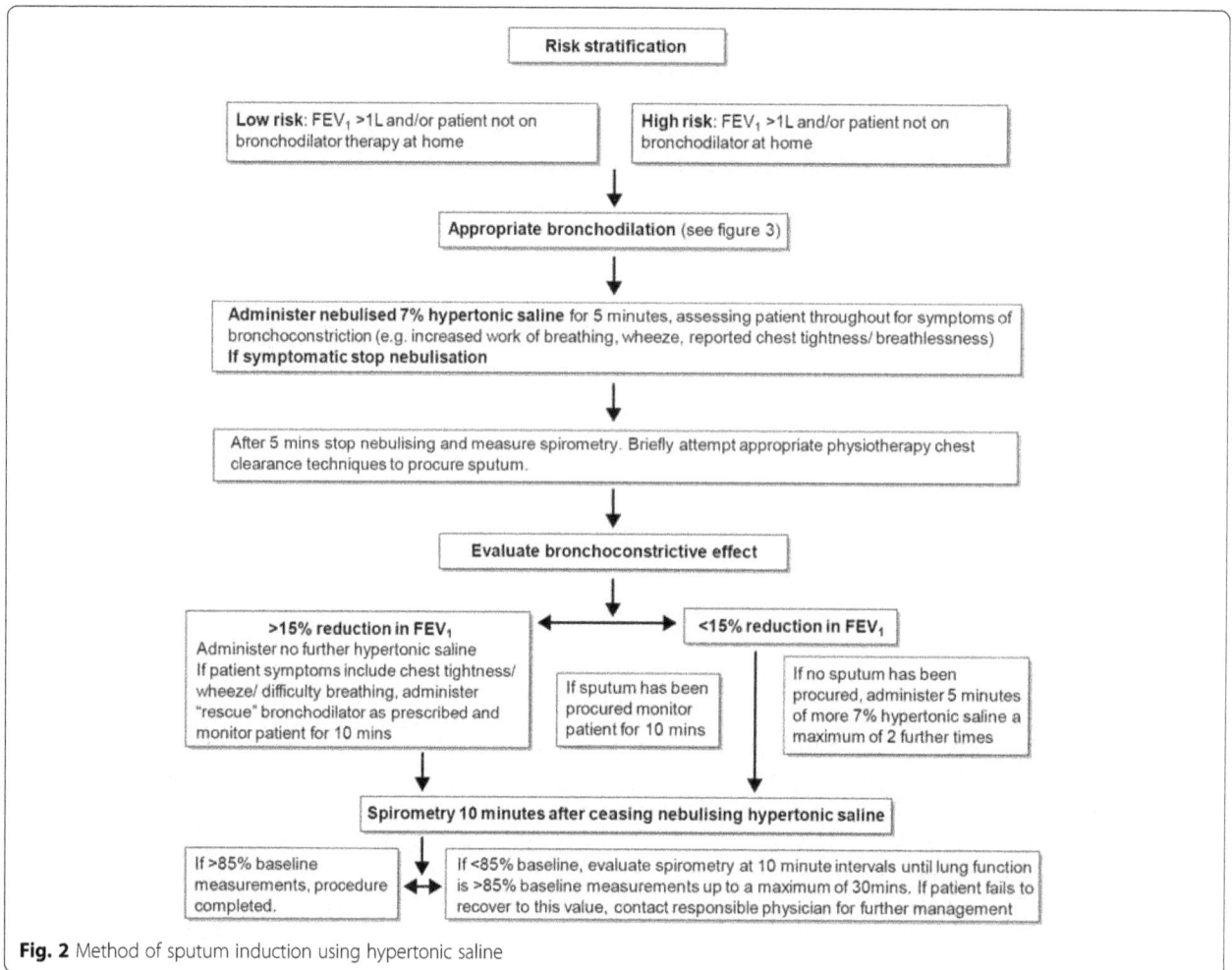

Fig. 2 Method of sputum induction using hypertonic saline

were fully susceptible. One *A. fumigatus* strain was solely resistant to voriconazole (MIC >8 mg/L) and two were panazole resistant, with MICs to all 3 azoles of >8 mg/L, and susceptible to amphotericin B. Overall, therefore 4 (31 %) isolates were resistant to one or more drugs.

Discussion

The interventions from the specialist physiotherapists were well tolerated and successful in procuring sputum for testing. On site sampling led to timely processing. Eight patients failed to produce sputum using physiotherapeutic techniques but were unsuitable to go on to have sputum induction using hypertonic saline (e.g. time constraints, high clinical risk, lack of consent). Our fall-back position for these patients is to given them a sterile pot for expectoration, with special packaging, pre-paid addressed plastic envelope and request form ("postal pack for sputum"), which is also successful, although slower.

Little has been published about induced sputum and resultant bacterial culture. One study of 48 children with CF showed that in 2 cases samples induced with nebulised 7 % saline grew additional organisms compared with the prior spontaneous sample [16]. Positive bacterial culture may alter empirical antibiotic treatment or prompt further investigation. For example, gram negative cultures may prompt intravenous antibiotic treatment or further investigation for bronchiectasis diagnosis.

Empirical antifungal therapy for *Aspergillus* is rarely given in the outpatient setting. Arguably finding *Aspergillus* (by whatever method) has a potentially profound impact on management. While colonization of the airway is more common in certain settings such as COPD or cystic fibrosis, finding *Aspergillus* usually means some form of aspergillosis [17, 18]. Here culture was positive in 16 patients, whereas PCR was positive 72 patients, with a strong signal in 59, an improved yield of 360 %. Monitoring sputum fungal loads with the strength of PCR signal aids treatment efficacy monitoring [19]. Unlike with PCP, [20] the cost-effectiveness of sputum induction for *Aspergillus*-related disease has not been

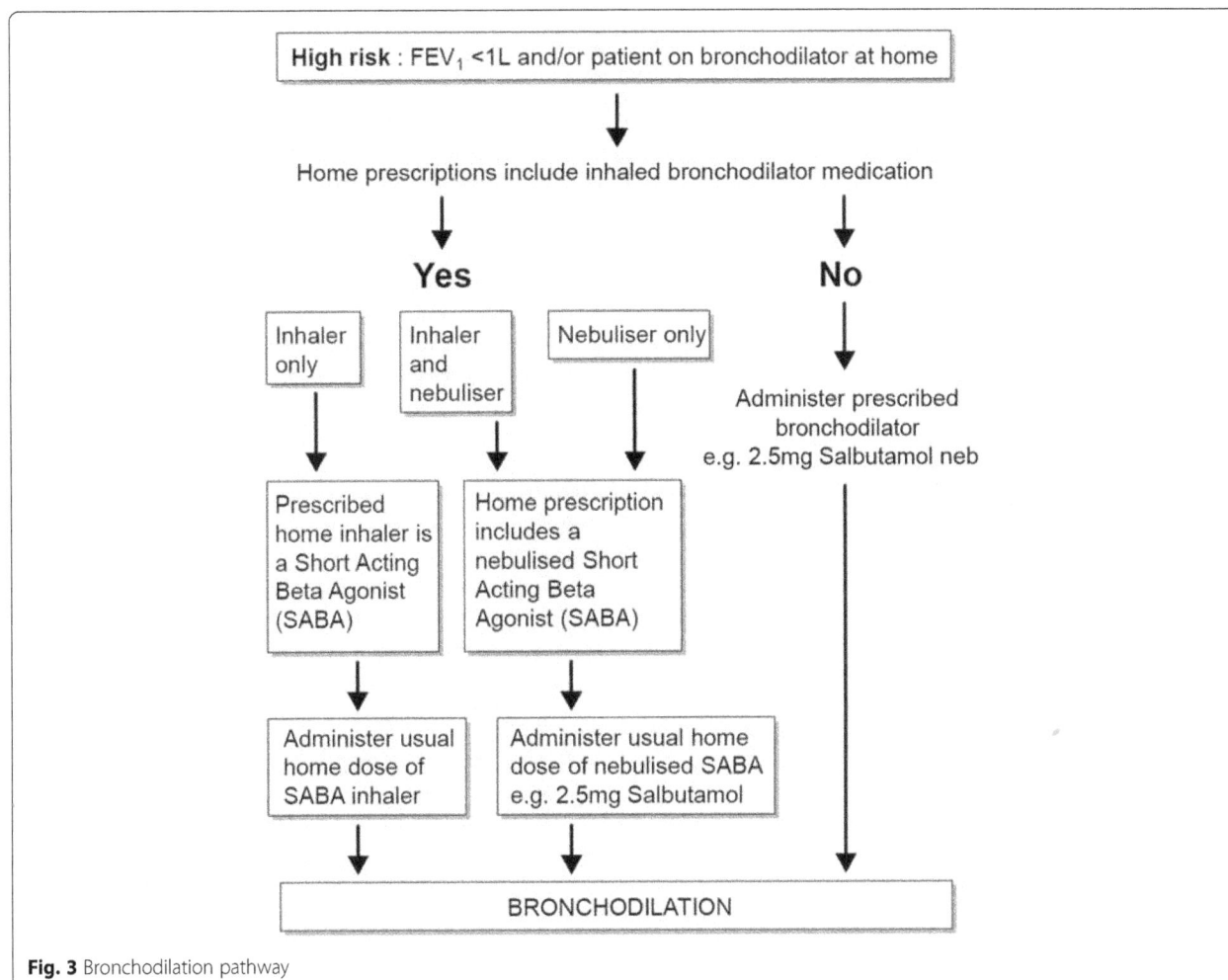

Fig. 3 Bronchodilation pathway

estimated. It is expected that sputum induction in the management of *Aspergillus*-related disease is likely to be cost-effective when compared to bronchoalveolar lavage, and may have a higher yield [4].

Adverse effects
Non-pharmacological physiotherapy airway clearance techniques were extremely well tolerated with no reported problems. Two hundred and thirty nine patients needed only this intervention to produce sputum, which required short treatment times of up to 10 min.

One hundred and twenty five patients underwent hypertonic saline challenge for sputum induction. Three (2 %) of those induced with hypertonic saline experienced bronchospasm, all of whom required rescue with nebulised bronchodilator. All patients returned home safely the same day of their clinic appointment. In a previous service evaluation, of those adult non-CF patients challenged with 4 ml 7 % saline, 17 % of subjects showed an initial >15 % drop in FEV_1 reaction to inhalation of

4 ml 7 % saline. Makris *et al.* [6] report an incidence of bronchospasm of approximately 27 % when performing sputum induction with COPD patients. They found 31 % presented with a hyperresponsive (>20 % drop in FEV_1) reaction to inhalation of 4.5 % saline, despite a preceding dose of 200 µg salbutamol via metered dose inhaler. This may be partly accounted for by the fact that in their study there was a 4 week washout period with no inhaled/oral steroid use, and long acting bronchodilators and short acting bronchodilators were omitted 12 and 8 h respectively before interventions. In our service evaluation, patients had taken their usual steroid/ bronchodilator medication which accounts for the low rate of associated bronchospasm. Also, in our service evaluation the patients received 5 min inhalations of 7 % saline, approximating to a dose of 2 ml over the 5 min. This lower dose, although sufficient to yield sputum for sampling, may not have been enough to precipitate bronchospasm. Some patients, however, received 5 min of 7 % saline inhalations repeated 3 times (total approximate dose 6 ml) with no duly associated increased adverse effects.

Table 2 Microbiological (culture) yield by organism

	Non-pharmacological physiotherapy airway clearance techniques	Hypertonic saline
Probably significant organisms		
Aspergillus fumigatus complex	12	3
Aspergillus terreus	1	0
Haemophilus influenzae	9	5
Haemophilus parainfluenzae	1	0
Staphylococcus aureus	2	2
Methicillin resistant Staphylococcus aureus	2	0
Escherichia coli	1	1
Pseudomonas aeruginosa	16	3
Pseudomonas eurefenosa	1	0
Mycobacterium Intracellulare	0	1
Moraxella catarrhalis	1	1
Enterobacter cloacae	0	1
Streptococcus pneumoniae	3	0
Citrobacter koseri	1	1
Serratia marcescens	1	0
Stenotrophomononas maltophilia	2	0
Acinetobacter haemolyticus	1	0
Probably insignificant organisms		
Saccharomyces cerevisiae	2	0
Candida albicans	16	7
Candida glabrata	7	3
Candida lusitaniae	0	1
Candida tropicalis	1	1
Candida parapsilosis	1	0
Unidentified fungus	5	1
Yeasts unspecified	4	2
Total	91	33

Clinical impact of sputum testing

Patients with MRSA ($n = 2$), *Pseudomonas aeruginosa* ($n = 19$) and *Stenotrophomonas maltophilia* ($n = 2$) require alternative antibiotics and often dose escalation for successful eradication. These are therefore important findings. The diagnosis of *Aspergillus* bronchitis requires repeated identification of *Aspergillus* species in the airway, by whatever means (13). Forty one patients studied had this diagnosis. A stronger PCR signal implies disease rather than colonisation [17]. In the context of patients taking oral antifungal azole therapy with therapeutic antifungal levels, a strong PCR signal probably signifies triazole antifungal resistance.

Tolerance of nebulised hypertonic saline in the context of sputum induction may provide helpful reassurance about long term use for patient's needing this intervention of chronic disease management (e.g. bronchiectasis and ABPA) [21].

Limitations

The patients had mixed respiratory diagnoses, reflecting real life clinic experience. It was impractical to retrospectively evaluate the clinical impact of 364 physiotherapy interventions without additional resources. It was not noted *a priori* what samples were obtained per patient at time of collection: the results were examined retrospectively from an electronic pathology reporting system (SunQuest ICE). For the first year of the study date, the sputum requesting was done using paper forms so there is no accessible audit trail to differentiate what was sent for processing and what results actually were: there may have been lost and/or insufficient samples. Very few samples were submitted for mycobacterial culture and acid fast bacillus microscopy.

The ACBT, when used, was tailored specifically to the clinical presentation at the time by the physiotherapist so that the interventions may differ subtly in terms of techniques used, repetitions etc. Also, the dose of hypertonic saline administered did vary between patients according to when sputum was produced.

Choice of nebuliser/compressor may influence delivery of hypertonic saline [22]. However, a recommendation that ultrasonic nebulisers should be used due to usually inadequate outputs from other nebulisers [23, 24] no longer necessarily applies [25, 26]: the output from the Pari Sprint nebuliser is 590 mg/min, mass median diameter 2.9 μg and 75 % particles below 5 μm (when driven by PARI Boy® SX compressor). Practicalities inherent to ultrasonic nebulisers (e.g. access, cleaning, cost) may steer clinicians to other equipment, especially when doing so still results in the desired outcome *viz.* sputum sample procurement.

The equipment used was what was readily accessible in the clinic. When routinely tested by the medical engineering department, the compressor flow rates varied between 7.5 and 9.5 Lpm despite being the same makes/

Table 3 Success in yielding sputum from 364 patients with the 2 techniques used and the microbiological results obtained

	Physiotherapy techniques (%)	Induced sputum (%)	Totals (%)
Total number patients treated	239	125*	364
Unable to procure sputum from patient	8 (3)[a]	3 (2)[a]	353 (97
Sputum induction discontinued due to adverse effects	0	3 (2)[b]	3 (1)
Positive bacterial and/or fungal culture	76 (32)	29 (23)	105 (30)
Positive *Aspergillus* PCR	54 (23 %)	28 (22 %)	82 (23)
Strongly positive *Aspergillus* PCR (Ct <36)	41 (76 %)	18 (64 %)	58 (16)
Aspergillus cultured	13 (5 %)	3 (2 %)	16 (5)
Hyphae consistent with *Aspergillus* spp. seen on sputum microscopy	11 (5 %)	7 (6 %)	18 (5)

* 1 patient required N-acetylcysteine. [a] patient declined; [b] patients wheezy
PCR polymerase chain reaction

models. This variance in flow rate would result in varying nebuliser outputs [27].

The goal of the interventions was to elicit sputum from those who could not spontaneously produce. It is not known whether sputum gained from ACBT yielded more clinically-relevant information than that elicited after inhalation of 7 % hypertonic saline. Neither is it known whether unsuccessful airway clearance techniques reduced the time or dose required for subsequent nebulised hypertonic saline to produce a sputum sample. Elkins *et al* [20] evaluated the effect of airway clearance techniques as part of sputum induction: they showed organism identification did not improve with them, but the difference in sensitivities of the tests was 7 % better with airway clearance techniques. It is also not known from this evaluation if there is an order effect on success of testing: if 2 sputum samples were produced the first one could have been sent for culture, the second for PCR or vice-versa. It is also not known how spontaneous samples tested compared to physiotherapist-collected samples. It is recommended that future work investigates the order effect of sputum sampling and that physiotherapist-collected samples are compared to spontaneously-produced ones when subjected to fungal testing.

Conclusion

Physiotherapeutic interventions safely and effectively procured sputum from patients unable to spontaneously produce. The method for sputum induction was well-tolerated and time-efficient, with important microbiological results. Molecular detection of *Aspergillus* spp. was superior to culture, although resistance was found in 31 % of those that were cultured. Sputum from 34 % patients cultured other potentially pathogenic organisms which justified specific therapy.

Abbreviations
ABPA: allergic bronchopulmonary aspergillosis; ACBT: active cycle of breathing technique; CF: cystic fibrosis; CPA: chronic pulmonary aspergillosis; Lpm: Litres per minute; MIC: minimum inhibitory concentration; MRSA: methicillin resistant *Staphylococcus aureus*; NTM: non-tuberculous mycobacterial infection; PCP: *Pneumocystis* pneumonia; PCR: polymerase chain reaction; SAFS: severe asthma with fungal sensitization.

Competing interests
PJL and RLS have no potential conflicts of interest. Dr Denning holds Founder shares in F2G Ltd a University of Manchester spin-out antifungal discovery company, in Novocyt which markets the Myconostica real-time molecular assays and has current grant support from the National Institute of Allergy and Infectious Diseases, National Institute of Health Research, North-West Lung Centre Charity, Medical Research Council, Astellas and the Fungal Infection Trust. He acts or has recently acted as a consultant for Basilea, Astellas, Sigma Tau and Pulmicort. In the last 3 years, he has been paid for talks on behalf of Astellas, Dynamiker, Gilead, Merck and Pfizer. He is also a member of the Infectious Disease Society of America Aspergillosis Guidelines and European Society for Clinical Microbiology and Infectious Diseases Aspergillosis Guidelines groups.

Authors' contributions
RLS and PJL completed the physiotherapeutic procedures concerned with sputum procurement as well as collation and interpretation of data and drafting and editing the manuscript. DWD participated in the study design and manuscript editing, and data retrieval on resistance. All authors read and approved the final manuscript.

Acknowledgements
We are indebted to the patients who graciously submitted to physiotherapy assessment and diagnostic sputum induction. We are also indebted to the specialist nurses Georgina Powell, Deborah Kennedy and Deborah Hawker for facilitating each patient's journey in clinic.

Funding
This work was completely funded by the National Health Service via national specialised commissioning to the National Aspergillosis Centre.

References
1. Leigh TR, Hume C, Gazzard B, et al. Sputum induction for diagnosis of *Pneumocystis carinii* pneumonia. Lancet. 1989;2:205–6.
2. Wark PAB, Saltos N, Simpson J, Slater S, Hensley MJ, Gibson PG. Induced sputum eosinophils and neutrophils and bronchiectasis severity in allergic bronchopulmonary aspergillosis. Eur Respir J. 2000;16:1095–101.
3. Denning DW, Park S, Lass-Florl C, Fraczek MG, Kirwan M, Gore R, et al. High frequency triazole resistance found in non-culturable *Aspergillus fumigatus* from lungs of patients with chronic fungal disease. Clin Infect Dis. 2011;52: 1123–9.
4. Fraczek MG, Kirwan MB, Moore CB, Morris J, Denning DW, Richardson MD. Volume dependency for culture of fungi from respiratory secretions and increased sensitivity of *Aspergillus* quantitative PCR. Mycoses. 2014;57:69–78.
5. Pashley CH, Fairs A, Morley JP, Tailor S, Agbetile J, Bafadhel M, et al. Routine processing procedures for isolating filamentous fungi from respiratory

sputum samples may underestimate fungal prevalence. Med Mycol. 2012;50: 433–8.

6. Makris D, Tzanakis N, Moschandreas J, et al. Dyspnea assessment and adverse events during sputum induction in COPD. BMC Pulm Med. 2006;6: 1–9.

7. Fahey JV, Boushey HA, Lazarus SC, et al. Safety and reproducibility of sputum induction in asthmatic subjects in a multicenter study. Am J Respir Crit Care Med. 2001;163:1470–5.

8. Smith N, Denning DW. Underlying pulmonary disease frequency in patients with chronic pulmonary aspergillosis. Eur Resp J. 2011;37:865–72.

9. Denning DW, Riniotis K, Dobrashian R, Sambatakou H. Chronic cavitary and fibrosing pulmonary and pleural aspergillosis: Case series, proposed nomenclature and review. Clin Infect Dis. 2003;37 Suppl 3:S265–80.

10. Agarwal R, Chakrabarti A, Shah A, et al. Allergic bronchopulmonary aspergillosis: review of literature and proposal of new diagnostic and classification criteria. Clin Exp Allergy. 2013;43:850–73.

11. Denning DW, O'Driscoll BR, Powell G, et al. Randomized controlled trial of oral antifungal treatment for severe asthma with fungal sensitisation (SAFS), the FAST study. Am J Resp Crit Care Med. 2009;179:11–8.

12. Denning DW, Pashley C, Hartl D, et al. Fungal allergy in asthma–state of the art and research needs. Clin Transl Allergy. 2014;4:14. doi:10.1186/2045-7022-4-14. Published online 2014 April 15.

13. Chrdle A, Mustakim S, Bright-Thomas R, Baxter C, Felton T, Denning DW. *Aspergillus* bronchitis in non-immunocompromised patients – case series, response to treatment and criteria for diagnosis. Ann NY Acad Sci. 2012; 1272:73–85.

14. UK standards for microbiological investigations: Investigation of bronchoalveolar sputum and associated specimens. https://www.gov.uk/ government/uploads/system/uploads/attachment_data/file/343994/B_57i2. 5.pdf (Accessed 15th August 2015).

15. Bueid A, Howard SJ, Moore CB, et al. Azole antifungal resistance in *Aspergillus fumigatus* – 2008 and 2009. J Antimicob Chemother. 2010;65: 2116–8.

16. Suri R, Marshall LJ, Wallis C, et al. Safety and use of sputum induction in children with cystic fibrosis. Pediatr Pulmonol. 2003;35:309–13.

17. Lewis White P, Barnes RA. *Aspergillus* PCR. Platforms, strengths and weaknesses. Med Mycol. 2006;44:S191–8.

18. Bretagne S, Costa JM, Marmarot-Khuong A, et al. Detection of *Aspergillus* species DNA in bronchoalveolar lavage samples by competitive PCR. J Clin Microbiol. 1995;33:1164–8.

19. Kosmidis C, Denning DW. The clinical spectrum of pulmonary aspergillosis. Thorax. 2015;70:270–7.

20. Harris JR, Marston BJ, Sangrujee N, DuPlessis D, Park B. Cost-effectiveness analysis of diagnostic options for Pneumocystis Pneumonia (PCP). PLoS ONE. 2001;6:e23158.

21. Pasteur MC, Bilton D, Hill AT. British Thoracic Society guideline for non-CF bronchiectasis. Thorax. 2010;65:i1–58.

22. Elkins MR, Lane T, Goldberg H, et al. Effect of airway clearance techniques on the efficacy of the sputum induction procedure. Eur Respir J. 2005;26: 904–8.

23. Paggiaro PL, Chanez P, Holz O, Ind PW, Djukanovic R, Maestrelli P, et al. Sputum induction. Eur Respir J. 2002;37(Suppl):3s–8s.

24. Pizzichini MMM, Leigh R, Djukanovic R, Sterk PJ. Safety of sputum induction. Eur Respir J. 2002;27(Suppl):9s–18s.

25. Elkins M. Sputum induction - current practice in Australia & New Zealand. Respirology. 2003;7(Suppl):1–A63.

26. Khatri L, Taylor KMG, Craig DQM, Palin K. An assessment of jet and ultrasonic nebulisers for the delivery of lactate dehydrogenase solutions. Int J Pharm. 2001;227:121–31.

27. Hess D, Fisher D, Williams P, Pooler S, Kacmarek RM. Medication nebulizer performance- effects of diluent volume, nebulizer flow and nebulizer brand. Chest. 1996;110:498–505.

Observation management of pulmonary embolism and agreement with claims-based and clinical risk stratification criteria in United States patients: a retrospective analysis

Elaine Nguyen[1], Craig I. Coleman[1*], W. Frank Peacock[2], Philip S. Wells[3], Erin R. Weeda[1], Veronica Ashton[4], Concetta Crivera[4], Peter Wildgoose[4], Jeff R. Schein[4], Thomas J. Bunz[5] and Gregory J. Fermann[6]

Abstract

Background: Guidelines suggest observation stays are appropriate for pulmonary embolism (PE) patients at low-risk for early mortality. We sought to assess agreement between United States (US) observation management of PE and claims-based and clinical risk stratification criteria.

Methods: Using US Premier data from 11/2012 to 3/2015, we identified adult observation stay patients with a primary diagnosis of PE, ≥1 PE diagnostic test claim and evidence of PE treatment. The proportion of patients at high-risk was assessed using the In-hospital Mortality for PulmonAry embolism using Claims daTa (IMPACT) equation and high-risk characteristics (age > 80 years, heart failure, chronic lung disease, renal or liver disease, high-risk for bleeding, cancer or need for thrombolysis/embolectomy).

Results: We identified 1633 PE patients managed through an observation stay. Despite their observation status, IMPACT classified 46.4% as high-risk for early mortality and 33.3% had ≥1 high-risk characteristic. Co-morbid heart failure, renal or liver disease, high-risk for major bleeding, cancer and hemodynamic instability were low (each <4.5%), but 7.8% were >80 years-of-age and 19.4% had chronic lung disease.

Conclusion: Many PE patients selected for management in observation stay units appeared to have clinical characteristics suggestive of higher-risk for mortality based upon published claims-based and clinical risk stratification criteria.

Keywords: Pulmonary embolism, Observation stays, Resource utilization, Mortality

Background

Current guidelines suggest low-risk pulmonary embolism (PE) patients are candidates for treatment at home or with an abbreviated hospital stay versus ~5+ days of in-hospital management [1]. Prior studies suggest up to 50% of PE patients may be treated in such a fashion [2].

In the United States (US), observation stays are intended to manage patients for short periods to determine appropriateness for inpatient admission, with the determination of admission/discharge occurring within 2-midnights. Observation stays may serve as an alternative to inpatient management for low-risk PE patients. Reimbursement policy changes have led to an increasing use of observation stays [3–6]. We assessed agreement between observation management of PE and claims-based and clinical risk stratification criteria using administrative claims data.

* Correspondence: craig.coleman@hhchealth.org
[1]University of Connecticut School of Pharmacy, 69 North Eagleville Road, Unit 3092, Storrs, CT 06269, USA

Methods

We performed a retrospective analysis using Premier claims data from 11/2012 to 3/2015. Premier captures ~20% of all discharges from US acute care hospitals. This study was performed in accordance with the Declaration of Helsinki. All data included in the Premier Perspective Comparative Hospital Database are de-identified and are in compliance with the Health Insurance Portability and Accountability Act (HIPAA) of 1996 to preserve participant anonymity and confidentiality. For this reason, this study was exempt from institutional review board oversight and did not require an approval by an ethics committee. The data used in this study was under license from Premier Inc. and provided through the study sponsor, Janssen Scientific Affairs, LLC.

To be included, adult patients had to have undergone an observation stay (self-reported by hospitals) with an International Classification of Diseases, 9th-revision (ICD-9) diagnosis code for PE (415.1x) in the primary position, have a claim for ≥1 diagnostic test for PE on day 0–2 (computed tomography, ventilation-perfusion scan, pulmonary angiography) and received pharmacologic (anticoagulation, thrombolysis) and/or non-pharmacologic (pulmonary embolectomy, filter placement) PE treatment [1].

Patient risk for early post-PE mortality was assessed using the validated In-hospital Mortality for PulmonAry embolism using Claims daTa (IMPACT) equation [$1/(1 + \exp(-x)$); x = −5.833 + (0.026 × age) + (0.402 × myocardial infarction) + (0.368 × chronic lung disease) + (0.464 × stroke) + (0.638 × prior major bleeding) + (0.298 × atrial fibrillation) + (1.061 × cognitive impairment) + (0.554 × heart failure) + (0.364 × renal failure) + (0.484 × liver disease) + (0.523 × coagulopathy) + (1.068 × cancer)], with an estimated in-hospital mortality risk >1.5% deemed higher-risk [7–9]. We also determined the proportion of patients with characteristics placing them at higher-risk for early mortality or other complications included in the simplified PE severity index (sPESI) or Hestia criteria (age > 80 years, heart failure, chronic lung disease, renal impairment, liver disease, high-risk for major bleeding, cancer or a need for early thrombolysis/embolectomy [proxy for hemodynamic instability]) when assessable in the claims database [10, 11].

IMPACT mortality risk and patient characteristics were summarized using descriptive statistics. Percentages and means ± standard deviations or medians (25%, 75% range) were used to summarize categorical and continuous data. Statistical analysis was performed in IBM SPSS v22 (IBM Corp., Armonk, NY, USA).

Results

In total, 47,607 hospital encounters for PE were identified and 3.4% were coded as observation stays. Using IMPACT, ~46% of observation stay patients were at higher-risk for early post-PE mortality (Table 1). Over one-third of PE patients managed via an observation stay had ≥1 criteria placing them at high-risk for early mortality. The proportion of patients with co-morbid heart failure, renal or liver disease, high-risk for major bleeding, cancer and requiring thrombolysis/pulmonary embolectomy were low (<4.5% for each), but 7.8% patients were >80 years-of-age and 19.4% had chronic lung disease. One patient died during hospitalization (out-of-hospital mortality is not available in Premier) and 28% stayed >2-midnights. High-risk patients by IMPACT or those with ≥1 high-risk criteria had longer length-of-stay ($p \leq 0.005$ for both using a generalized linear model with a gamma distribution and log-link).

Discussion

Our study suggest anywhere from one-third to about half of PE patients managed via an observation stay in the US would be classified as higher-risk for early post-PE mortality according to claims-based or clinical risk stratification criteria [7–11]. Advanced age and chronic lung disease were the most frequent "high-risk" characteristics identified in observation stay-managed patients.

The substantial proportion of observation stay patients in our study classified at higher-risk by IMPACT and select components of the sPESI and the Hestia criteria highlights the lack of agreement between US observation management of PE and risk stratification tools. Whether this observed disagreement suggests inappropriate use of observation stays is unknown. It does suggest; however, that risk stratification tools may be used infrequently by practitioners in routine practice [12–14]. Studies have reported common clinician barriers to using risk stratification tools including difficulties in implementation in routine practice [12, 13], lack of training in their use, regulatory constraints and the nature of the physician-patient relationship [14]. Also of concern, risk stratification tools tend to oversimplify risk assessment (accurately identifying those at very low-risk, but classify a large majority who inevitably do not experience a complication as higher-risk) [12]. This overall lack of prognostic accuracy likely explains some inconsistencies between tool recommendations and clinical gestalt.

Whether clinical gestalt alone is optimal for identifying PE patients suitable for abbreviated stays is unclear. In a meta-analysis by Piran et al. [15], the pooled risk of recurrent venous thromboembolism in outpatient-treated PE patients was shown not to differ between clinical gestalt and risk stratification methods (1.9% vs. 1.4%). Of note, nearly all studies examined in this meta-analysis were conducted in non-US centers decreasing its generalizability to US practice. Future studies to determine the prognostic

Table 1 Characteristics of pulmonary embolism patients managed through observation stays

Characteristic	IMPACT low-risk patients, n (%) N = 876	IMPACT higher-risk patients, n (%) N = 757	No high-risk criteria patients, n (%) N = 1,090	≥1 High-risk criteria patients, n (%) N = 543
Age (mean ± SD)	43.7 ± 12.3	70.1 ± 10.7	52.3 ± 15.8	63.4 ± 18.5
Male gender	385 (43.9)	340 (44.9)	503 (46.1)	222 (40.9)
High-risk criteria included in sPESI or Hestia criteria				
Age >80 years	0 (0)	127 (16.8)	0 (0)	127 (23.4)
Heart failure	4 (0.5)	68 (9.0)	0 (0)	72 (13.3)
Chronic lung disease	91 (10.4)	226 (29.9)	0 (0)	317 (58.4)
Renal impairment	3 (0.3)	67 (8.9)	0 (0)	70 (12.9)
Severe liver disease	6 (0.7)	23 (3.0)	0 (0)	29 (5.3)
High risk for major bleeding[a]	1 (0.1)	9 (1.2)	0 (0)	10 (1.8)
Cancer	0 (0)	46 (6.1)	0 (0)	46 (8.5)
Required thrombolysis or embolectomy (days 0–2)	2 (0.2)	2 (0.3)	0 (0)	4 (0.7)
Estimated IMPACT[b] mortality risk, % (mean ± SD)	1.0 ± 0.3	3.2 ± 2.5	1.3 ± 0.7	3.4 ± 2.9
Myocardial infarction	1 (0.1)	0 (0)	0 (0)	1 (0.2)
Stroke	0 (0)	2 (0.3)	0 (0)	2 (0.4)
Atrial Fibrillation	3 (0.3)	85 (11.2)	31 (2.8)	57 (10.5)
Cognitive impairment	0 (0)	57 (7.5)	14 (1.3)	43 (7.9)
Coagulopathy	1 (0.1)	35 (4.6)	18 (1.7)	18 (3.3)
Length of stay, days (mean ± SD) (median [25%, 75% range])	2.1 ± 0.8 2.0 (2.0, 3.0)	2.4 ± 1.6 2.0 (2.0, 3.0)	2.2 ± 1.3 2.0 (2.0, 3.0)	2.3 ± 1.0 2.0 (2.0, 3.0)

IMPACT In-hospital Mortality for PulmonAry embolism using Claims daTa, *SD* standard deviation, *sPESI* simplified pulmonary embolism severity index
[a] Active or recent history of major bleed
[b] The multivariable IMPACT equation is: $1/(1 + \exp(-x)$; where $x = -5.833 + (0.026*age) + (0.402*myocardial\ infarction) + (0.368*chronic\ lung\ disease) + (0.464*stroke) + (0.638*prior\ major\ bleeding) + (0.298*atrial\ fibrillation) + (1.061*cognitive\ impairment) + (0.554*heart\ failure) + (0.364*renal\ failure) + (0.484*liver\ disease) + (0.523*coagulopathy) + (1.068*cancer)$

accuracy of clinical gestalt in comparison to accepted risk stratification tools are needed.

Our study has limitations worth noting. First, Premier does not provide access to clinical data including vital signs (e.g., blood pressure, heart or respiratory rate, oxygen saturation), out-of-hospital mortality or clot burden. Thus, we could not apply commonly used clinical criteria, tools such as PESI or assess all criteria included in the sPESI and Hestia tools. Inclusion of these data could have only increased the percentage of patients classified as higher-risk, and as a result, we likely underestimated the percentage of patients at high-risk of early post-PE mortality. However, nearly half of observation stay patients in our analysis were identified as high-risk according to the IMPACT equation, which was specifically designed for identification of low-risk PE patients using claims data and shown to have similar prognostic accuracy for both in-hospital and 30-day mortality as PESI, sPESI and Hestia [7–9]. Second, we did not have 30-day mortality data available and therefore cannot comment on

whether these observation stay and higher-risk patients had subsequent adverse outcomes after discharge. Finally, since the overall proportion of patients being managed through observations stays in the US is limited, it is possible that other unidentified factors (e.g., societal or economic) are influencing the generalizability of these findings.

Conclusion
Our analysis suggests patient selection for abbreviated stays is not consistent with claims-based risk stratification tools and accepted clinical criteria denoting higher-risk for early mortality.

Abbreviations
ICD-9: International Classification of Diseases 9th-revision; IMPACT: In-hospital Mortality for PulmonAry embolism using Claims daTa; PE: Pulmonary embolism; SPESI: Simplified pulmonary embolism severity index; US: United States

Acknowledgements
Not applicable.

Funding
This study was funded by Janssen Scientific Affairs, LLC, Raritan, NJ, USA.

Authors' contributions
Study concept and design: EN, CIC, WFP, ERW, VA, CC, JRS, TJB, GJF. Acquisition of data: EN, CIC, VA, CC, JRS. Analysis and interpretation of data: EN, CIC, WFP, PSW, ERW, VA, CC, PW, JRS, TJB, GJF. Drafting of the manuscript: EN, CIC. Critical revision of the manuscript for important intellectual content: EN, CIC, WFP, PSW, ERW, VA, CC, PW, JRS, TJB, GJF. Administrative, technical, or material support: EN, CIC, ERW, TJB, VA. Study supervision: CIC. EN, CIC and TJB had full access to all the data in the study and take responsibility for the integrity of the data and the accuracy of the data analysis. All authors read and approved the final manuscript. The authors meet criteria for authorship as recommended by the International Committee of Medical Journal Editors (ICJME) and were fully responsible for all content and editorial decisions, and were involved in all stages of manuscript development.

Competing interests
Dr. Coleman has received grant funding and consultancy fees from Janssen Pharmaceuticals; Bayer Pharma AG and Boehringer-Ingelheim Pharmaceuticals, Inc. Dr. Peacock has received grant funding and consultancy fees from Janssen Pharmaceuticals and Portola. Dr. Wells has received grant funding from Bristol Myers Squib and Pfizer, is on the advisory board and has received speaker's fees from Bayer Healthcare, has received consultancy fees from Janssen Pharmaceuticals, and served on a writing committee with Itreas. Ms. Ashton and Drs. Crivera, Schein, and Wildgoose are employees of Janssen Scientific Affairs LLC. Dr. Fermann has received grant funding for Pfizer and is on the advisory board and speaker's bureau for Janssen Pharmaceuticals. Drs. Nguyen, Weeda and Bunz have no competing interests germane to this article to report.

Author details
[1]University of Connecticut School of Pharmacy, 69 North Eagleville Road, Unit 3092, Storrs, CT 06269, USA. [2]Department of Emergency Medicine, Baylor College of Medicine, 1504 Taub Loop, Houston, TX, USA. [3]Department of Medicine, University of Ottawa, Ottawa Hospital Research Institute, 501 Smyth Road, Box 206, Ottawa, ON, Canada. [4]Janssen Scientific Affairs, LLC, 1000 Route 202, Raritan, NJ, USA. [5]New England Health Analytics, LLC, Granby, CT, USA. [6]Department of Emergency Medicine, University of Cincinnati, 231 Albert Sabin Way, Cincinnati, OH, USA.

References
1. Kearon C, Akl EA, Ornelas J, et al. Antithrombotic therapy for VTE disease: CHEST guideline and expert panel review. Chest. 2016;149:315–52.
2. Baglin T. Fifty per cent of patients with pulmonary embolism can be treated as outpatients. J Throm Haemost. 2010;8:2404–5.
3. Sheehy AM, Graf BK, Gangireddy S, Formisano R, Jacobs EA. Observation status: for hospitalized patients: implications of a proposed Medicare rules change. JAMA Intern Med. 2013;173:2004–6.
4. Wright S. Memorandum report: hospitals' use of observation stays and short inpatient stays for Medicare beneficiaries, OEI-02-12-00040. Washington DC: United States Department of Health and Human Services, Office of Inspector General; 2013. [Accessed 4 Mar 2016]. Available from: http://oig.hhs.gov/oei/reports/oei-02-12-00040.pdf.
5. Feng Z, Wright B, Mor V. Sharp rise in Medicare enrollees being held in hospitals for observation raises concerns about causes and consequences. Health Aff. 2012;31:1251–9.
6. Overman RA, Freburger JK, Assimon MM, Li X, Brookhart MA. Observation stays in administrative claims databases: underestimation of hospitalized cases. Pharmacoepidemiol Drug Saf. 2014;23:902–10.
7. Coleman CI, Kohn CG, Bunz TJ. Derivation and validation of the In-hospital Mortality for PulmonAry embolism using Claims daTa (IMPACT) prediction rule. Curr Med Res Opin. 2015;31:1461–8.
8. Coleman CI, Kohn CG, Crivera C, Schein JR, Peacock WF. Validation of the multivariable In-hospital Mortality for PulmonAry embolism using Claims data (IMPACT) prediction rule within an all-payer inpatient administrative claims database. BMJ Open. 2015;5:e009251.
9. Weeda ER, Kohn CG, Fermann GJ, et al. External validation of prognostic rules for early post-pulmonary embolism mortality: assessment of a claims-based and three clinical-based approaches. Thromb J. 2016;14:7.
10. Jimenez D, Aujesky D, Moores L, RIETE Investigators, et al. Simplification of the pulmonary embolism severity index for prognostication in patients with acute symptomatic pulmonary embolism. Arch Intern Med. 2010;170:1383–9.
11. Zondag W, den Exter PL, Crobach MJ, Hestia Study Investigators, et al. Comparison of two methods for selection of out of hospital treatment in patients with acute pulmonary embolism. Thromb Haemost. 2013;109:47–52.
12. Eichler K, Zoller M, Tschudi P, Steurer J. Barriers to apply cardiovascular prediction rules in primary care: a postal survey. BMC Fam Pract. 2007;8:1.
13. Graham ID, Logan J, Bennett CL, et al. Physicians' intentions and use of three patient decision aids. BMC Med Inform Decis Mak. 2007;7:20.
14. Muller-Riemenschneider F, Holmberg C, Rieckmann N, et al. Barriers to routine risk-score use for healthy primary care patients: survey and qualitative study. Arch Intern Med. 2010;170:719–24.
15. Piran S, Le Gal G, Wells PS, et al. Outpatient treatment of symptomatic pulmonary embolism: a systematic review and meta-analysis. Thromb Res. 2013;132:515–9.

Mechanical ventilation in idiopathic pulmonary fibrosis: a nationwide analysis of ventilator use, outcomes, and resource burden

Joshua J. Mooney[1], Karina Raimundo[2*], Eunice Chang[3] and Michael S. Broder[3]

Abstract

Background: Idiopathic pulmonary fibrosis (IPF) is associated with increased risk of respiratory-related hospitalizations. Studies suggest mechanical ventilation (MV) use in IPF does not improve outcomes and guidelines recommend against its general use. Our objective was to investigate MV use and association with cost and mortality in IPF.

Methods: This retrospective study, using a nationwide sample, included claims with IPF (ICD-9-CM: 516.3) in 2009–2011 and principal respiratory disease diagnosis (ICD-9-CM: 460–519); excluding lung transplant. Regression models were used to determine predictors of MV and association with cost, LOS, and mortality. Domain analysis was used to account for use of subpopulation. Costs were adjusted to 2011. Data on patient severity not available.

Results: Twenty two thousand three hundred fifty non-transplant IPF patients were admitted with principal respiratory disease diagnosis: Mean age 70.0 (SD 13.9), 49.1% female, mean LOS 7.4 (SD 8.2). MV was used in 11.4% of patients with a non-significant decline over time. In regression models, MV was associated with an increased stay of 9.78 days (95% CI 8.38–11.18) and increased cost of $36,583 (95% CI $32,021–41,147). MV users had significantly increased mortality (OR 15.55, 95% CI 12.13–19.95) versus nonusers.

Conclusions: Mechanical ventilation use has not significantly changed over time and is mostly used in younger patients and those admitted for non-IPF respiratory conditions. MV was associated with a 4-fold admission cost increase ($49,924 versus $11,742) and a 7-fold mortality increase (56% versus 7.5%), although patients who receive MV may differ from those who do not. Advances in treatment and decision aids are needed to improve outcomes in IPF.

Keywords: Mechanical ventilation, Mortality, Outcomes, Cost of illness, Idiopathic pulmonary fibrosis, Noninvasive ventilation

Background

Idiopathic pulmonary fibrosis (IPF), a form of interstitial pneumonia, affects 0.5% of US adults over age 65 [1]. The disease is characterized by progressive lung fibrosis [2] and unpredictable episodes of disease worsening, which may lead to hospitalization and frequently death [3–5]. The median survival from diagnosis is 3–5 years [6]. Although two pharmacologic treatments that slow physiologic decline are now available [7, 8], limited options remain for IPF patients hospitalized with respiratory-related symptoms or failure.

Management of respiratory failure in IPF is challenging as patients can develop acute disease episodes that necessitate ventilator support. In select IPF patients, ventilator support can be used as a bridge to lung transplant [9, 10] or could allow for treatment of reversible non-IPF causes of respiratory failure. However, overall outcomes of IPF patients who require non-invasive ventilation or mechanical ventilation (MV) are poor [11–16]. A systematic review [17] summarizing 9 single-center studies reported an 87% in-hospital mortality rate for IPF patients who received MV. Given this evidence, IPF treatment guidelines recommend the majority of IPF patients with respiratory failure not receive MV, and when used should occur

* Correspondence: raimundo.karina@gene.com
[2]Genentech, Inc, South San Francisco, CA, USA
Full list of author information is available at the end of the article

after assessing patient-specific goals of care or lung transplant candidacy [10].

While studies have repeatedly demonstrated high mortality with MV, the nationwide pattern of its use in IPF patients has not been well characterized. In this study, we investigated US trends in the use of non-invasive ventilation and MV for IPF, predictors of use, and association with hospital cost, length of stay (LOS), and mortality. We also examined whether MV had a direct effect on mortality, or whether the effect was entirely mediated by the patients' underlying disease and comorbid conditions.

Methods
Design and data sources
We conducted a retrospective cohort study using the Nationwide Inpatient Sample (NIS), the largest publicly available US inpatient database that includes individuals covered by Medicare, Medicaid, or private insurance, as well as the uninsured. Data elements include diagnoses, procedures, demographics, hospital characteristics, payment source, charges, discharge status, LOS, and severity measures [18]. The study used de-identified data and was exempt from institutional review board review.

Patient Population
We included all hospitalizations from 2009–2011 with claims for IPF (International Classification of Diseases, 9th Revision, Clinical Modification [ICD-9-CM] code 516.3) and a principal diagnosis of respiratory disease (ICD-9-CM: 460–519). Hospital discharge records may contain multiple diagnoses, with the primary cause for admission listed as "principal." A hospitalization for a patient with IPF admitted with pneumonia as the principal diagnosis would have been included in our study, as pneumonia is a respiratory disease, as would a hospitalization with a principal diagnosis of IPF (also a respiratory disease). An admission with a principal diagnosis of hip fracture would not be included, even if IPF was listed as a secondary diagnosis. Included patients had ≥ 1 inpatient claim with IPF as a discharge diagnosis between 2009–2011. We excluded lung transplant admissions (ICD-9-CM: 33.5×, 33.6).

Variables
Outcome variables of interest were non-invasive (ICD-9-CM: 93.90) and MV (ICD-9-CM: 96.7×) use, hospital LOS, total inpatient costs, and in-hospital mortality. Other study variables include demographics, primary payer type, hospital characteristics, and all patient refined diagnosis-related group (APR-DRG) severity of illness. APR-DRG assigns patients to severity and mortality subclasses using comorbidities, age, procedures, and principal diagnosis [19]. We looked for evidence of concomitant acute and chronic pulmonary conditions, including chronic obstructive pulmonary disease (COPD), bacterial pneumonia, and lung

cancer. Cardiovascular conditions were identified, including ischemic heart disease, myocardial infarction (MI), congestive heart failure, and pulmonary hypertension. The number of chronic conditions for each patient, calculated using the Chronic Condition Indicator, was reported. This indicator uses 5 digit ICD-9-CM codes to categorize conditions as chronic or not chronic [20]. Admissions were characterized as elective, emergency, urgent, or other non-elective. Discharge disposition was reported as routine, transfer to short-term hospital, transfer to other facilities, home health care, died in hospital, or unknown.

Statistical analysis
Variables were weighted to represent national estimates and rounded to the nearest integer. NIS reports only charges, so cost-to-charge ratios were used to estimate costs. These ratios are constructed using costs and charge information from hospital reports to CMS. Hospital-specific ratios were used if available; otherwise a weighted group average was used. Costs were adjusted to 2011 US\$ using the medical care component of the consumer price index [21]. For categorical variables, Rao-Scott chi-square goodness-of-fit tests adjusting for sampling design were used, relevant p-values reported. We calculated variance using domain analysis to account for subpopulations. Linear regression models were used for LOS and cost, logistic regression models for MV and mortality. Models were adjusted for age, gender, race, principal diagnosis of IPF, lung cancer, selected cardiovascular conditions, hospital region, hospital teaching status, and MV use, as appropriate. Adjusted mean LOS and hospital cost, and adjusted inpatient mortality rate (and 95% confidence intervals) were reported for MV users and nonusers.

Patients with certain characteristics may have a higher risk of inpatient mortality and MV use. To investigate whether MV use was a mediator between clinical characteristics and mortality (rather than directly related), we followed the approach described by Baron and Kenny [22]. We conducted additional regression models to examine the association of clinical conditions/characteristics (the causal variables) on both the MV use (the mediator) and mortality (the outcome variable). Model results were compared to determine whether mediation effects were identifiable. Data transformations and statistical analyses were performed using SAS® version 9.4.

Results
From 2009–2011 42,924 IPF patients were admitted to US short-stay hospitals; 23,739 admissions had a principal diagnosis of respiratory disease. The remainder of admissions for these IPF patients were for non-respiratory conditions. After excluding 1,379 lung transplant admissions and 10 with missing age, final sample size was 22,350: 7,346 in 2009, 6,643 in 2010, and 8,362 in 2011. MV was

used in 11.4% (2,546) of admissions: 12.1% (887) in 2009, 11.5% (764) in 2010, and 10.7% (894) in 2011 ($p = 0.578$). Non-invasive ventilation was used in 8.9% (1,995) of admissions: 7.9% (583) in 2009, 8.3% (550) in 2010, and 10.3% (862) in 2011 ($p = 0.112$) (Fig. 1).

Unadjusted analysis

Mean age was 65.9 (+/−0.62) for MV users and 70.5 (+/−0.34) for nonusers ($p < 0.001$). Overall, 49.1% (10,976) of patients were female: 40.2% (1,024) of MV users and 50.3% (9,953) of nonusers ($p < 0.001$). The majority (64.4%, $n = 14,404$) of patients were White, 9.4% Hispanic, 7.6% Black, with no significant difference by MV use. The primary payer was Medicare for 58.9% of admissions at which MV was used, compared to 69.7% where it was not ($p < 0.001$). A principal diagnosis of IPF was present in 31.5% of admissions at which MV was used vs. 44.6% where it was not ($p < 0.001$) (Table 1).

ICD-9-CM diagnoses of pneumonia (49.2% vs. 37.1%, $p < 0.001$) and MI (10.5% vs. 5.4%, $p < 0.001$) were more common in patients requiring MV, while COPD (28.9% vs. 39.4%, $p < 0.001$) was less common. As is the case for all diagnoses in this study, these conditions were not confirmed clinically. MV users had significantly fewer chronic conditions (4.2 vs. 4.3, $p < 0.001$) (Table 2). Patients who used MV had longer hospital stays (16.5 days [+/−0.73] vs. 6.2 [+/−0.10], $p < 0.001$), were more likely to have died in the hospital (55.3% vs. 8.8%) and less likely to have a routine home discharge (9.3% vs. 51.2%) ($p < 0.001$). Costs ($49,924 vs. $11,742, $p < 0.001$) were higher in MV users compared to nonusers (Table 3).

Adjusted analysis

MV was associated with an adjusted LOS of 16.1 days (95% CI: 15; 17.5) versus 6.3 days (95% CI: 6; 6.5) for nonusers. The adjusted cost associated with MV was $48,772 (95% CI: 43,979; 53,565) versus $11,861 (95% CI: 11,292; 12,431) for nonusers. The adjusted in-hospital death rate for MV users and nonusers was 55.7% (95% CI: 50.3; 61.0) and 7.5% (95% CI: 6.6; 8.4) (Table 4). Each year of increased age was associated with shorter LOS (−0.03; 95% CI: −0.06; −0.01) and lower cost (-143; 95% CI: −208; −78) but greater in-hospital death (OR 1.02; 95% CI: 1.01; 1.03). The use of non-invasive ventilation was associated with increased LOS (2.03 days; 95% CI: 0.93; 3.14), cost ($5,119; 95% CI: 2,000; 8,238) and death (OR 4.77; 95% CI: 3.48; 6.55) (Fig. 2). A principal diagnosis of IPF was associated with increased cost ($1,731; 95%CI: 636; 2,827) and death (OR 1.78; 95% CI: 1.42; 2.24) but no change in LOS (Fig. 2).

To investigate the association among clinical conditions/characteristics, MV use, and inpatient mortality, we conducted two additional logistic regression models. In the model for risk of MV, we controlled for patient and hospital characteristics. In this model, decreasing age (OR 0.97, 95% CI: 0.97; 0.98), female gender (OR 0.68, 95% CI: 0.55; 0.85), Hispanic ethnicity (OR 0.66, 95% CI: 0.45; 0.97) and principal diagnosis of IPF (OR 0.60, 95% CI: 0.48; 0.76) were associated with a lower risk of MV. Cardiovascular conditions (OR 1.34, 95% CI: 1.08; 1.65; $p = 0.007$), bacterial pneumonia (OR 1.55, 95% CI: 1.27; 1.90; $p < 0.001$), and teaching hospital admission (OR 1.58, 95% CI 1.26; 1.98; $p < 0.001$) were associated with higher risk of MV. In the model for in-hospital death that excluded MV as a predictor, female gender was associated with a lower risk of death (OR 0.62, 95% CI: 0.52; 0.74; $p < 0.001$), whereas principal diagnosis of IPF (OR 1.26, 95% CI: 1.03; 1.55; $p = 0.026$), teaching hospital admission (OR 1.37, 95% CI 1.11; 1.69; $p = 0.003$), cardiovascular conditions (OR 1.26, 95% CI: 1.04; 1.51; $p = 0.017$), and

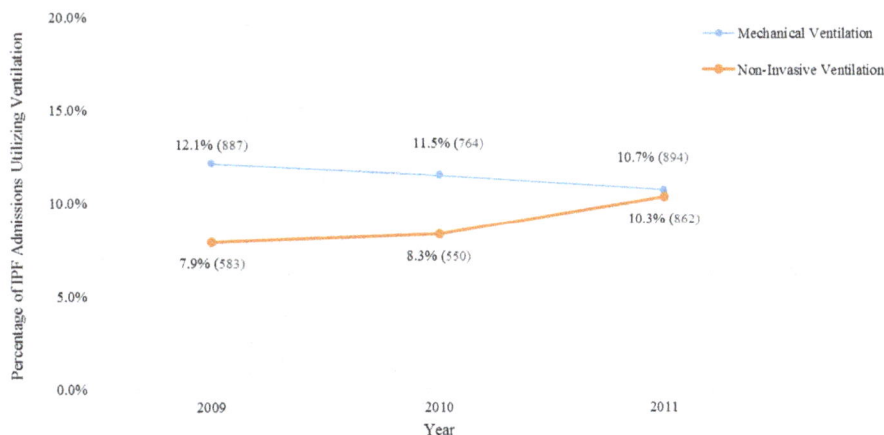

Fig. 1 Trend in Ventilation Use in IPF Hospitalizations. The proportion of IPF hospitalizations where mechanical ventilation was used declined each year, going from 12.1% (887) in 2009, to 11.5% (764) in 2010, and 10.7% (894) in 2011 ($p = 0.578$). The use of non-invasive ventilation increased over the same period: 7.9% (583) in 2009, 8.3% (550) in 2010, and 10.3% (862) in 2011 ($p = 0.112$)

Table 1 Patient Demographics, Hospital Characteristics, and Admission Type

	Mean (+/−SE)/no.(%)			P Value
	MV N = 2,546	No MV N = 19,805	All N = 22,350	
Age	65.9 (+/−0.62)	70.5 (+/−0.34)	70.0 (+/−0.32)	<.001
Female	1,024 (40.2%)	9,953 (50.3%)	10,976 (49.1%)	<.001
Race				0.657
White	1,639 (64.4%)	12,764 (64.5%)	14,404 (64.4%)	
Black	224 (8.8%)	1,483 (7.5%)	1,707 (7.6%)	
Hispanic	200 (7.8%)	1,910 (9.6%)	2,110 (9.4%)	
Other	129 (5.1%)	999 (5.0%)	1,128 (5.0%)	
Missing	353 (13.9%)	2,649 (13.4%)	3,002 (13.4%)	
Primary payer type				<.001
Medicare	1,499 (58.9%)	13,798 (69.7%)	15,297 (68.4%)	
Medicaid	231 (9.1%)	1,300 (6.6%)	1,531 (6.9%)	
Private (including HMO)	710 (27.9%)	3,880 (19.6%)	4,590 (20.5%)	
Self-pay	41 (1.6%)	408 (2.1%)	448 (2.0%)	
Missing/No charge/Other	65 (2.5%)	420 (2.1%)	484 (2.2%)	
Hospital region				0.845
Northeast	433 (17.0%)	3,465 (17.5%)	3,897 (17.4%)	
Midwest	607 (23.8%)	5,037 (25.4%)	5,644 (25.3%)	
South	1,055 (41.4%)	8,114 (41.0%)	9,169 (41.0%)	
West	452 (17.8%)	3,189 (16.1%)	3,641 (16.3%)	
Teaching hospital	1,332 (52.3%)	8,354 (42.2%)	9,687 (43.3%)	<.001
Bed size				0.022
Small	229 (9.0%)	2,581 (13.0%)	2,811 (12.6%)	
Medium	499 (19.6%)	4,309 (21.8%)	4,807 (21.5%)	
Large	1,771 (69.6%)	12,676 (64.0%)	14,447 (64.6%)	
Missing	47 (1.8%)	239 (1.2%)	286 (1.3%)	
Evidence of ED services[a]	1,650 (64.8%)	13,262 (67.0%)	14,912 (66.7%)	0.363
Principal diagnosis of IPF	802 (31.5%)	8,823 (44.6%)	9,626 (43.1%)	<.001
Elective admission[b]	361 (14.2%)	3,152 (15.9%)	3,512 (15.7%)	0.307

[a]Defined by NIS as having either an ED revenue code, charge, CPT procedure code, or admission source, or being on a state-defined ED record
[b]Defined by NIS as admission other than emergency, urgent, newborn, delivery, trauma center, or other-non elective

bacterial pneumonia (OR 1.42. 95% CI: 1.18; 1.71; $p < 0.001$) were associated with increased risk (Table 5).

Discussion

Our study of IPF patients admitted to a nationwide sample of acute care hospitals found 11-12% of IPF patients admitted with a respiratory condition used MV, with no significant change from 2009–2011. Younger, male patients with fewer comorbidities and/or with a non-IPF principal diagnosis (e.g., pneumonia) were more likely to use MV. MV was associated with nearly 10-day longer hospital stays, $37,000 higher cost, and a more than 7-fold increase in mortality (56% versus 7.5%). Less than 10% of patients who used MV were discharged home routinely, compared to more than half of nonusers. Non-invasive

ventilation was associated with increased LOS and cost, although to a lesser extent than MV.

The unchanging nationwide use of MV over time, despite IPF treatment guidelines conditionally recommending against MV use, reflects the limited options available to clinicians treating acute worsening of IPF and the difficulty of advance care planning in IPF. As acute worsening leading to respiratory failure can occur quickly and unexpectedly, MV can provide time to evaluate for possible treatable conditions, to assess patient preferences and/or to support gas-exchange while awaiting lung transplant. Lung transplantation remains the only curative and life-prolonging option for select patients with advanced IPF and respiratory failure. Notably, IPF patients who received MV were younger with fewer chronic medical conditions,

Table 2 Patient Clinical Characteristics and Treatment

	Mean (+/−SE)/no.(%)			P Value
	MV N = 2,546	No MV N = 19,805	All N = 22,350	
No. of chronic conditions	4.2 (+/−0.06)	4.3 (+/−0.03)	4.3 (+/−0.03)	<.001
Chronic obstructive pulmonary disease	736 (28.9%)	7,800 (39.4%)	8,535 (38.2%)	<.001
Bacterial pneumonia	1,252 (49.2%)	7,352 (37.1%)	8,604 (38.5%)	<.001
Lung cancer	59 (2.3%)	348 (1.8%)	407 (1.8%)	0.380
Cardiovascular conditions	1,229 (48.3%)	8,835 (44.6%)	10,063 (45.0%)	0.137
Ischemic heart disease	717 (28.2%)	5,622 (28.4%)	6,339 (28.4%)	0.913
Myocardial infarction	267 (10.5%)	1,078 (5.4%)	1,345 (6.0%)	<.001
Congestive heart failure	793 (31.1%)	5,427 (27.4%)	6,219 (27.8%)	0.119
Pulmonary hypertension	19 (0.8%)	65 (0.3%)	84 (0.4%)	0.146
APR-DRG severity of illness				<.001
Minor loss of function	5 (0.2%)	443 (2.2%)	447 (2.0%)	
Moderate loss of function	16 (0.6%)	5,042 (25.5%)	5,058 (22.6%)	
Major loss of function	341 (13.4%)	10,197 (51.5%)	10,538 (47.1%)	
Extreme loss of function	2,184 (85.8%)	4,123 (20.8%)	6,307 (28.2%)	

more often admitted at a teaching hospital, and more frequently coded with a non-IPF principal respiratory diagnosis (e.g., pneumonia). This suggests a nationwide preference for MV use in younger, somewhat healthier, IPF patients or in those with a clinical suspicion of a reversible condition. Possible explanations for this finding are that younger patients with less chronic comorbidity may be potential lung transplant candidates or clinicians may feel compelled to offer them a trial of ventilator support. We cannot ascertain from the data if patients were awaiting transplant or later transferred for transplant evaluation.

The overall economic and health care burden of IPF is well-recognized [23–27]. This study uniquely highlights the burden associated with MV use in IPF, while reinforcing with nationwide data the poor outcomes reported in prior smaller studies. Hospital cost was more than 4-fold greater and mortality 7-fold greater in IPF patients hospitalized with a respiratory problem requiring MV. While in-hospital mortality (55.3%) was lower than previously reported, this underestimates mortality as a significant number of patients were transferred to short-term hospitals (6.9%) or other facilities (20.8%) where their final vital status is unknown. Only 16.4% of MV users were discharged home. The high

Table 3 Patient Discharge Status, LOS, and Total Costs

	Mean (+/−SE)/no.(%)			P Value
	MV Use N = 2,546	No MV Use N = 19,805	All N = 22,350	
Discharge status				<.001
Routine	236 (9.3%)	10,131 (51.2%)	10,367 (46.4%)	
Transfer to short-term hospital	175 (6.9%)	548 (2.8%)	724 (3.2%)	
Transfer to other facilities	531 (20.8%)	3,353 (16.9%)	3,883 (17.4%)	
Home health care	181 (7.1%)	3,937 (19.9%)	4,118 (18.4%)	
Died in hospital	1,408 (55.3%)	1,738 (8.8%)	3,146 (14.1%)	
Other[a]	15 (0.6%)	98 (0.5%)	112 (0.5%)	
Days of stay (among all IPF patients)	16.5 (+/−0.73)	6.2 (+/−0.10)	7.4 (+/−0.15)	<.001
Died in hospital	1,408 (55.3%)	1,738 (8.8%)	3,146 (14.1%)	<.001
Total inpatient costs (2011 US$)	$49,924 (+/−2,490)	$11,742 (+/−390)	$16,042 (+/−631)	<.001

[a]Against medical advice, discharged alive, or destination unknown

Table 4 Adjusted LOS, Inpatient Costs, and In-Hospital Death Rate[a]

IMV Use	Adjusted[a] in-Hospital Death Rate (95% CI)	Adjusted[a] OR (95% CI)	P Value
Yes	55.7% (50.3 – 61.0)	15.55 (12.13 – 19.95)	<.001
No	7.5% (6.6 – 8.4)	ref	

CI Confidence interval; *OR* Odds ratio
[a]Adjusted by age, gender, race, hospital region, teaching hospital, principal diagnosis of IPF, lung cancer, selected cardiovascular conditions (ischemic heart disease, myocardial infarction, and congestive heart failure), and non-invasive ventilatio4n use

mortality and economic burden associated with MV in IPF stresses the need to improve the quality of medical care for IPF patients, including advances in prevention, treatment, and patient-clinician shared decision-making. While recently approved pharmacologic therapies slow disease progression and may reduce acute exacerbations [7, 8, 28], the course of IPF remains unpredictable. Therefore, early patient-centered discussions on treatment expectations, appropriate referrals for transplant and/or palliative care, and coordination of care across providers, remain integral to honoring patients' values while ensuring high value care. IPF-specific decision aids are needed to help guide patients.

Some conditions that lead to MV may themselves be associated with greater mortality, confounding the interpretation of our findings. We used a method similar to that of Baron and Kenny [22] to test whether MV simply

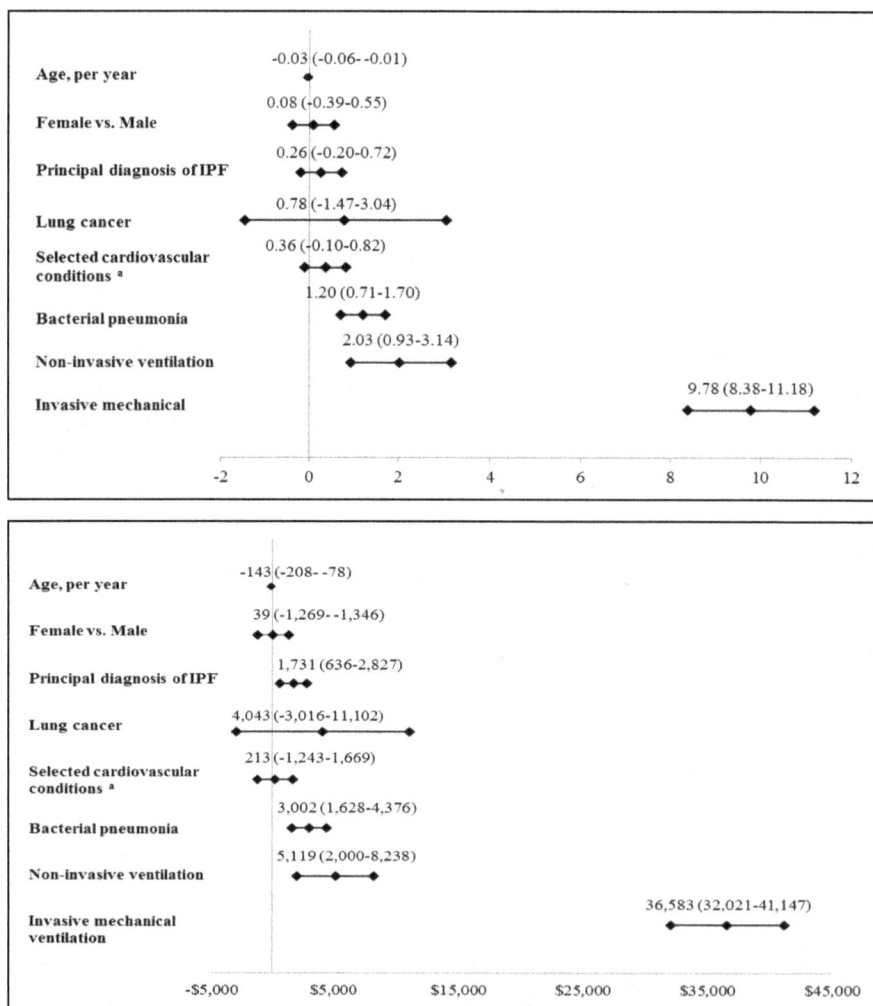

Fig. 2 Linear Regression Model for LOS and Costs. Age, bacterial pneumonia, and use of mechanical ventilation were statistically significantly (p < 0.001) associated with cost and LOS. Admission with a principal diagnosis of IPF was significantly associated with cost but not LOS. Use of mechanical ventilation had the largest effect on LOS and cost, with an increase of 9.78 days [95% CI: 8.38 - 11.18] and $36,583 [32,021 – 41,147] respectively. Non-invasive ventilation was associated with an increase of 2.03 days [0.93 – 3.14] in LOS and $5,119 [2,000 – 8,238] in cost. Point estimates and 95% CI for LOS and cost are adjusted for all listed variables. *CI* Confidence interval; [a] Ischemic heart disease, myocardial infarction, and congestive heart failure

Table 5 Logistic Regression Model Results for Risk of Mechanical Ventilation and Death

Parameter	Logistic Regression Model			
	Risk of In-Hospital Death		Risk of Invasive Mechanical Ventilation	
	OR (95% CI)	P Value	OR (95% CI)	P Value
Age, per year	1.00 (1.00 – 1.01)	0.562	0.97 (0.97 – 0.98)	<.001
Female vs. Male	0.62 (0.52 – 0.74)	<.001	0.68 (0.55 – 0.85)	<.001
Race				
Black vs. White	0.70 (0.47 – 1.04)	0.081	0.98 (0.68 – 1.39)	0.896
Hispanic vs. White	0.80 (0.56 – 1.15)	0.235	0.66 (0.45 – 0.97)	0.036
Other vs. White	1.05 (0.68 – 1.62)	0.836	0.86 (0.52 – 1.42)	0.547
Missing vs. White	1.09 (0.78 – 1.52)	0.627	0.99 (0.71 – 1.39)	0.966
Hospital region				
Northeast vs. West	0.95 (0.65 – 1.37)	0.776	0.75 (0.50 – 1.11)	0.151
Midwest vs. West	0.85 (0.60 – 1.20)	0.362	0.77 (0.53 – 1.11)	0.161
South vs. West	0.92 (0.68 – 1.25)	0.605	0.82 (0.59 – 1.12)	0.207
Teaching hospital	1.37 (1.11 – 1.69)	0.003	1.58 (1.26 – 1.98)	<.001
Principal diagnosis of IPF	1.26 (1.03 – 1.55)	0.026	0.60 (0.48 – 0.76)	<.001
Lung cancer	1.71 (0.99 – 2.94)	0.053	1.12 (0.57 – 2.20)	0.750
Selected cardiovascular conditions [a]	1.26 (1.04 – 1.51)	0.017	1.34 (1.08 – 1.65)	0.007
Bacterial pneumonia	1.42 (1.18 – 1.71)	<.001	1.55 (1.27 – 1.90)	<.001

OR Odds ratio, *CI* Confidence interval
[a]Ischemic heart disease, myocardial infarction, and congestive heart failure

mediated the mortality effects of other variables. Our results suggest that this was not true of a principal IPF diagnosis, as it remains associated with mortality in the models both with and without MV use. Both cardiovascular conditions and bacterial pneumonia had statistically significant effects in the model that did not include MV, and smaller, not statistically significant, effects in the model that included it. This suggests the association between these characteristics and in-hospital death results, at least in part, from their association with MV, which independently increases the risk of death. However, some residual confounding by indication likely still exists.

This study has limitations. First, there is debate on how to identify IPF patients using claims data. The ICD-9-CM code we used has been used before in several publications [1, 6, 23, 24], however a recent validation study (not in the NIS) found it had a positive predictive value of 30-60% [29]. While less than desirable, this positive predictive value is within the range reported in study of ICD-9-CM codes for 32 conditions (median 80.7%, mean 77%, range 23-100%) [30]. Similarly, none of the conditions we identified (e.g., COPD) were confirmed clinically. Identification relied on ICD-9-CM codes, which are designed and used primarily for billing. Our study was further limited in that the NIS does not allow patients to be followed through subsequent outpatient care, repeat

hospitalizations, or transfer to other facilities. We could not determine whether a subject died, received a transplant, or was discharged home after being transferred. The study relied on secondary data collected at discharge for administrative purposes, so no clinical information, including disease severity, was available. We could not determine whether medical conditions were present on admission or developed during hospitalization, nor could we determine the order in which diagnoses were made or treatments were given. Further, less severe comorbid conditions common to patients with IPF (e.g., obesity and gastroesophageal reflux) may be undercoded. Finally, as in prior studies [23, 24] we excluded transplant-related expenditures. This exclusion allows for a close look at direct costs of IPF-related care, but underestimates the complete cost of IPF.

A strength of the study is the use of the Nationwide Inpatient Sample, which was designed to inform policy decisions regarding health and health care at national and regional levels. Previous evaluations of IPF MV use and cost have been limited to specific centers or populations (e.g., Medicare and select private insurers) and their findings may be less generalizable. The NIS includes patients with Medicare, Medicaid, and private insurance, as well as the uninsured, making this dataset the best way to produce estimates valid for the overall US population.

Conclusion

In a nationwide sample of IPF patients, MV was used in 11-12% of those hospitalized due to a respiratory diagnosis with no significant change in its use over time. Mechanical ventilation was more frequent in younger male IPF patients, those admitted at teaching hospitals, and those with fewer chronic medical conditions or a non-IPF respiratory diagnosis. Its use was associated with a 4-fold increase in admission cost ($49,924 compared to $11,742) and a 7-fold increase in admission mortality (56% compared to 7.5%). Further advances in IPF treatment and development of IPF-specific decision aids are needed to improve the resource burden, outcomes, and use of MV in IPF.

Abbreviation
APR-DRG: All patient refined diagnosis-related group; CI: Confidence interval; COPD: Chronic obstructive pulmonary disease; CPT: Current procedural terminology; ED: Emergency department; ICD-9-CM: International classification of diseases, 9th revision, clinical modification; IPF: Idiopathic pulmonary fibrosis; LOS: Length of stay; MI: Myocardial infarction; MV: Mechanical ventilation; NIS: Nationwide inpatient sample; OR: Odds ratio; Revision: Clinical modification; SD: Standard deviation

Acknowledgments
Not applicable.

Funding
This study was funded by Genentech, Inc. The sponsor was involved in the study design, interpretation, and manuscript writing. K. Raimundo is an employee of Genentech, Inc. E. Chang and M. Broder are employees of Partnership for Health Analytic Research, LLC, a health services research company paid by Genentech to conduct this research.

Authors' contributions
All authors meet the ICMJE criteria for authorship. All authors were equally involved in the design of the study. EC conducted the statistical analyses and all authors contributed equally in the interpretation of results and writing of the manuscript. All authors read and approved the final manuscript.

Competing interests
K. Raimundo is an employee of Genentech, Inc. E. Chang and M. Broder are employees of Partnership for Health Analytic Research, LLC, a health services research company paid by Genentech to conduct this research.

Author details
[1]Stanford University, Stanford, CA, USA. [2]Genentech, Inc, South San Francisco, CA, USA. [3]Partnership for Health Analytic Research, LLC, Beverly Hills, CA, USA.

References
1. Raghu G, Chen S-Y, Yeh W-S, Maroni B, Li Q, Lee Y-C, et al. Idiopathic pulmonary fibrosis in US Medicare beneficiaries aged 65 years and older: incidence, prevalence, and survival, 2001–11. Lancet Respir Med. 2014;2:566–72.
2. Ryu JH, Moua T, Daniels CE, Hartman TE, Yi ES, Utz JP, et al. Idiopathic Pulmonary Fibrosis: Evolving Concepts. Mayo Clin Proc. 2014;89:1130–42.
3. Ley B, Collard HR, King TE. Clinical Course and Prediction of Survival in Idiopathic Pulmonary Fibrosis. Am J Respir Crit Care Med. 2011;183:431–40.
4. Martinez FJ, Safrin S, Weycker D, et al. The clinical course of patients with idiopathic pulmonary fibrosis. Ann Intern Med. 2005;142:963–7.
5. Song JW, Hong S-B, Lim C-M, et al. Acute exacerbation of idiopathic pulmonary fibrosis: incidence, risk factors and outcome. Eur Respir J. 2011;37:356–63.
6. Raghu G, Weycker D, Edelsberg J, et al. Incidence and Prevalence of Idiopathic Pulmonary Fibrosis. Am J Respir Crit Care Med. 2006;174:810–6.
7. King TE, Bradford WZ, Castro-Bernardini S, et al. A Phase 3 Trial of Pirfenidone in Patients with Idiopathic Pulmonary Fibrosis. N Engl J Med. 2014;370:2083–92.
8. Richeldi L, du Bois RM, Raghu G, et al. Efficacy and Safety of Nintedanib in Idiopathic Pulmonary Fibrosis. N Engl J Med. 2014;370:2071–82.
9. Weill D, Benden C, Corris PA, et al. A consensus document for the selection of lung transplant candidates: 2014—An update from the Pulmonary Transplantation Council of the International Society for Heart and Lung Transplantation. J Heart Lung Transplant. 2015;34:1–15.
10. Raghu G. Idiopathic pulmonary fibrosis: guidelines for diagnosis and clinical management have advanced from consensus-based in 2000 to evidence-based in 2011. Eur Respir J. 2011;37:743–6.
11. Simon-Blancal V, Freynet O, Nunes H, et al. Acute Exacerbation of Idiopathic Pulmonary Fibrosis: Outcome and Prognostic Factors. Respiration. 2012;83:28–35.
12. Vianello A, Arcaro G, Battistella L, et al. Noninvasive ventilation in the event of acute respiratory failure in patients with idiopathic pulmonary fibrosis. J Crit Care. 2014;29:562–7.
13. Blivet S, Philit F, Sab JM, et al. Outcome of patients with idiopathic pulmonary fibrosis admitted to the ICU for respiratory failure. Chest. 2001; 120:209–12.
14. Stern JB, Mal H, Groussard O, et al. Prognosis of patients with advanced idiopathic pulmonary fibrosis requiring mechanical ventilation for acute respiratory failure. Chest. 2001;120:213–9.
15. Fumeaux T, Rothmeier C, Jolliet P. Outcome of mechanical ventilation for acute respiratory failure in patients with pulmonary fibrosis. Intensive Care Med. 2001;27:1868–74.
16. Saydain G, Islam A, Afessa B, et al. Outcome of Patients with Idiopathic Pulmonary Fibrosis Admitted to the Intensive Care Unit. Am J Respir Crit Care Med. 2002;166:839–42.
17. Mallick S. Outcome of patients with idiopathic pulmonary fibrosis (IPF) ventilated in intensive care unit. Respir Med. 2008;102:1355–9.
18. Houchens R, Ross D, Elixhauser A, et al. Nationwide Inpatient Sample (NIS) Redesign Final Report. U.S. Agency for Healthcare Research and Quality. 2014 Apr. Report No.: 2014–04. http://www.hcup-us.ahrq.gov/reports/methods/methods.jsp
19. APR DRG Software. 3 M Health Information Systems – US. http://solutions.3m.com/wps/portal/3M/en_US/Health-Information-Systems/HIS/Products-and-Services/Products-List-A-Z/APR-DRG-Software/. Accessed 25 April 2016.
20. Hwang W, Weller W, Ireys H, et al. Out-of-pocket medical spending for care of chronic conditions. Health Aff (Millwood). 2001;20:267–78.
21. Inflation Calculator. Bureau of Labor Statistics. http://www.bls.gov/data/inflation_calculator.htm. Accessed 25 April 2016.
22. Baron RM, Kenny DA. The moderator-mediator variable distinction in social psychological research: conceptual, strategic, and statistical considerations. J Pers Soc Psychol. 1986;51:1173–82.
23. Collard HR, Ward AJ, Lanes S, et al. Burden of illness in idiopathic pulmonary fibrosis. J Med Econ. 2012;15:829–35.
24. Collard HR, Chen S-Y, Yeh W-S, et al. Health care utilization and costs of idiopathic pulmonary fibrosis in U.S. Medicare beneficiaries aged 65 years and older. Ann Am Thorac Soc. 2015;12:981–7.
25. Raimundo K, Chang E, Broder MS, et al. Clinical and economic burden of idiopathic pulmonary fibrosis: a retrospective cohort study. BMC Pulm. Med. 2016. http://www.biomedcentral.com/1471-2466/16/2. Accessed 22 Jan 2016

26. Wu N, Yu YF, Chuang C-C, et al. Healthcare resource utilization among patients diagnosed with idiopathic pulmonary fibrosis in the United States. J Med Econ. 2015;18:249–57.

27. Yu YF, Wu N, Chuang C-C, et al. Patterns and Economic Burden of Hospitalizations and Exacerbations Among Patients Diagnosed with Idiopathic Pulmonary Fibrosis. J Manag Care Spec Pharm. 2016;22:414–23.

28. Azuma A, Nukiwa T, Tsuboi E, et al. Double-blind, Placebo-controlled Trial of Pirfenidone in Patients with Idiopathic Pulmonary Fibrosis. Am J Respir Crit Care Med. 2005;171:1040–7.

29. Esposito DB, Lanes S, Donneyong M, et al. Idiopathic Pulmonary Fibrosis in United States Automated Claims. Incidence, Prevalence, and Algorithm Validation. Am J Respir Crit Care Med. 2015;192:1200–7.

30. Quan H, Li B, Duncan Saunders L, et al. Assessing Validity of ICD-9-CM and ICD-10 Administrative Data in Recording Clinical Conditions in a Unique Dually Coded Database: Assessing Validity of ICD-9-CM and ICD-10. Health Serv Res. 2008;43:1424–41.

Effect of sivelestat sodium in patients with acute lung injury or acute respiratory distress syndrome

Shenglan Pu[1], Daoxin Wang[1*], Daishun Liu[2], Yan Zhao[1], Di Qi[1], Jing He[1] and Guoqi Zhou[1]

Abstract

Background: Sivelestat is widely used in treating acute lung injury (ALI)/acute respiratory distress syndrome (ARDS), although the clinical efficacy of sivelestat remains controversial. This study aimed to evaluate the impact of sivelestat in patients with ALI/ARDS.

Methods: Electronic databases, PubMed, Embase, and the Cochrane Library, were searched to identify trials through April 2017. Randomized controlled trials (RCTs) were included irrespective of blinding or language that compared patients with and without sivelestat therapy in ALI/ARDS. A random-effects model was used to process the data, and the relative risk (RR) and standard mean difference (SMD) with corresponding 95% confidence intervals (CIs) were used to evaluate the effect of sivelestat.

Results: Six RCTs reporting data on 804 patients with ALI/ARDS were included. Overall, no significant difference was found between sivelestat and control for the risk of 28–30 days mortality (RR: 0.94; 95% CI: 0.71–1.23; $P = 0.718$). Sivelestat therapy had no significant effect on ventilation days (SMD: 0.05; 95% CI: −0.27 to 0.38; $P = 0.748$), arterial oxygen partial pressure (PaO2)/fractional inspired oxygen (FiO2) level (SMD: 0.48; 95% CI: −0.45 to 1.41; $P = 0.315$), and intensive care unit (ICU) stays (SMD: −9.87; 95% CI: −24.30 to 4.56; $P = 0.180$). The results of sensitivity analysis indicated that sivelestat therapy might affect the PaO_2/FiO_2 level in patients with ALI/ARDS (SMD: 0.87; 95% CI: 0.39 to 1.35; $P < 0.001$).

Conclusions: Sivelestat therapy might increase the PaO_2/FiO_2 level, while it had little or no effect on 28–30 days mortality, ventilation days, and ICU stays. These findings need to be verified in large-scale trials.

Keywords: Sivelestat sodium, Patients, Acute lung injury, Acute respiratory distress syndrome

Background

Acute lung injury (ALI) or acute respiratory distress syndrome (ARDS) is characterized by abnormal pulmonary physiology and gas exchange properties [1, 2], which are common complications in various diseases, and is related to higher morbidity and mortality [3, 4]. Generally, the process of gas exchange is completed by mechanical ventilation. However, mechanical ventilation does not significantly reduce the mortality caused by ALI/ARDS.

Rather, the lung injury could aggravated by ventilator due to surfactant deficiency and dysfunction, which associated with the exacerbation of atelectasis, increased formation of oedema, and impairment of local host defence [4–7]. Until now, the effect of most-employed treatment strategies, including high dose of steroids, aspirin, and ulinastain, in patients with ALI/ARDS remains limited [8].

Sivelestat is a neutrophil elastase inhibitor, which induces competitive inhibition of neutrophils, inhibition of neutrophil activation, and reduction of inflammation in the lungs [9, 10]. Currently, the use of sivelestatis already approved in Japan [11, 12]. However, the effectiveness of

* Correspondence: wanwhnj@sina.com; wangdaoxin163@163.com
[1]Department of Respiratory Medicine, Second Affiliated Hospital of Chongqing Medical University, Chongqing 400010, China

sivelestat in clinical needs is yet to be interpreted. Several randomized controlled trials (RCTs) have indicated that sivelestat therapy can improve ventilation days and arterial oxygen partial pressure (PaO2)/fractional inspired oxygen (FiO2), while the efficacy of sivelestat therapy on other outcomes in patients with ALI/ARDS remains controversial. Therefore, a systematic review and meta-analysis of available RCTs were conducted to evaluate the treatment effect of sivelestat.

Methods

Data sources, search strategy, and selection criteria

This review was conducted and reported according to the Preferred Reporting Items for Systematic Reviews and Meta-analysis Statement issued in 2009 (Additional file 1: Checklist S1) [13].

A systematic review and meta-analysis of RCTs published through April 2017 were conducted to identify trials of sivelestat for patients with ALI/ARDS. Electronic databases PubMed, Embase, and the Cochrane Library were searched using the following key words: ("sivelestat" OR "elaspol") AND ("ARDS" OR "adult respiratory distress syndrome" OR "acute respiratory distress syndrome" OR "noncardiogenic pulmonary edema" OR "respiratory insufficiency" OR "systemic inflammatory response syndrome" OR "shock lung" OR "respiratory failure" OR "lung injury*" OR "septic shock" OR "sepsis"). Manual searches of the reference lists were also conducted from all relevant original and review articles to identify additional eligible studies. No language restriction was applied. Unpublished trials were excluded. The medical subject heading, methods, patient disease status, study design, intervention, and outcome variables were used to identify relevant studies.

The literature search was independently performed by two authors using a standardized approach. Any inconsistencies were settled by a group discussion until a consensus was reached. The included studies met the following criteria. (1) RCTs, (2) patients confirmed with ALI/ARDS, (3) patients received sivelestat, and (4) data included 28–30 days mortality, improved ventilation days, PaO_2/FiO_2 level, and intensive care unit (ICU) stays. All retrospective clinical studies that could affect the treatment effects due to various confounding biases were excluded.

The ethical approval and written consent are not necessary for the meta-analysis, because the data of meta-analysis is collected from published literature.

Data collection and quality assessment

The data collected included the first author's name, publication year, country, sample size, mean age, percentage of male, disease status, intervention, baseline PaO_2/FiO_2 ratio, baseline acute physiology and chronic health evaluation (APACHE II) score, reported endpoints, and study design variables. The authors independently scanned the titles and abstracts of the studies for eligibility and relevance. Potentially relevant articles were retrieved and reviewed for selection based on the inclusion and exclusion criteria. Any discrepancies were resolved by discussion. Further, the Jadad scale was employed to evaluate the methodological quality, based on randomization, concealment of treatment allocation, blinding, completeness of follow-up, and use of intention-to-treat analysis [14].

Statistical analysis

Relative risks (RRs) and standard mean differences (SMDs) with 95% confidence intervals (CIs) were calculated using outcomes extracted from each study before data pooling. The random-effects model was used to calculate pooled RRs with 95% CI to estimate the effect of sivelestat on the risk of 28–30 days mortality, and SMDs were employed to estimate the efficacy of sivelestat therapy on the ventilation days, PaO_2/FiO_2 level, and ICU stays [15, 16]. Heterogeneity among trials was investigated using the Q statistic, and P values <0.10 were indicative of significant heterogeneity [17, 18]. Sensitivity analyses were conducted for ventilation days and PaO_2/FiO_2 level by removing each individual study from the meta-analysis [19]. The subgroup analysis was also performed for 28–30 days mortality based on publication year, mean age, percentage of male, disease status, baseline PaO_2/FiO_2 ratio, and Jadad score. The visual inspection of funnel plots for 28–30 days mortality was conducted. The Egger [20] and Begg [21] tests were also used to statistically assess the publication bias for 28–30 days mortality. All reported P values were two sided, and P values <0.05 were considered as statistically significant. Statistical analyses were performed using the STATA software (version 10.0; Stata Corporation, TX, USA).

Results

The results of the study-selection process are shown in Fig. 1. A total of 541 potentially relevant articles were identified after systematically searching electronic databases, professional journals, and other sources. After reviewing the titles or abstracts, 527 were excluded as they did not meet the inclusion criteria, leaving 14 articles for further full-text reviews. Six RCTs were finally identified and included for the analysis of treatment effect of sivelestat in patients with ALI/ARDS [22–27], and the rest were excluded for the following reasons: conference abstracts without full text, retrospective study, and no desirable outcomes. A manual search of the reference lists of these trials did not yield any new eligible studies. The general characteristics of the included studies are presented in Table 1.

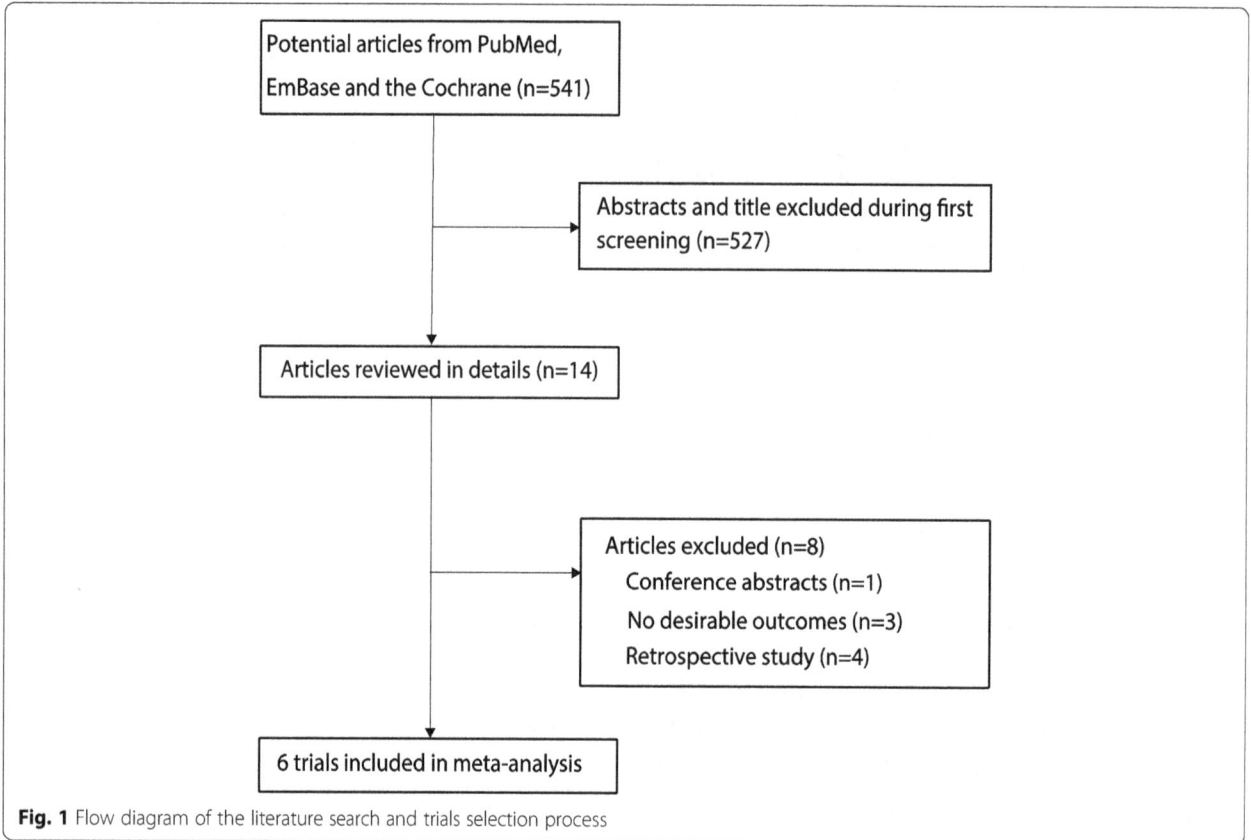

Fig. 1 Flow diagram of the literature search and trials selection process

Six RCTs involving a total of 804 patients with ALI/ARDS were included. The mean age of the patients was 56.0–73.1 years. Each trial included 22–487 individuals. Further, the percentage of included males ranged from 59.3%–76.0%. Five trials were conducted in Japan [22–25, 27], and the remaining one trial in multiple countries [26]. Four of the included trials reported patients with ALI [22, 24, 26, 27], one trial included patients with ARDS [25], and the remaining one trial included patients with both ALI and ARDS [23]. Moreover, five trials included patients who received 0.2 mg/kg/h sivelestat [22–25, 27], and one trial included those who received 0.16 mg/kg/h sivelestat [26]. The study quality was assessed using the Jadad score and is presented in Table 1. Overall, four trials had a score of 3 [22, 24, 26, 27], and the remaining two had a score of 2 [23, 25].

All included trials reported the effect of sivelestat on the risk of 28–30 days mortality. The summary results indicated no significant difference between sivelestat and control for the risk of 28–30 days mortality (RR: 0.94; 95% CI: 0.71–1.23; $P = 0.643$; Fig. 2), and without evidence of heterogeneity. The sensitivity analysis found that the risk of 28–30 days mortality was reduced by 42%, but was not statistically significant when excluding the study by Zeiher et al. (RR: 0.58; 95% CI: 0.29–1.18;

$P = 0.131$; Fig. 2). This trial specifically included a higher incidence of mortality within 28–30 days and included patients who received low-dose sivelestat therapy.

A total of five trials reported the effect of sivelestat therapy on ventilation days in patients with ALI/ARDS. No significant difference was found between sivelestat and control for ventilation days (SMD: 0.05; 95% CI: −0.27 to 0.38; $P = 0.748$; Fig. 3). Although substantial heterogeneity was observed in the magnitude of the effect across the studies ($P = 0.028$), the conclusion was not affected by the exclusion of any specific study after the sequential exclusion of each study from all of the pooled analyses (Table 2).

A total of four trials reported the effect of sivelestat therapy on PaO_2/FiO_2 in patients with ALI/ARDS. It was noted that the PaO_2/FiO_2 level in patients with ALI/ARDS who received sivelestat therapy had increased by 0.48, although it was not statistically significant (SMD: 0.48; 95% CI: −0.45 to 1.41; $P = 0.315$; Fig. 4), and the potential evidence of significant heterogeneity was detected ($P < 0.001$). According to the sensitivity analysis, the study by Tamakuma et al. was excluded because it specifically included patients with higher baseline PaO_2/FiO_2 level and might affect the treatment effect of sivelestat therapy. After this exclusion, it was concluded that sivelestat therapy significantly increased the level of

Table 1 Baseline characteristic of studies included in the systematic review and meta-analysis

Study	Publication year	Country	Sample size	Mean age	Percentage male (%)	Disease status	Intervention	Baseline PaO$_2$/FiO$_2$ ratio	Baseline APACHE II score	Jadad scale
Endo [22]	2006	Japan	26	NA	NA	ALI	0.2 mg/kg/h for 14 days	NA	NA	3
Sato [23]	2008	Japan	24	69.0	75.0	ALI/ARDS	0.2 mg/kg/h for 14 days	196.5	NA	2
Morimoto [24]	2011	Japan	22	73.1	63.6	ALI	0.2 mg/kg/h huntil weaning from mechanical ventilation	<150.0	NA	3
Kadoi [25]	2004	Japan	24	64.0	75.0	ARDS	0.2 mg/kg/h for 14 days	148.5	20.1	2
Zeiher [26]	2004	Multiple countries	487	56.0	59.3	ALI	0.16 mg/kg/h for 14 days	148.7	20.8	3
Tamakuma [27]	2004	Japan	221	57.8	76.0	ALI	0.2 mg/kg/h for 14 days	199.0	NA	3

ALI Acute lung injury, *APACHE II* acute physiology and chronic health evaluation, *ARDS* acute respiratory distress syndrome, *FiO$_2$* fractional inspired oxygen, *PaO$_2$* arterial oxygen partial pressure

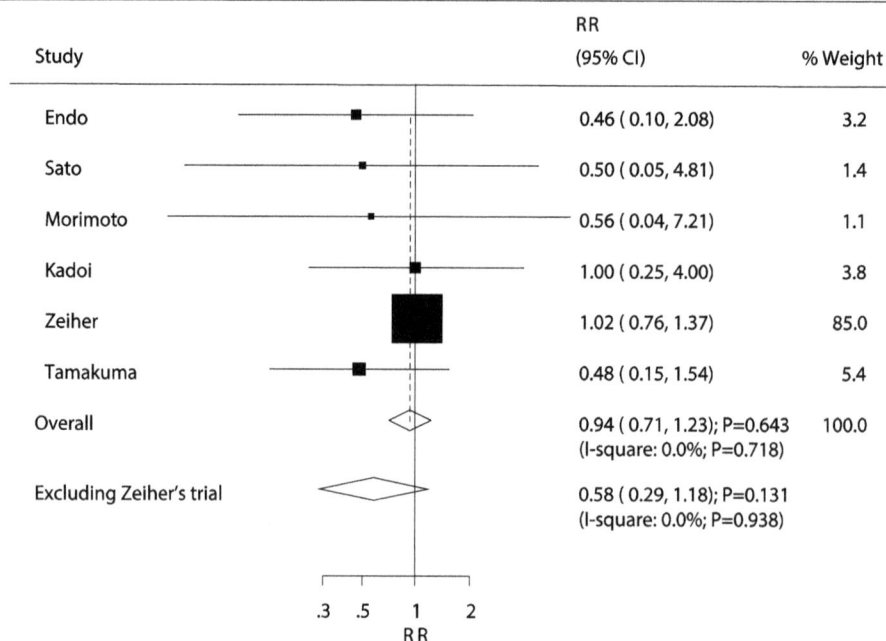

Fig. 2 Effect of sivelestat on the risk of 28–30 days mortality

PaO$_2$/FiO$_2$ in patients with ALI/ARDS (SMD: 0.87; 95% CI: 0.39 to 1.35; $P < 0.001$; Table 2). Moreover, sivelestat therapy had little or no effect on ICU stays in patients with ALI/ARDS (SMD: –9.87; 95% CI: –24.30 to 4.56; $P = 0.180$; Fig. 5) (Table 3).

The publication bias was assessed using the funnel plot for 28–30 days mortality (Fig. 6). Although the Begg test showed no evidence of publication bias for 28–30 days mortality, the Egger test showed potential evidence of publication bias. However, the results were not influenced after adjustment for publication bias using the trim-and-fill method [28].

Discussion

The objective of the present meta-analysis was to evaluate the effect of sivelestat therapy in patients with ALI/ARDS. Six trials including 804 patients with ALI/ARDS were included. The summary results showed that sivelestat therapy had little or no significant effect on 28–30 days mortality, ventilation days, PaO$_2$/FiO$_2$ level, and ICU stays.

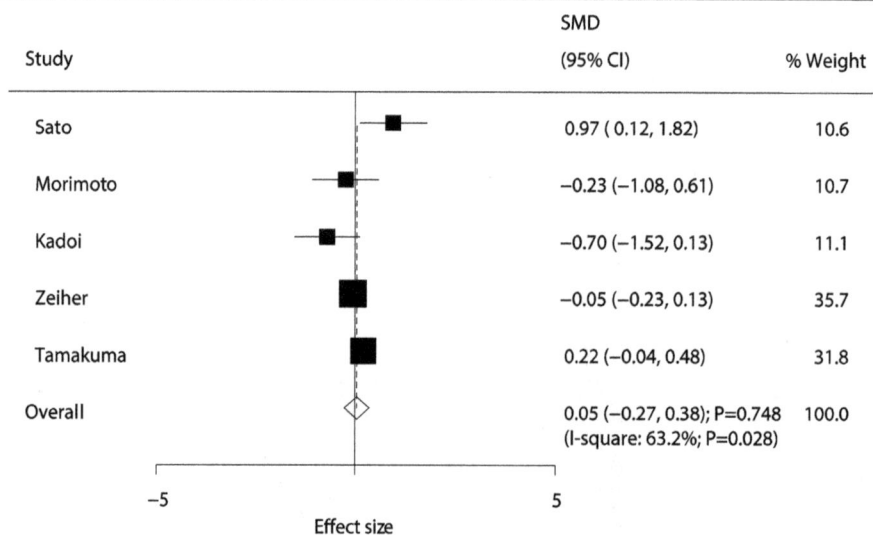

Fig. 3 Effect of sivelestat therapy on ventilation days

Table 2 Sensitivity analysis for ventilation days and PaO_2/FiO_2

Outcomes	Excluding study	SMD (95% CI)	P value	Heterogeneity (%)	P value for heterogeneity
Ventilation days	Sato	−0.02 (−0.29 to 0.25)	0.865	50.7	0.107
	Morimoto	0.09 (−0.27 to 0.45)	0.633	71.4	0.015
	Kadoi	0.14 (−0.17 to 0.45)	0.388	61.3	0.052
	Zeiher	0.08 (−0.48 to 0.64)	0.766	65.4	0.034
	Tamakuma	−0.02 (−0.54 to 0.50)	0.950	62.9	0.044
PaO_2/FiO_2	Morimoto	0.37 (−0.73 to 1.47)	0.507	97.4	<0.001
	Kadoi	0.53 (−0.58 to 1.64)	0.350	97.4	<0.001
	Zeiher	0.18 (−0.53 to 0.89)	0.623	73.2	0.024
	Tamakuma	0.87 (0.39 to 1.35)	<0.001	49.1	0.140

CI confidence interval, FiO_2 fractional inspired oxygen, PaO_2 arterial oxygen partial pressure, SMD standard mean difference, RR relative risk

The findings of the sensitivity analysis indicated that sivelestat therapy might play a beneficial effect on the level of PaO_2/FiO_2. These results might help better define the treatment effect of sivelestat therapy in patients with ALI/ARDS and help physicians to select appropriate treatment strategies.

A previous meta-analysis including eight trials suggested that sivelestat therapy was not associated with 28–30 days mortality and mechanical ventilation days, while it was associated with lower PaO_2/FiO_2 ratio in patients with ALI/ARDS [29]. The study did not recommend its routine use in patients with ALI/ARDS. The effect of sivelestat therapy on ICU stays was not conducted, and the treatment effects according to different baseline characteristics were not performed. Therefore, the present study conducted a comprehensive systematic review and meta-analysis to evaluate the effect of sivelestat therapy in patients with ALI/ARDS.

The findings of the present study suggested that sivelestat therapy had no significant effect on 28–30 days mortality. All included trials reported that sivelestat therapy did not affect the risk of mortality within 28–30 days. However, nearly all trials reported that the incidence of 28–30 days mortality reduced but was not statistically significant. Moreover, Zeiher et al. found that sivelestat therapy was associated with a nonsignificant increase in the risk of 28 days mortality by 2% [26]. The possible reason could be the efficacy of sivelestat on 28 days mortality which might be affected by specific clinical conditions [30]. Meanwhile, sivelestat has maximum efficacy in patients with mild to moderate ARDS [31]. Further, the treatment effects of sivelestat were correlated with age, disease status, haemodialysis, and methylprednisoline use [32]. Furthermore, subgroup analyses for 28 days mortality, excluding the study conducted by Zeiher et al., were performed [26]. The

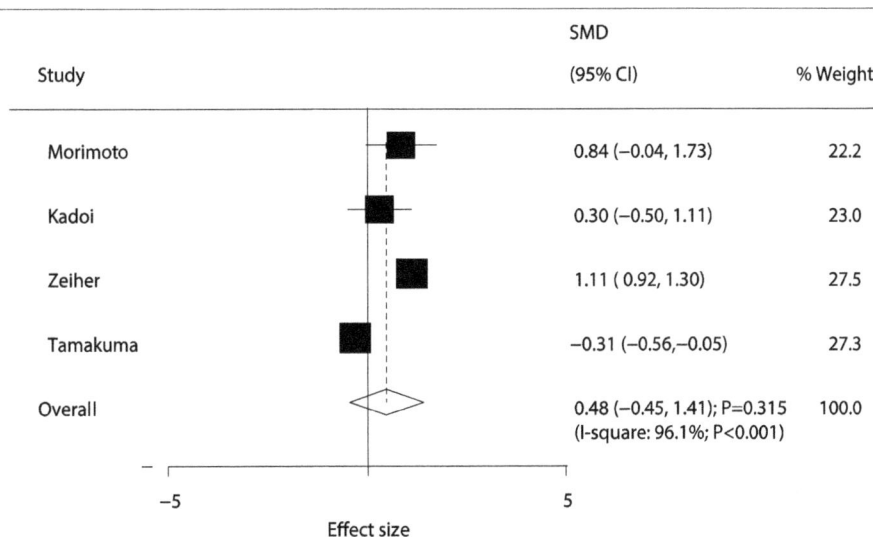

Study		SMD (95% CI)	% Weight
Morimoto		0.84 (−0.04, 1.73)	22.2
Kadoi		0.30 (−0.50, 1.11)	23.0
Zeiher		1.11 (0.92, 1.30)	27.5
Tamakuma		−0.31 (−0.56,−0.05)	27.3
Overall		0.48 (−0.45, 1.41); P=0.315 (I-square: 96.1%; P<0.001)	100.0

Fig. 4 Effect of sivelestat therapy on PaO_2/FiO_2

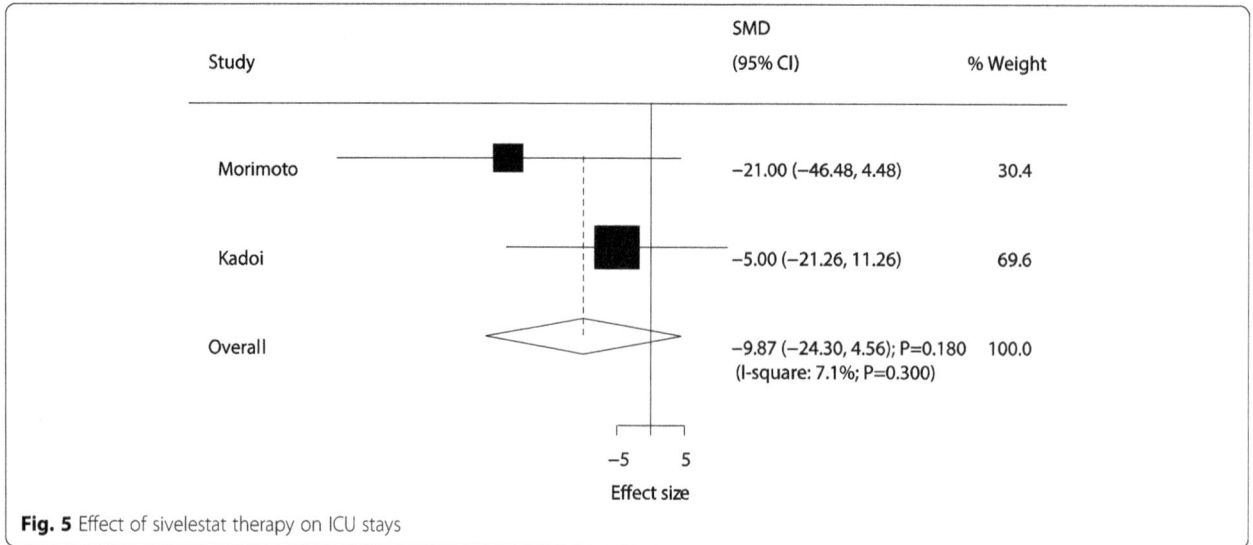

Fig. 5 Effect of sivelestat therapy on ICU stays

findings of subgroup analysis were consistent with the overall analysis.

No significant difference was found between sivelestat therapy and control for ventilation days. Mostly included trials indicated that sivelestat therapy had no significant effect on ventilation days, while the trial conducted by Sato et al. reported inconsistent results [23]. This study specifically included patients with both ALI and ARDS, which might affect ventilation days. Further, the Sato's study might include more severe ALI/ARDS patients,

which was associated with lower respiratory function so that sivelestat became less effective [33]. Finally, sivelestat therapy did not affect the PaO_2/FiO_2 level, and ICU stays in ALI/ARDS patients. However, these conclusions may be variable since a smaller number of trials were included. Therefore, the present study gave a relative result and provided a synthetic and comprehensive review.

The strengths of this meta-analysis were as follows: (1) the large sample size allowed the quantitative assessment of the efficacy of sivelestat, and thus these findings were

Table 3 Subgroup analyses for 28–30 days mortality excluding the study conducted by Zeiher et al.

Group	RR (95% CI)	P value	Heterogeneity (%)	P value for heterogeneity	P value for interaction test
Publication year					
2005 or after	0.49 (0.16–1.52)	0.215	0.0	0.992	0.696
Before 2005	0.65 (0.27–1.59)	0.344	0.0	0.427	
Mean age (years)					
≥ 65.0	0.53 (0.09–2.92)	0.462	0.0	0.949	0.897
< 65.0	0.60 (0.28–1.28)	0.186	0.0	0.677	
Percentage male (%)					
≥ 70.0	0.63 (0.27–1.44)	0.272	0.0	0.713	0.741
< 70.0	0.48 (0.13–1.79)	0.277	0.0	0.898	
Disease status					
ALI	0.48 (0.20–1.15)	0.100	0.0	0.992	0.468
ALI/ARDS or ARDS	0.83 (0.25–2.71)	0.757	0.0	0.611	
Baseline PaO_2/FiO_2 ratio					
≥ 150	0.48 (0.17–1.37)	0.170	0.0	0.975	0.634
< 150	0.68 (0.26–1.77)	0.430	0.0	0.751	
Jadad score					
3	0.48 (0.20–1.15)	0.100	0.0	0.992	0.468
2	0.83 (0.25–2.71)	0.757	0.0	0.611	

ALI Acute lung injury, *ARDS* acute respiratory distress syndrome, *CI* confidence interval, *FiO2* fractional inspired oxygen, *PaO2* arterial oxygen partial pressure, *RR* relative risk

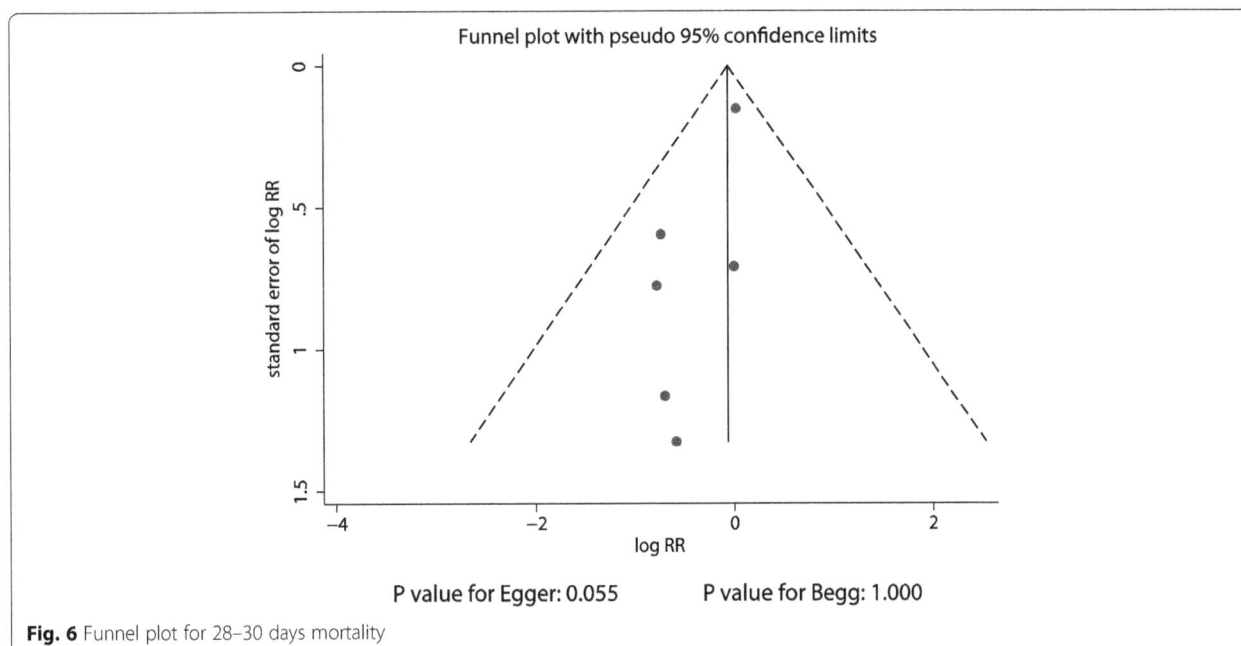

Fig. 6 Funnel plot for 28–30 days mortality

potentially more robust than any individual study. Second, the results of ICU stays were summarized, as the previous meta-analysis was not conducted. Third, the treatment effect of sivelestat in patients with ALI/ARDS according to different baseline characteristics was conducted, which provided any potential effect of sivelestat therapy in specific subpopulations.

The limitation of this study were as follows: (1) the number of included studies was smaller than expected, which always acquired broad CIs, that is, no statistically significant difference; (2) data on baseline APACHE score of the enrolled patients were available in two trials, which might affect the treatment effect of sivelestat in ALI/ARDS patients [25, 26]; (3) the information about ALI/ARDS classification were available in two trials [26, 27] and other trials could not provide diagnosis criteria of ALI/ARDS patients, which was correlated with the treatment effects of sivelestat; (4) mostly included trials were conducted in Japan, which might induce ethnic biases; (5) in a meta-analysis of published studies, publication bias is inevitable; and (6) the analysis used pooled data (individual data were not available), which prevented a detailed analysis to obtain more comprehensive results.

Conclusion
The findings of this study suggested that sivelestat therapy might play an important role on the PaO_2/FiO_2 level, while it had no significant effect on 28–30 days mortality, ventilation days, and ICU stays. Future large-scale trials should focus on different disease status, patient characteristics, and trials from other countries to analyze any possible efficacy and safety of sivelestat therapy.

Abbreviations
ALI: Acute lung injury; ARDS: Acute respiratory distress syndrome; CIs: Confidence intervals; FiO2: Fractional inspired oxygen; ICU: Intensive care unit; PaO2: Arterial oxygen partial pressure; RCTs: Randomized controlled trials; RR: Relative risk; SMD: Standard mean difference

Acknowledgements
None

Funding
None

Authors' contributions
SLP and DXWcontributed to conception and design; SLP, DXW, DSL, YZ, DQ, JH and GQZcontributed to acquisition of data, or analysis and interpretation of data; SLP, DXW, DSL, YZ, DQ, JH and GQZhave been involved in drafting the manuscript or revising it critically for important intellectual content; all authors have given final approval of the version to be published.

Competing interests
The authors declare that they have no competing interests.

Author details
[1]Department of Respiratory Medicine, Second Affiliated Hospital of Chongqing Medical University, Chongqing 400010, China. [2]Department of Respiratory and Critical Care Medicine, The First People's Hospital of Zunyi, Zunyi, China.

References

1. Lynch JE, Cheek JM, Chan EY, Zwischenberger JB. Adjuncts to mechanical ventilation in ARDS. Semin Thorac Cardiovasc Surg. 2006;18:20–7.

2. Ashbaugh DG, Bigelow DB, Petty TL, Levine BE. Acute respiratory distress in adults. Lancet. 1967;2:319–23.

3. Janz DR, Ware LB. Approach to the patient with the acute respiratory distress syndrome. Clin Chest Med. 2014;35:685–96.

4. Tu X, Wang X, Chen W. Nursing care of patients with acute respiratory distress syndrome accepting NO inhalation. Chin Nurs Res. 2008;

5. Liao P, Whitehead T, Evans T, Griffiths M. Ventilator-associated lung injury. Lancet. 2003;361:332–40.

6. Chiumello D, Pristine G, Slutsky AS. Mechanical ventilation affects local and systemic cytokines in an animal model of acute respiratory distress syndrome. Am J Respir Crit Care Med. 1999;160:109–16.

7. Tremblay L, Valenza F, Ribeiro SP, Li J, Slutsky SA. Injurious ventilatory strategies increase cytokines and c-fos m-RNA expression in an isolated rat lung model. J Clin Invest. 1997;99:944–52.

8. Adhikari N, Burns KE, Meade MO. Pharmacologic treatments for acute respiratory distress syndrome and acute lung injury: systematic review and meta-analysis. Treat Respir Med. 2004;3:307–28.

9. Hagio T, Matsumoto S, Nakao S, Abiru T, Ohno H, Kawabata K. Elastase inhibition reduced death associated with acid aspiration-induced lung injury in hamsters. Eur J Pharmacol. 2004;488:173–80.

10. Chai JK, Cai JH, Deng HP, Zou XF, Liu W, Hu QG, et al. Role of neutrophil elastase in lung injury induced by burn-blast combined injury in rats. Burns. 2013;39:745–53.

11. Hayakawa M, Katabami K, Wada T, Sugano M, Hoshino H, Sawamura A, et al. Sivelestat (selective neutrophil elastase inhibitor) improves the mortality rate of sepsis associated with both acute respiratory distress syndrome and disseminated intravascular coagulation patients. Shock. 2010;33:14–8.

12. Okayama N, Kakihana Y, Setoguchi D, Imabayashi T, Omae T, Matsunaga A, et al. Clinical effects of a neutrophil elastase inhibitor, sivelestat, in patients with acute respiratory distress syndrome. J Anesth. 2006;20:6–10.

13. Moher D, Liberati A, Tetzlaff J, Altman DG, Group TP. Preferred reporting items for systematic reviews and meta-analyses: the PRISMA statement. Revista Española De Nutrición Humana Y Dietética. 2010;18:889–96.

14. Jadad AR, Moore RA, Carroll D, Jenkinson C, Reynolds DJ, Gavaghan DJ, et al. Assessing the quality of reports of randomized clinical trials: is blinding necessary? Control Clin Trials. 1996;17:1–12.

15. Dersimonian R, Laird N. Meta-analysis in clinical trials. Control Clin Trials. 1986;7:177–88.

16. Ades AE, Lu G, Higgins JPT. The interpretation of random-effects meta-analysis in decision models. Med Decis Mak. 2005;25:646–54.

17. Deeks JJ, Higgins JPT, Altman DG. Analysing Data and Undertaking Meta-Analyses. In: Higgins J, Green S, editors. Cochrane handbook for systematic reviews of interventions 5.0.1, vol. 2008. Oxford: The Cochrane Collaboration; 2008. p. 243–96.

18. Higgins JP, Thompson SG, Deeks JJ, Altman DG. Measuring inconsistency in meta-analyses. Br Med J. 2003;327:557–60.

19. Tobias A. Assessing the influence of a single study in meta-analysis. Stata Tech Bull. 1999;47:15–7.

20. Egger M, Smith GD, Schneider M, Minder C. Bias in meta-analysis detected by a simple, graphical test. BMJ. 1997;315:629–34.

21. Begg CB, Mazumdar M. Operating characteristics of a rank correlation test for publication bias. Biometrics. 1994;50:1088–101.

22. Endo S, Sato N, Yaegashi Y, Suzuki Y, Kojika M, Yamada Y, et al. Sivelestat sodium hydrate improves septic acute lung injury by reducing alveolar dysfunction. Res Commun Mol Pathol Pharmacol. 2006;119:53–65.

23. Sato N, Imai S, Yaegashi Y. The effect of use of Elaspol on acute lung injury (ALI) with sepsis. Prog Med. 2003;23:915–9.

24. Morimoto K, Nishimura K, Miyasaka S, Maeta H, Taniguchi I. The effect of sivelestat sodium hydrate on severe respiratory failure after thoracic aortic surgery with deep hypothermia. Ann Thorac Cardiovasc Surg. 2011;17:369–75.

25. Kadoi Y, Hinohara H, Kunimoto F, Saito S, Goto F, Kosaka T, et al. Pilot study of the effects of ONO-5046 in patients with acute respiratory distress syndrome. Anesth Analg. 2004;99:872–7.

26. Zeiher BG, Artigas A, Vincent JA, Jackson K, Thompson BT, Bernard G. Neutrophil elastase inhibition in acute lung injury: results of the STRIVE study. Crit Care Med. 2004;32:1695 702.

27. Tamakuma S, Ogawa M, Aikawa N, Kubota T, Hirasawa H, Ishizaka A, et al. Relationship between neutrophil elastase and acute lung injury in humans. Pulm Pharmacol Ther. 2004;17:271.

28. Duval S, Tweedie R. A nonparametric "trim and fill" method of accounting for publication bias in meta-analysis. J Am Stat Assoc. 2000;95:89–98.

29. Iwata K, Doi A, Ohji G, Oka H, Oba Y, Takimoto K, et al. Effect of neutrophil elastase inhibitor (sivelestat sodium) in the treatment of acute lung injury (ALI) and acute respiratory distress syndrome (ARDS): a systematic review and meta-analysis. Intern Med. 2010;49:2423–32.

30. Aikawa N, Kawasaki Y. Clinical utility of the neutrophil elastase inhibitor sivelestat for the treatment of acute respiratory distress syndrome. Ther Clin Risk Manag. 2014;10:621–9.

31. Tsushima K, Yokoyama T, Matsumura T, Koizumi T, Kubo K, Tatsumi K. The potential efficacy of noninvasive ventilation with administration of a neutrophil elastase inhibitor for acute respiratory distress syndrome. J Crit Care. 2014;29:420–5.

32. Kido T, Muramatsu K, Yatera K, Asakawa T, Otsubo H, Kubo T, et al. Efficacy of early sivelestat administration on acute lung injury and acute respiratory distress syndrome. Respirology. 2017;22:708–13.

33. Ozawa T, Mihara K, Yasuno N. Predictors of the therapeutic effect of sivelestat in patients with acute lung injuryassociated with systemic inflammatory response syndrome. J Pharm Health Care Sci. 2016;2:19.

5

Impact of rapid investigation clinic on timeliness of lung cancer diagnosis and treatment

Nicole Ezer[1,2], Asma Navasakulpong[3], Kevin Schwartzman[1,2], Linda Ofiara[2] and Anne V. Gonzalez[1,2*]

Abstract

Background: Guidelines recommend timely evaluation of patients with suspected lung cancer. We evaluated the impact of a Rapid Investigation Clinic (RIC) on timeliness of lung cancer diagnosis and treatment between February 2010 and December 2011.

Methods: Investigation within the RIC was conducted by a pulmonologist and a nurse clinician. Controls were patients with lung cancer, investigated outside the RIC at the same institution during the same time period. The primary outcome was time between first contact with a local physician for suspected lung cancer (T0) and first treatment. Factors associated with the delay from T0 to first treatment were examined using multivariate analysis. Completeness of lung cancer staging according to guidelines was assessed.

Results: A total of 195 patients were investigated within the RIC vs. 132 patients outside the RIC. The median delay between T0 and first treatment was 65 days (interquartile range [IQR] 46–92 days) in the RIC and 78 days (IQR 49–119 days) in the non-RIC patients ($p \leq 0.01$). Time from T0 to pathological diagnosis was shorter in the RIC (median 26 days; IQR 14–42 days) vs. non-RIC patients (median 40 days; IQR 16–68 days). In multivariate analysis, investigation in the RIC was associated with a reduction in time to first treatment of 24 days (95% confidence interval [CI] 12–35 days) when adjusted for relevant confounders. Guideline-concordant investigation occurred more frequently in RIC patients, based on the quality indicators examined.

Conclusions: A Rapid Investigation Clinic reduces delays to lung cancer diagnosis and treatment, and impacts quality of care.

Keywords: Lung cancer diagnosis, Neoplasm staging, Timeliness, Delay

Background

Lung cancer remains the leading cause of cancer death for both men and women [1]. Timeliness of lung cancer care is an important quality indicator; however, standards for investigation of new lung cancer patients vary. With the advent of Computed tomography (CT) screening for lung cancer [2] the number of patients requiring investigation is likely to increase. This will require evidence-based strategies aimed at improving guideline-concordant care and minimizing delays.

Accurate lung cancer diagnosis and staging requires various imaging studies and procedures. Positron Emission Tomography (PET) scanning detects unsuspected metastatic disease and reduces non-curative surgical resections [3]. Minimally invasive needle techniques such as endobronchial ultrasound-guided needle aspiration (EBUS) are now considered the test of first choice to confirm mediastinal disease [4]. Work-up of patients with suspected lung cancer requires ready access to these tests and adequate coordination of care, in addition to multi-disciplinary input.

The 2011 National Institute for Health and Clinical Excellence (NICE) guidelines recommend that rapid access clinics should be provided, where possible, for the investigation of patients with suspected lung cancer [5]. The most recent American College of Chest Physicians

---

* Correspondence: anne.gonzalez@mcgill.ca
[1]Respiratory Epidemiology and Clinical Research Unit, Montreal Chest Institute, McGill University Health Centre, Montreal, QC, Canada
[2]Respiratory Division, McGill University Health Centre, Montreal, QC, Canada

(ACCP) lung cancer guidelines suggest that efforts be made to deliver "timely" care [6]. At the McGill University Health Centre (MUHC), a Rapid Investigation Clinic (RIC) was established to coordinate and accelerate the workup of patients with suspected lung cancer. The aim of the study was to assess the impact of this model of care on timeliness of lung cancer diagnosis, staging and treatment. The impact of the RIC on the delivery of a guideline-concordant investigation was also examined.

Methods

The Rapid Investigation Clinic (RIC) was established in February 2010. The RIC operates twice a week, and is staffed by a rotating pulmonary physician and nurse-clinician. The nurse-clinician monitors the investigation progress, assists with coordination of care, and provides patients with the necessary psychosocial support. At initial encounter, preference is given to the invasive diagnostic procedure felt to have the best yield/risk ratio based on CT findings. Procedures that allow simultaneous diagnosis and staging are favored. Patients are staged according to the 2009 staging system [7], and the 2007 American College of Chest Physicians guidelines for lung cancer diagnosis and staging were followed during the study period [8]. Patients in the RIC and non-RIC groups had access to the same imaging studies and diagnostic procedures within the institution.

An institutional database of all patients with a pathological diagnosis of lung cancer was established in November 2008. A prospective database of patients evaluated in the RIC was established in 2010 and maintained by a registrar, to facilitate delays surveillance. Patients investigated within the RIC between February 2010 and December 2011, in whom a diagnosis of lung cancer was confirmed, are included in this analysis (RIC patients). Patients investigated within our institution but outside the RIC, whether by other "non-RIC" pulmonologists or thoracic surgeons, and in whom a diagnosis of lung cancer was confirmed, constituted the comparison group. The "non-RIC" physicians elected to continue investigation of patients with suspected lung cancer within their own clinics, as was being done prior to RIC implementation. Patients with a second lung cancer diagnosis, patients partially investigated outside the institution (e.g. referred only for a specific diagnostic procedure or for surgery), patients undergoing re-staging after initial treatment for lung cancer, and patients investigated during a hospitalization were excluded.

The data extracted from electronic health records included patient demographics, date and type of imaging studies and invasive procedures, histopathological diagnosis, disease stage, date and type of treatments. Performance status was extracted from consultation notes.

Time 0 (T0) refers to the first visit with any MUHC physician for suspected lung cancer, and was defined as follows: 1) In symptomatic patients T0 was the first visit in the ER which triggered further testing for lung cancer; 2) If lung cancer was suspected from imaging, T0 was the visit date after the imaging study, which prompted further investigation; 3) If the patient was followed by a pulmonary physician for an alternate diagnosis or a lung nodule and there was a suspicion of lung cancer, T0 was considered the visit that triggered additional tests; 4) In patients referred to the RIC by any physician, T0 was considered the date of referral. Hence, T0 was not the date of first visit to the RIC, but rather the visit that triggered the lung cancer investigation and/or RIC referral. All delays were measured from T0. The specialty of the physician who evaluated the patient at T0 was recorded.

All invasive diagnostic procedures performed were reviewed. These included bronchoscopy, EBUS (linear or radial), transthoracic needle aspiration (TTNA), endoscopic ultrasound (EUS) and mediastinoscopy. Procedures aimed at sampling a peripheral lung nodule or mass, and procedures aimed at sampling hilar and/or mediastinal nodes were examined separately. The number of non-diagnostic procedures was documented in RIC and non-RIC patients. The invasive diagnostic procedure that first provided a pathological diagnosis of lung cancer was recorded.

The primary outcome was the time interval (in days) between first contact with a local physician for suspected lung cancer (T0) and date of first treatment. First treatment encompassed surgery or radiosurgery for early stage lung cancer, and chemotherapy or combined chemo-radiotherapy for advanced stage disease. The time interval from T0 to date of tissue diagnosis (i.e. date of a pathology report that confirms the diagnosis), and the interval from T0 to the date all staging investigations are completed were also examined. "Staging completed" refers to the date of the last test (imaging study or invasive procedure) that completes the lung cancer investigation according to the ACCP 2007 guidelines [8]. Quality indicators of guideline-concordant investigation were compared in the RIC and non-RIC groups. These included: PET scanning in stage I-II patients treated with surgical resection, brain imaging prior to curative-intent treatment in stage III non-small cell lung cancer (NSCLC), and brain imaging for small cell lung cancer (SCLC). The proportion of patients referred to multidisciplinary lung cancer clinic and/or the lung cancer tumor board was recorded.

Time intervals are reported as median and interquartile range, and were compared using the Wilcoxon rank sum test. Linear regression analysis was used to examine factors thought to be associated with delay from T0 to first treatment. A multivariate model was constructed with the following covariates: age (≤ 75 or >75 years), sex, performance status (Eastern Cooperative Oncology Group (ECOG) 0–1 versus ≥2), lung cancer type (NSCLC versus SCLC), investigation in the RIC versus outside the RIC, inclusion of EBUS and PET scan in the lung cancer investigation, and number of non-diagnostic tests (0, 1 or ≥2). To examine the impact of disease stage, the multivariate analysis was repeated in the subgroup of patients with NSCLC. Quality metrics were compared using a chi-squared test or Fisher's exact test, as appropriate.

The study was approved by the Research Ethics Board of the MUHC. All analyses were performed using SAS version 9.3. Graphs were designed using GraphPad Prism.

Results

There were 195 patients in the RIC group and 132 patients in the non-RIC group. Baseline characteristics are detailed in Table 1. The RIC group included a higher proportion of patients with SCLC (13%) compared to the non-RIC group (5%). Performance status was similar in both groups. Among RIC patients, the physician who initiated the lung cancer investigation and referred to the RIC (type of 0 physician) was more likely to be a pulmonologist (93%), while the investigation of non-RIC patients was initiated by both pulmonologists (67%) and

thoracic surgeons (27%). During the study period, 103 patients evaluated within the RIC ultimately did not have a diagnosis of lung cancer. These patients were excluded from the analysis. The majority were diagnosed with non-malignant lung pathologies (including sarcoidosis); 14 patients had other primary malignancies; 28 patients did not pursue investigation due to poor performance status; and one patient was diagnosed with a carcinoid tumor.

The number of invasive diagnostic procedures performed was similar in RIC and non-RIC patients (Table 2). The invasive procedures providing the first pathological evidence of lung cancer were directed at lung masses or nodules in 60% of patients in the RIC and 56% of the non-RIC groups ($p = 0.42$). These were directed at lymph nodes in 26% of the RIC and 23% of the non-RIC patients ($p = 0.22$) (Table 3). The last test performed to complete lung cancer diagnosis and staging was most frequently an imaging study. In particular, PET scan was the last test in 48% of RIC and 36% of non-RIC patients (Table 4).

The median delay between T0 and first lung cancer treatment was 65 days (interquartile range [IQR] 46–92 days) for RIC versus 78 days (IQR 49–119) for non-RIC patients ($p = 0.01$). The median delay to first chemotherapy or radiotherapy was significantly reduced in RIC patients ($p = 0.01$), while time to surgery was similar in RIC and non-RIC patients (p = ns). There was no significant difference in time to staging being completed ($p = 0.39$), however time to pathological diagnosis of lung cancer was reduced significantly in the RIC patients ($p < 0.01$) (Fig. 1).

In the multivariate logistic regression analysis, significant predictors of longer intervals to first treatment were being investigated outside the RIC, a pathological diagnosis of small cell lung cancer, age > 75 years, inclusion of PET scan in the work-up, and increasing numbers of non-diagnostic tests (Table 5). Worse performance

Table 1 Baseline characteristics of patients investigated within the Rapid Investigation Clinic (RIC) and those investigated at the same institution (Non-RIC)

Characteristics	RIC (N = 195)	Non-RIC (N = 132)	p-value[a]
Age in years (mean ± SD)	69 (9)	68 (10)	0.55
Male, N (%)	94 (48)	68 (52)	0.57
NSCLC, N (%)	169 (87)	125 (95)	<0.01
Stage I-II	51 (26)	55 (42)	
Stage III-IV	118 (61)	70 (53)	
SCLC, N (%)	26 (13)	7 (5)	0.29
Extensive Stage	14 (7)	3 (2)	
Limited Stage	12 (6)	4 (3)	
Performance Status, N (%)			0.13
ECOG 0–1	162 (83)	118 (90)	
ECOG 2–3	33 (17)	14 (11)	
Type of T0 Physician, N (%)			<0.01
Pulmonologist	181 (93)	89 (67)	
Thoracic surgeon	–	35 (27)	
Medical oncology	4 (2)	4 (3)	
Internal medicine	6 (3)	–	
Other	4 (2)	4 (3)	

[a]Baseline characteristics were compared using the chi-squared test for categorical variables, and the Student t-test for continuous variables

Table 2 Number and type of invasive diagnostic procedures performed in RIC versus non-RIC patients

	Patients who underwent a given number of invasive diagnostic procedures (%)	
	RIC (N = 195)	Non-RIC (N = 132)
Total number of invasive diagnostic procedures performed		
0[a]	9 (5)	10 (8)
1	99 (51)	68 (51)
2	67 (34)	41 (31)
≥3	20 (10)	13 (9)

[a]Includes patients with no invasive procedure performed, and those with pathology only confirmed at the time of surgical resection (wedge resection, lobectomy or pneumonectomy)

Table 3 Type of invasive procedures providing the first tissue diagnosis, in RIC versus non-RIC patients

	Number of patients in whom a given type of procedure provided the tissue diagnosis (%)	
	RIC (N = 195)	Non-RIC (N = 132)
Lung mass or peripheral nodule sampling	**118 (60)**	**74 (56)**
Conventional Bronchoscopy	59 (30)	22 (17)
TTNA	51 (26)	48 (36)
Radial EBUS	8 (4)	4 (3)
Lymph Node sampling	**53 (27)**	**28 (21)**
Linear EBUS	48 (25)	16 (12)
Mediastinoscopy	2 (1)	2 (1)
EUS	0 (0)	4 (3)
Chamberlain	2 (1)	0 (0)
Lymph Node FNA	1 (<1)	6 (<1)
Surgical Sampling[a]	**13 (7)**	**20 (15)**
Biopsy of Metastases[b]	**5 (3)**	**6 (5)**
No pathologic confirmation	**6 (3)**	**4(3)**

[a]At time of lobectomy or wedge resection
[b]Includes thoracentesis, medical thoracoscopy, liver biopsy, brain biopsy, and bone biopsy

Table 4 Last imaging test or procedure performed to complete the lung cancer investigation (diagnosis and staging) among patients who received treatment

	Number of patients in whom a given test is the last test to complete the investigation, among treated patients (N = 283)	
	RIC (N = 167)	Non-RIC (N = 116)
Lung mass or peripheral nodule sampling	**12 (7)**	**27 (23)**
Conventional Bronchoscopy	4 (2)	4 (3)
TTNA	7 (4)	23 (20)
Radial EBUS	1 (1)	–
Lymph Node sampling	**26 (16)**	**19 (16)**
Linear EBUS	12 (7)	9 (8)
Mediastinoscopy	10 (6)	8 (7)
EUS	2 (1)	1 (1)
Chamberlain	2 (1)	0 (0)
Lymph Node FNA	1 (<1)	1 (1)
Imaging study	**115 (69)**	**64 (55)**
CT scan	19 (11)	14 (12)
PET scan	80 (48)	42 (36)
MRI	9 (5)	4 (3)
Ultrasound	1 (1)	–
Bone scan	6 (4)	4 (3)
Biopsy of Metastases[a]	**14 (8)**	**6 (5)**
N/A	**1 (–)**	–

[a]Includes thoracentesis, medical thoracoscopy, liver biopsy, brain biopsy, and bone biopsy

status and use of EBUS were not associated with longer delays ($p > 0.05$). After adjustment for these variables, investigation within the RIC was associated with a shorter time to treatment (−24 days, 95% confidence interval [CI] -35 to −12 days). Among the subset of patients with NSCLC, patients with stage I −IIB tumors had significantly longer delays to treatment (15 days, 95% CI 3−28) compared to those with later stage tumors when adjusted for investigation within vs. outside RIC, and other confounders.

Quality indicators were compared in the RIC and non-RIC groups (Table 6). PET scans were performed more frequently in early stage patients investigated within the RIC (94% vs. 82%, $p = 0.05$). Brain imaging in the context of stage IIIA NSCLC was performed in 51% of RIC and 38% of non-RIC patients ($p = $ ns). Neuroimaging for SCLC was performed in 92% of RIC and 72% of non-RIC patients ($p = $ ns). A larger proportion of patients investigated via the RIC were discussed at tumor board or evaluated in the multidisciplinary lung cancer clinic (74% vs. 55%, $p < 0.01$).

Discussion

Implementation of a rapid investigation clinic was associated with decreased time between the first visit for suspected lung cancer and first treatment. In multivariate analysis, the difference in time to treatment related to

RIC was 24 days, when adjusted for relevant confounders such as sex, age, performance status, inclusion of EBUS and/or PET scan in the investigation, and number of non-diagnostic procedures. The factors associated with significantly longer delays were advanced age, early

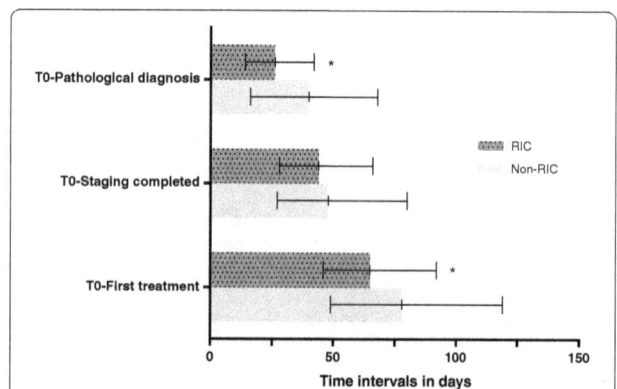

Fig. 1 Time intervals from T0 to lung cancer diagnosis, staging and first treatment. * $p \leq 0.01$

Table 5 Multivariate model of time interval from T0 to first treatment (in days)

All patients (N = 283)			Patients with NSCLC only (N = 254)		
Characteristic	Beta (days)	p-value	Characteristic	Beta (days)	p-value
RIC	−24 (−35 to −12)	<0.01	RIC	−24 (−37 to −11)	<0.01
Male	−4 (−15 to 8)	0.53	Male	−2 (−14 to 11)	0.77
Age ≥ 75 years	16 (3 to 30)	0.02	Age ≥ 75 years	14 (0–29)	0.05
ECOG ≥ 2[a]	1 (−16 to 16)	0.98	ECOG ≥ 2[a]	3 (−14 to 11)	0.77
NSCLC (vs. SCLC)	10 (4 to 43)	0.02	Stage I-II (vs. Stage III-IV)	15 (3–28)	0.02
PET	17 (2 to 31)	0.03	PET	13 (−4 to 29)	0.14
EBUS	2 (−11 to 14)	0.20	EBUS	−1 (−14 to 12)	0.90
Number of non-diagnostic procedures			Number of non-diagnostic procedures		
0	Reference	–	0	Reference	–
1	20 (6 to 33)	<0.01	1	18 (5 to 33)	<0.01
≥1	37 (15 to 60)	<0.01	≥1	38 (14 to 60)	<0.01

Patients treated with palliative intent, patients receiving treatment outside the McGill University Health Centre, and patients with time to treatment greater than 1 year were excluded from this analysis. [a]Reference category is patients with ECOG of 0 or 1
NSCLC; SCLC

stage NSCLC, and patients with a first invasive test that was non-diagnostic. Patients investigated within the RIC were more likely to undergo PET scan for early stage lung cancer; they were more likely to be referred to the multidisciplinary lung cancer clinic or have their case reviewed at tumor board. Thus, the rapid investigation clinic improved timeliness of care while improving certain aspects of guideline-concordant care.

The study was based at a single university-affiliated center, which limits the generalizability of the results. The database for RIC patients was maintained prospectively by a trained registrar, with the goal of monitoring investigation delays in real time. In contrast, controls were individuals with a pathological diagnosis of lung cancer identified from the institutional tumor registry, and the investigation path was reviewed retrospectively. However, this definition allowed identification of a comparison group of patients who had access to similar imaging and procedural resources during the study timeframe. The dates and type of tests were easily identified from the institution's clinical information system, so

Table 6 Pre-specified indicators of guideline-concordant investigation

	RIC (%)	Non-RIC (%)	p-value[a]
PET scans in stage I/II NSCLC	48/51 (94)	45/ 55(82)	0.05[a]
Brain imaging in stage IIIA NSCLC	26/ 51(51)	14/ 37(38)	0.22[a]
Brain imaging in SCLC	24/26 (92)	5/7 (72)	0.13[b]
Patient seen in multi-disciplinary lung cancer clinic, or case reviewed at Tumor Board	144/ 195 (74)	73/132 (55)	<0.01[a]

Chi-squared[a] or Fisher's exact test[b] were used

that delays could be accurately measured and compared. Previous authors have reported that advanced disease may be associated with more prompt investigation and treatment [9, 10]. It is unlikely that sicker patients would be systematically referred to the RIC. In fact, baseline performance status was not significantly different between RIC and non-RIC patients. A larger number of non-RIC patients had early stage NSCLC; however, the RIC-related reduction in delays remained significant after adjustment for stage in the multivariate model of NSCLC patients.

The time required to complete lung cancer staging was comparable in the RIC and non-RIC patients. Several factors may be responsible for lack of change in this regard. EBUS was introduced at our institution at the end of 2008, and was performed by only two operators during the study period. Traditional practice patterns and/or ready availability of certain tests, conventional diagnostic bronchoscopy for example, led to their frequent use in both the RIC and non-RIC patients. In addition, limited access to PET scan delayed completion of staging in both RIC and non-RIC patients. PET scan was the last test needed to complete staging in 48% or RIC vs. 36% of non-RIC patients (Table 4). Despite these challenges, the RIC had a positive impact on time to lung cancer treatment.

Previous studies have evaluated delays to diagnosis or treatment of lung cancer. Olsson et al. systematically reviewed studies describing timeliness of care in patients with lung cancer [11]. Time to diagnosis and treatment of lung cancer were frequently longer than recommended. Salomaa et al. examined delays for 132 patients with NSCLC at a Finnish hospital and reported a median delay from specialist visit to diagnosis of 15 days (mean

55 days), and from diagnosis to treatment of 15 days [12]. More recently a United Kingdom (UK) administrative study of 28,733 patients found that only 43% of patients were treated within 1 month of diagnosis of lung cancer [13]. A United States of America (USA) study of veterans reported median delays of 42 days for diagnosis and 84 days for first treatment [10]. Wait times for diagnosis and treatment in Canada vary across provinces. In Ontario, median time to diagnosis of lung cancer was 37 days (IQR 29–49 days) [14]; in Manitoba median time from abnormal chest x-ray to tissue diagnosis was 26 days, with more than 25% of patients waiting longer than 55 days for diagnosis [15]. In Quebec, median time from initial contact with a physician for lung cancer and surgery was 109 days [16]. The variability in measures is partly due to different definitions of "time 0".

Guidelines for timeliness of care vary among countries. The 2011 NICE guidelines suggest an acceptable delay is 2 months from urgent general practitioner (GP) referral to beginning of treatment [5]. In this study, the median delay from T0 to first treatment was 81 days, thus not within the recommended 8 weeks. Significant challenges remain in meeting these targets, as highlighted by additional recent studies from Canada and the USA [17–19]. Avoiding diagnostic delays may be increasingly difficult, as accurate staging requires specific procedures and imaging tests [4]. The goal of the RIC was to centralize management of referrals, improve access to specialized providers and diagnostic tests, and standardize the workup of lung cancer. In essence, we attempted to modify both structure and process elements in order to reduce time to treatment.

A systematic review of studies evaluating diagnostic assessment units in patients with solid tumors reported reduced time to first treatment and greater patient satisfaction [20]. When reviewed systematically in patients with lung cancer, factors associated with improved delays included nurse-led coordination of care and use of a "two-stop" investigation pathway, while a multidisciplinary clinic approach did not result in more timely care [11]. Two studies from the UK prospectively implemented a two-stop pathway at centralized hospitals with a team dedicated to investigation and staging; both decreased time to diagnosis and increased radical treatment rates by scheduling patients for procedures the same day as physician evaluations [21, 22]. A single-center, Veterans' Administration (VA) study from the USA retrospectively reviewed timeliness of care provided in a multidisciplinary clinic with "usual" care provided after the clinic closed. The comparison revealed similar intervals to diagnosis and treatment with a multidisciplinary approach; the authors hypothesized this may have been due in part to absence of a surgeon in the multidisciplinary setting, and existing infrastructure from the previous multidisciplinary clinic [23]. A VA study in Birmingham reported improved lung cancer resection rates after implementation of a "Lung Mass Clinic" staffed by specialists in lung cancer, although the median time to resection was longer than expected (104 days) [24]. These conflicting results highlight the complexity of lung cancer care. Medical complexity was shown to increase delays to treatment in a recent Norwegian study, yet too few of even the least complex patients received timely treatment [25].

The impact of timeliness of care on lung cancer outcomes is unclear. In the systematic review of Olsson et al., the association between timely lung cancer care and patient outcomes were mixed and, at times, paradoxical [11]. A large population-based study of surgical patients demonstrated no influence of time to surgery on survival [26]. A Swedish study of 466 patients treated with curative or palliative intent showed that those with shortest time to treatment had worse survival [27]. Gould et al. investigated 129 veterans with NSCLC and found that more timely care was not associated with better survival. More advanced patients may require more urgent evaluation, thereby decreasing overall survival in patients treated sooner. However, in the subgroup of patients with solitary pulmonary nodules, there was a trend toward improved survival with shorter time to treatment [10]. O'Rourke et al. reported tumor growth while patients waited for radiotherapy treatment by comparing diagnostic and CT simulation scans, suggesting that delays to treatment may be associated with worse outcomes [28].

No study may be sufficiently powered to assess the survival benefit of a rapid access clinic model, and efforts to improve more scalable quality outcomes may be more realistic. Quality gaps have been defined as differences between health-care processes observed in clinical practice and those recommended by evidence-based guidelines [29]. Ost and colleagues examined quality gaps in lung cancer diagnosis and staging, using the Surveillance Epidemiology and End Results (SEER) database and the Texas Cancer Registry. Patients with lung cancer with regional spread and no distant metastases were classified as receiving guideline-consistent care if they underwent mediastinal lymph node sampling as the first invasive test; only 21% of patients had guideline-consistent diagnostic evaluations [30]. In the current study, implementation of a rapid access clinic was associated with more frequent guideline-concordant care, based on the quality indicators examined.

Conclusion

The implementation of a rapid investigation clinic for patients with lung cancer reduced delays to diagnosis and treatment and improved quality of care. Continued monitoring of investigation pathways and wait times is necessary to ensure barriers and quality gaps are addressed in a timely manner.

Abbreviations
ACCP: American College of Chest Physicians; CI: Confidence interval; CT: Computed tomography; EBUS: Endobronchial ultrasound; ECOG : Eastern Cooperative Oncology Group; EUS: Endoscopic ultrasound; GP: General Practitioner; IQR: Interquartile range; MUHC: McGill University Health Centre; NICE: National Institute for Health and Clinical Excellence; NSCLC: Non-small cell lung cancer; PET: Positron emission tomography; RIC: Rapid Investigation Clinic; SCLC: Small cell lung cancer; SEER: Surveillance Epidemiology and End Results; TTNA: Transthoracic needle aspiration; USA: United States of America; UK: United Kingdom; VA: Veterans' Administration

Acknowledgements
The authors gratefully acknowledge Ms. Chantal Savard, nurse-clinician for the Rapid Investigation Clinic and Ms. Julie Latreille, registrar. We would like to thank Ms. Pei Zhi Li for assistance with statistical analyses.

Funding
This project was supported by the Montreal General Hospital Foundation. Dr. Gonzalez is the recipient of an FRQS chercheur-boursier-clinicien award, and a Réseau en Santé Respiratoire du FRQS (RSR) award.

Authors' contributions
NE and AVG designed the study, interpreted the results and wrote the manuscript. NE was primarily responsible for data collection and analysis. AN participated in data collection and interpretation of the results. KS and LO participated in study design and interpretation of the results. All authors read and approved the final manuscript.

Competing interests
The authors declare that they have no competing interests.

Author details
[1]Respiratory Epidemiology and Clinical Research Unit, Montreal Chest Institute, McGill University Health Centre, Montreal, QC, Canada. [2]Respiratory Division, McGill University Health Centre, Montreal, QC, Canada. [3]Respiratory and Respiratory Critical Care Medicine, Faculty of Medicine, Prince of Songkla University, Songkhla, Thailand.

References
1. Surveillance Epidemiology and End Results Database: National Cancer Institute; Accessed 10 Dec 10, 2013. Available from: http://seer.cancer.gov/.
2. National Lung Screening Trial Research T, Aberle DR, Adams AM, Berg CD, Black WC, Clapp JD, et al. Reduced lung-cancer mortality with low-dose computed tomographic screening. N Engl J Med. Aug 4;365(5):395–409. PubMed PMID: 21714641. Epub 2011/07/01. eng.
3. Fischer B, Lassen U, Mortensen J, Larsen S, Loft A, Bertelsen A, et al. Preoperative staging of lung cancer with combined PET-CT. N Engl J Med 2009 Jul 2;361(1):32-9. PubMed PMID: 19571281. Epub 2009/07/03. eng.
4. Silvestri GA, Gonzalez AV, Jantz MA, Margolis ML, Gould MK, Tanoue LT, et al. Methods for staging non-small cell lung cancer: diagnosis and management of lung cancer, 3rd ed: American College of Chest Physicians evidence-based clinical practice guidelines. Chest 2013 May;143(5 Suppl): e211S-50S. PubMed PMID: 23649440. Epub 2013/05/10. eng.
5. NICE. Lung Cancer: Diagnosis and Management CG121 National Institute for Health Care Excellence 2011 21 April 2011.
6. Ost DE, Yeung SC, Tanoue LT, Gould MK. Clinical and organizational factors in the initial evaluation of patients with lung cancer: diagnosis and management of lung cancer, 3rd ed: American College of Chest Physicians evidence-based clinical practice guidelines. Chest 2013 May;143(5 Suppl): e121S-41S. PubMed PMID: 23649435. Epub 2013/05/10. eng.
7. Detterbeck FC, Boffa DJ, Tanoue LT. The new lung cancer staging system. Chest 2009 Jul;136(1):260-71. PubMed PMID: 19584208. Epub 2009/07/09. eng.
8. Detterbeck FC, Jantz MA, Wallace M, Vansteenkiste J, Silvestri GA, American College of Chest P. Invasive mediastinal staging of lung cancer: ACCP evidence-based clinical practice guidelines (2nd edition). Chest 2007 Sep; 132(3 Suppl):202S-20S. PubMed PMID: 17873169. Epub 2007/10/06. eng.
9. Powell AA, Schultz EM, Ordin DL, Enderle MA, Graham BA, Partin MR, et al. Timeliness across the continuum of care in veterans with lung cancer. J. Thorac. Oncol. 2008 Sep;3(9):951-7. PubMed PMID: 18758295. Epub 2008/09/02. eng.
10. Gould MK, Ghaus SJ, Olsson JK, Schultz EM. Timeliness of care in veterans with non-small cell lung cancer. Chest 2008 May;133(5):1167-73. PubMed PMID: 18263676. Epub 2008/02/12. eng.
11. Olsson JK, Schultz EM, Gould MK. Timeliness of care in patients with lung cancer: a systematic review. Thorax 2009 Sep;64(9):749-56. PubMed PMID: 19717709. Epub 2009/09/01. eng.
12. Salomaa ER, Sallinen S, Hiekkanen H, Liippo K. Delays in the diagnosis and treatment of lung cancer. Chest 2005 Oct;128(4):2282-8. PubMed PMID: 16236885. Epub 2005/10/21. eng.
13. Forrest LF, Adams J, White M, Rubin G. Factors associated with timeliness of post-primary care referral, diagnosis and treatment for lung cancer: population-based, data-linkage study. Br J Cancer 2014 Oct 28;111(9):1843-51. PubMed PMID: 25203519. Pubmed Central PMCID: Pmc4453730. Epub 2014/09/10. eng.
14. Grunfeld E, Watters JM, Urquhart R, O'Rourke K, Jaffey J, Maziak DE, et al. A prospective study of peri-diagnostic and surgical wait times for patients with presumptive colorectal, lung, or prostate cancer. Br J Cancer 2009 Jan 13;100(1):56-62. PubMed PMID: 19088720. Epub 2008/12/18. eng.
15. Cheung WY, Butler JR, Kliewer EV, Demers AA, Musto G, Welch S, et al. Analysis of wait times and costs during the peri-diagnostic period for non-small cell lung cancer. Lung Cancer. 2011;72(1):125–31. PubMed PMID: 20822826.
16. Liberman M, Liberman D, Sampalis JS, Mulder DS. Delays to surgery in non-small-cell lung cancer. Can J Surg 2006 Feb;49(1):31-6. PubMed PMID: 16524140. Epub 2006/03/10. eng.
17. Kim JO, Davis F, Butts C, Winget M. Waiting Time Intervals for Non-small Cell Lung Cancer Diagnosis and Treatment in Alberta: Quantification of Intervals and Identification of Risk Factors Associated with Delays. Clin. Oncol. (R. Coll. Radiol.). 2016 Dec; 28(12):750–9. PubMed PMID: 27357099.
18. Nadpara P, Madhavan SS, Tworek C. Guideline-concordant timely lung cancer care and prognosis among elderly patients in the United States: a population-based study. Cancer Epidemiol 2015 Dec;39(6):1136-1144 PubMed PMID: 26138902. Pubmed Central PMCID: 4679644.
19. Vidaver RM, Shershneva MB, Hetzel SJ, Holden TR, Campbell TC. Typical time to treatment of patients with lung cancer in a multisite, US-based study. J. Oncol. Pract. 2016 Jun;12(6):e643-53. PubMed PMID:27143146.
20. Brouwers M, Oliver TK, Crawford J, Ellison P, Evans WK, Gagliardi A, et al. Cancer diagnostic assessment programs: standards for the organization of care in Ontario. Curr Oncol 2009 Dec;16(6):29-41. PubMed PMID: 20016744. Epub 2009/12/18. eng.
21. Murray PV, O'Brien ME, Sayer R, Cooke N, Knowles G, Miller AC, et al. The pathway study: results of a pilot feasibility study in patients suspected of having lung carcinoma investigated in a conventional chest clinic setting compared to a centralised two-stop pathway. Lung Cancer 2003 Dec;42(3): 283-90. PubMed PMID: 14644515. Epub 2003/12/04. eng.
22. Laroche C, Wells F, Coulden R, Stewart S, Goddard M, Lowry E, et al. Improving surgical resection rate in lung cancer. Thorax 1998 Jun;53(6):445-9. PubMed PMID: 9713441. Pubmed Central PMCID: 1745249. Epub 1998/08/26. eng.
23. Riedel RF, Wang X, McCormack M, Toloza E, Montana GS, Schreiber G, et al. Impact of a multidisciplinary thoracic oncology clinic on the timeliness of care. J. Thorac. Oncol. 2006 Sep;1(7):692-6. PubMed PMID: 17409938.

24. Dransfield MT, Lock BJ, Garver RI, Jr. Improving the lung cancer resection rate in the US Department of veterans affairs health system. Clin. Lung Cancer 2006 Jan;7(4):268-72. PubMed PMID: 16512981. Epub 2006/03/04. eng.

25. Stokstad T, Sorhaug S, Amundsen T, Gronberg BH. Medical complexity and time to lung cancer treatment - a three-year retrospective chart review. BMC Health Serv Res 2017 Jan 17;17(1):45. PubMed PMID: 28095840. Pubmed Central PMCID: 5240346.

26. Aragoneses FG, Moreno N, Leon P, Fontan EG, Folque E. Influence of delays on survival in the surgical treatment of bronchogenic carcinoma. Lung Cancer 2002 Apr;36(1):59-63. PubMed PMID: 11891034. Epub 2002/03/14. eng.

27. Myrdal G, Lambe M, Hillerdal G, Lamberg K, Agustsson T, Stahle E. Effect of delays on prognosis in patients with non-small cell lung cancer. Thorax 2004 Jan;59(1):45-9. PubMed PMID: 14694247. Epub 2003/12/25. eng.

28. O'Rourke N, Edwards R. Lung cancer treatment waiting times and tumour growth. Clin. Oncol. (R. Coll. Radiol.). 2000;12(3):141–4. PubMed PMID: 10942328. Epub 2000/08/15. eng.

29. Shojania K MK, Wachter R. Owens DK, eds. Closing The Quality Gap: A Critical Analysis of Quality Improvement Strategies. Volume 1—Series Overview and Methodology. Agency for Health Care Research and Quality Publication. 2004 (04–0051-1).

30. Ost DE, Niu J, Elting LS, Buchholz TA, Giordano SH. Quality gaps and comparative effectiveness in lung cancer staging and diagnosis. Chest 2014 Feb 1;145(2):331-45. PubMed PMID: 24091637. Epub 2013/10/05. eng.

6

High-flow nasal cannula oxygen therapy versus conventional oxygen therapy in patients with acute respiratory failure

Youfeng Zhu[1†] (iD), Haiyan Yin[1†], Rui Zhang[1] and Jianrui Wei[2*]

Abstract

Background: Acute respiratory failure (ARF) is a common and life-threatening medical emergency in patients admitted to the hospital. Currently, there is a lack of large-scale evidence on the use of high-flow nasal cannulas (HFNC) in patients with ARF. In this systematic review and meta-analysis, we evaluated whether there were differences between HFNC therapy and conventional oxygen therapy (COT) for treating patients with ARF.

Methods: The EMBASE, Medline, and Wanfang databases and the Cochrane Library were searched. Two investigators independently collected the data and assessed the quality of each study. Randomized controlled trials that compared HFNC therapy with COT in patients with ARF were included. RevMan 5.3 was used to conduct the meta-analysis.

Results: Four studies that involved 703 patients with ARF were included, with 371 patients in the HFNC group and 332 patients in the COT group. In the overall estimates, there were no significant differences between the HFNC and COT groups in the rates of escalation of respiratory support (RR, 0.68; 95% CI, 0.37, 1.27; $z = 1.20$, $P = 0.23$), intubation (RR, 0.74; 95% CI, 0.55, 1.00; $z = 1.95$, $P = 0.05$), mortality (RR, 0.82; 95% CI, 0.36, 1.88; $z = 0.47$, $P = 0.64$), or ICU transfer (RR, 1.09; 95% CI, 0.57, 2.09; $z = 0.26$, $P = 0.79$) during ARF treatment. However, the subgroup analysis showed that HFNC therapy may decrease the rate of escalation of respiratory support (RR, 0.71; 95% CI, 0.53, 0.97; $z = 2.15$, $P = 0.03$) and the intubation rate (RR, 0.71; 95% CI, 0.53, 0.97; $z = 2.15$, $P = 0.03$) when ARF patients were treated with HFNC therapy for ≥24 h compared with COT.

Conclusions: HFNC therapy was similar to COT in ARF patients. The subgroup analysis showed that HFNC therapy may decrease the rate of escalation of respiratory support and the intubation rate when ARF patients were treated with HFNC for ≥24 h compared with COT. Further high-quality, large-scale studies are needed to confirm our results.

Keywords: High-flow nasal cannula, Mortality, Acute respiratory failure, Treatment

* Correspondence: Jianruiw@163.com
†Equal contributors
2Department of Cardiology, Guangzhou Red Cross Hospital, Medical College,
Jinan University, Guangzhou, Guangdong province 510220, China

Background

Acute respiratory failure (ARF) is a common and life-threatening medical emergency in patients admitted to hospitals [1]. It is caused by a variety of diseases, including heart failure, pneumonia, and exacerbations of chronic obstructive pulmonary disease. Many patients with ARF require oxygen therapy. The devices for oxygen therapy include unassisted oxygen delivery devices and assisted ventilation devices [2]. Unassisted oxygen therapy is also called conventional oxygen therapy (COT). It is the main supportive treatment administered to patients with ARF and is usually delivered with nasal prongs or facemasks. Assisted ventilation devices that are commonly used in hospitals include noninvasive ventilation (NIV, e.g., continuous positive airway pressure and biphasic positive airway pressure) and invasive mechanical ventilation (IMV). Previous studies have shown that avoiding IMV significantly decreases the risk of death [3, 4]. Therefore, choosing an optimal oxygen therapy device is very important for reducing the rates of IMV and mortality while also ensuring patients' safety and comfort.

The effect of COT is limited. The maximal flow rate that these COT devices can deliver is typically only 15 L/min (except for the Venturi mask), which is far lower than the demands of patients with ARF. This discrepancy leads

to a significant decrease in the fraction of inspired oxygen (FiO_2) that ultimately reaches a patient's lungs [5].

ARF patients admitted to the hospital may receive NIV. However, currently, the effects of NIV for these patients with respect to improvements in outcomes are conflicting and the use of NIV in hypoxemic ARF has recently been questioned [6–8]. Furthermore, NIV is not without limitations. The effect of NIV is highly dependent on a patient's cooperation, which is also called patient-ventilator synchrony. Additionally, there are many factors that affect the comfort of patients undergoing NIV that may lead to NIV failure, such as the interface, the amount of air leaks, the ventilator settings, pressurization and triggering performances [9]. Moreover, NIV is associated with gastric distension, which may further reduce the functional residual capacity and is poorly tolerated in some patients. [10, 11] Therefore, IMV may still be needed [11].

The high-flow nasal cannula (HFNC) is a recently developed oxygen therapy device in adult patients that can deliver a humidified and heated mixture of air and oxygen at a very high flow rate. It can provide a maximal flow rate of up to 60 l per minute with an FiO_2 of 100% [5]. The use of an HFNC has been demonstrated to generate positive airway pressure at

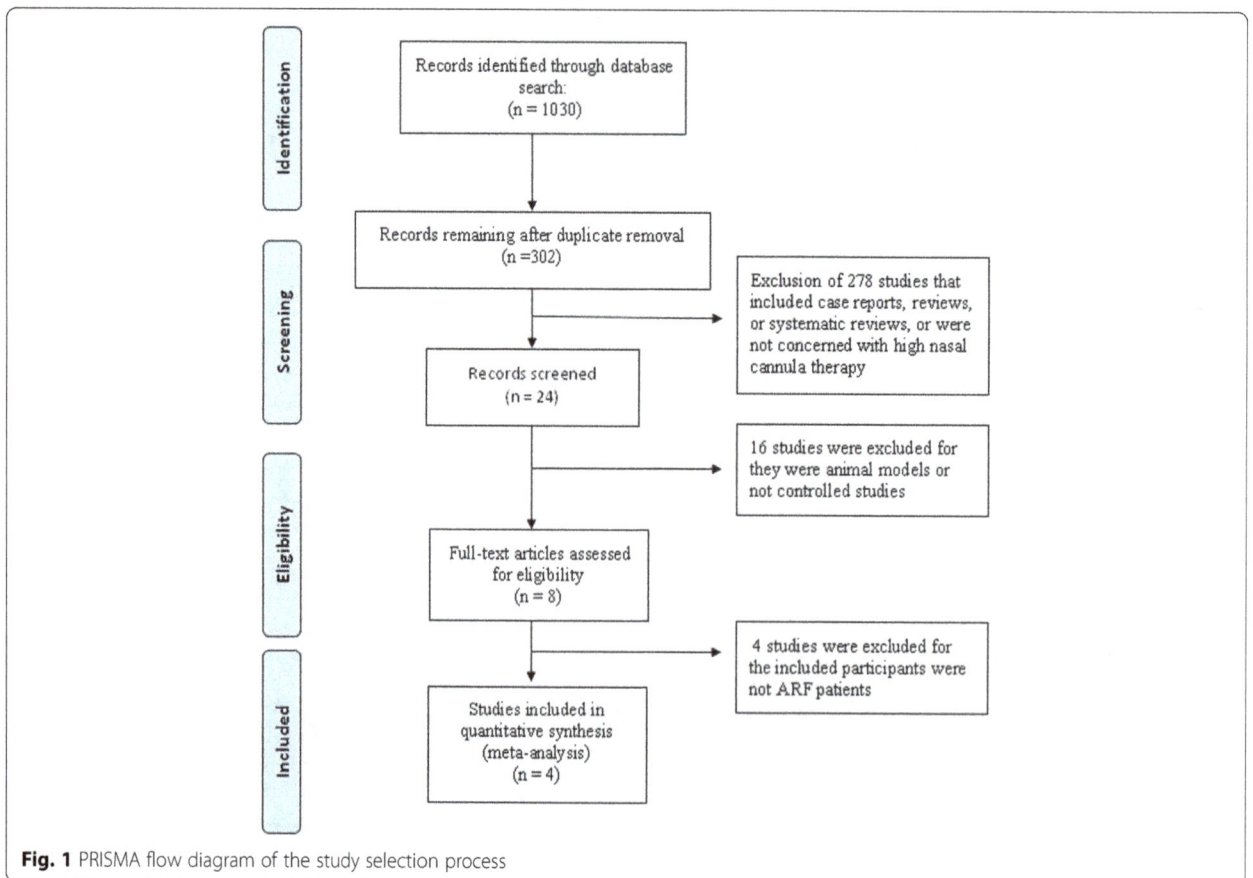

Fig. 1 PRISMA flow diagram of the study selection process

Table 1 Quality of the included studies

Study	Randomization method	Blind method	Allocation concealment	Withdrawals/Dropouts (NG/NJ)	Jadad score
Bell 2015	Computer-generated random numbers	Not used	An opaque, sealed envelope system	Yes	5
Frat 2015	Permuted-block randomization	Not used	Centralized web based management system	Yes	5
Lemiale 2015	Permuted-block randomization	Not used	An opaque, sealed envelope system	Yes	5
Jones 2016	Computer-generated random numbers	Not used	An opaque, sealed envelope system	Yes	5

The modified Jadad score was used to evaluate the quality of the included trials

end-expiration, ameliorate oxygenation and dyspnea, reduce the work of breathing and the respiratory rate, and be more comfortable for patients [5, 12–19]. These benefits are attributed to the mechanisms of HFNCs, including their ability to more adequately meet the peak flow of inspiration, flush the anatomical dead space, and deliver warm and humidified gas, thereby promoting mucociliary function [20, 21].

The use of HFNCs has become increasing popular in the treatment of many diseases and conditions, such as post-extubation, pre-intubation, sleep-related hypoventilation, cardiac surgery, and heart failure, and as an alternative to NIV [20]. However, currently, whether ARF patients benefit from this therapy is unclear and there is a lack of large-scale evidence on the use of HFNCs in patients with ARF. Some studies have shown that HFNC therapy is associated with an improved respiratory state or mortality rate in patients with ARF [2, 22]. However, other studies have not found significant differences between HFNC and COT groups [23, 24].

Recently, some meta-analyses tried to assess the efficiency of HFNC therapy in ARF patients. However, there were controversial results between these studies. [25, 26] After fully reviewing these meta-analyses, we found some studies that evaluated HFNC therapy in post-extubation patients were also involved in these studies. Though some post-extubation patients may suffer reintubation due to ARF, they constitute a different patient population rather than actual ARF patients. In the present systematic review and meta-analysis, we sought to evaluate whether there were differences between HFNC therapy and COT in treating ARF patients rather than post-extubation patients regarding the escalation of respiratory support and other aspects.

Methods

We performed this systematic review and meta-analysis according to the guidelines described in the Cochrane Handbook for Systematic Reviews of Interventions [27] and PRISMA statements.

Table 2 Basic demographic parameters of patients in the included studies

Study	n	Age (years)	Gender (M/F)	Patients	Duration of HFNC or COT	Starting flow of HFNC	RRs (breaths/min)	P/F (mmHg)
Bell 2015								
HFNC group	48	72.9 ± 15.1	20/28	Emergency patients with ARF	2 h	50 L/min	>25	Unknown
COT group	52	74.5 ± 14.0	24/28		2 h			
Frat 2015								
HFNC group	106	61 ± 16	75/31	ICU patients with hypoxemic ARF	At least 48 h	50 L/min	>25	≤300
COT group	94	59 ± 17	63/31		At least 48 h			
Lemiale 2015								
HFNC group	52	59.3(43-70)*	38/14	Immunocompromised ICU patients with hypoxemic ARF	2 h	40-50 L/min	>30	Unknown
COT group	48	64.5(53.25-72)*	32/16		2 h			
Jones 2016								
HFNC group	165	74.6 ± 15.6	73/94	Emergency patients with ARF	24 h	40 L/min	≥22	Unknown
COT group	138	72.2 ± 16.8	71/67		24 h			

Plus–minus values are means ± SD; * values are median (25th–75th percentile); *M* male, *F* female. *ARF* acute respiratory failure, *HFNC* high flow nasal cannula, *COT* conventional oxygen therapy, *L/min* liter per minute, *RRs* respiratory rates, *P/F* PaO_2/FiO_2

Study selection criteria

Types of studies

Randomized controlled trials (RCTs) comparing HFNC therapy and COT in the treatment of ARF patients were included. As described previously, RCTs comparing HFNC therapy and COT in post-extubation patients were excluded.

Types of participants

Adult patients who had ARF, as defined by the authors of each study, were included.

Types of interventions

Trials comparing HFNC therapy with COT were eligible.

The intervention for the HFNC group was oxygen therapy provided through HFNCs and the control group received COT through nasal prongs, facemasks or Venturi masks. In addition, NIV was not included in the COT group in the present meta-analysis.

Types of outcome measures

Our primary outcome was the rate of escalation of respiratory support and the secondary outcomes included the following variables: intubation rate, mortality at the longest study follow-up, transfers to the ICU and complications.

Data sources and search strategy

We searched for relevant studies published in the EMBASE, Medline, and Wanfang databases and the Cochrane Library.We also reviewed the references of relevant articles to avoid a loss of studies. We searched all relevant articles published from inception to June 2016. We used the following keywords and Emtree and MeSH terms in different combinations for the searches: "oxygen therapy", "Oxygen inhalation therapy", "Oxygen delivery devices", "standard oxygen", "high flow nasal cannula", "high flow oxygen therapy", "nasal high flow oxygen therapy", "Nasal Cannula", "acute respiratory failure", and "respiratory failure". No limits on the location of the trial, gender, age, sample size, or language were entered for the search. The full search strategies are shown in Additional file 1.

Data extraction and quality assessment

Two investigators independently screened the titles and abstracts using a standardized data extraction form. Disagreements were resolved by consensus or by consulting a third author. We extracted the following data: authors' names, the title of the article, the year and country of the study, the journal in which the study was published, laboratory results and clinical outcomes. The modified Jadad score was used to assess the quality of the included studies. Two independent investigators evaluated the risk

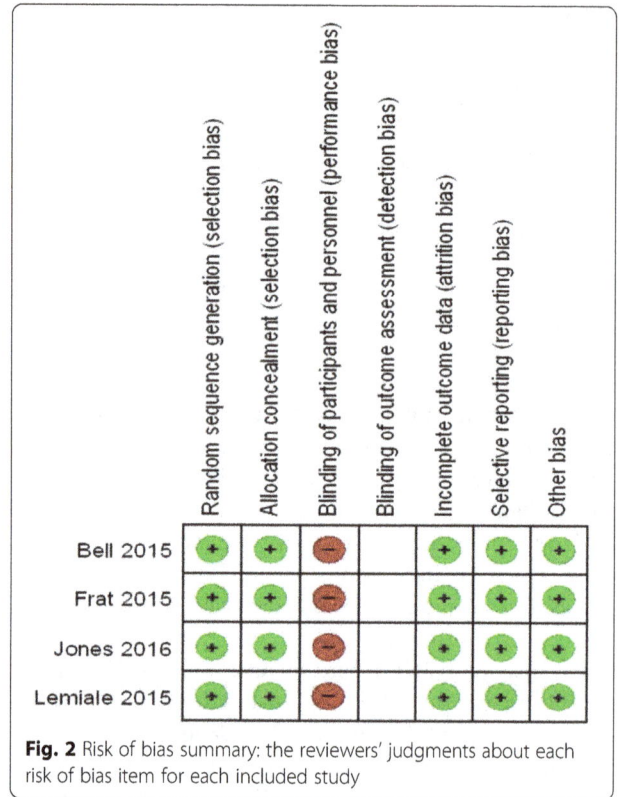

Fig. 2 Risk of bias summary: the reviewers' judgments about each risk of bias item for each included study

of bias of the included studies according to the methods described in the Cochrane Handbook [25]. Studies were assessed according to the following domains: participant and personnel blinding, random sequence generation, allocation concealment, incomplete outcome data, blinding for outcome assessments, selective outcome reporting and other sources of bias. According to the Cochrane Handbook, other sources of bias were related to the specific study design or to the early termination of the involved trials because of extreme baseline imbalances in the selected samples. Blinding could not be implemented due to the nature of these studies.

Statistical analysis

We used Review Manager Software 5.3 (RevMan 5.3, The Cochrane Collaboration, Oxford, United Kingdom) for the

Table 3 Strategies for escalation of respiratory support among included studies

Study	COT group	HFNC group
Bell 2015	HFNC, Noninvasive or invasive ventilation	Noninvasive or invasive ventilation
Frat 2015	Invasive ventilation	Invasive ventilation
Lemiale 2015	Noninvasive or invasive ventilation	Noninvasive or invasive ventilation
Jones 2016	Noninvasive or invasive ventilation	Noninvasive or invasive ventilation

COT conventional oxygen therapy, *HFNC* high flow nasal cannula oxygen therapy

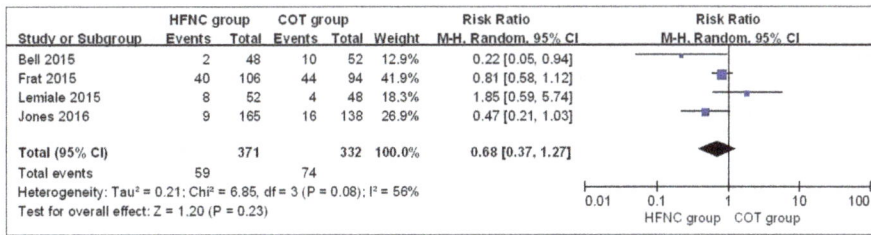

Fig. 3 Escalation of respiratory support in the HFNC and COT groups

meta-analysis. Data were obtained by direct extraction or by indirect calculation. Binary data such as the rate of escalation of respiratory support and the intubation rate were expressed as risk ratios (RRs) and 95% confidence intervals (CIs). Heterogeneity between the studies was evaluated using the chi-square test and $P < 0.05$ with I^2 greater than 50% indicated significant heterogeneity. A fixed effects model and a random effects model were used in the absence and presence of statistical heterogeneity, respectively. The results were graphically displayed using forest plots and the potential publication bias was analyzed by visual inspection of the funnel plot.

Because the durations of HFNC treatment were different in each study, we conducted a subgroup analysis according to the duration of HFNC therapy (< 24 h v. ≥24 h).

Sensitivity analysis
To test the reliability of the results, sensitivity analyses were also performed by repeating the present meta-analysis after removing one RCT at a time.

Results
The selection process of the eligible studies is shown in Fig. 1. Initially, 1030 potentially relevant records were identified. By screening the titles and evaluating the abstracts, we removed duplicate studies, reviews, case reports, animal studies, comments, and studies that were not randomized controlled studies, resulting in 8 studies that remained for assessment. Of these, 1 study compared HFNC therapy with NIV [28], 1 study evaluated the effect of HFNC therapy during endotracheal intubation [29], and 2 studies were conducted to prevent ARF after planned extubation [12, 30]. These studies were excluded. Finally, 4 studies were included in the present meta-analysis [2, 22–24]. The quality of the included studies is shown in Table 1.

A total of 703 patients with ARF were included in this meta-analysis. Of these patients, 371 were randomly assigned to the HFNC group and 332 were assigned to the COT group. Table 2 shows the basic demographic characteristics of all included patients.

Risk of bias in the included studies
The risk of bias of each study was evaluated according to the methods described in the Cochrane Handbook and the details of the results are presented in Fig. 2.

Escalation of respiratory support
When initial treatment (HFNC therapy or COT) failed, an escalation of respiratory support was needed. All the

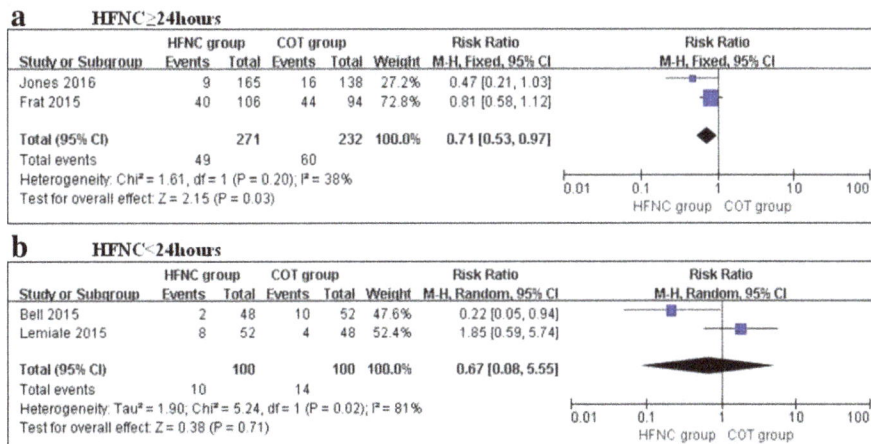

Fig. 4 Subgroup analysis of escalation for respiratory support in the HFNC and COT groups: (a) HFNC ≥ 24hours; (b) HFNC < 24hours

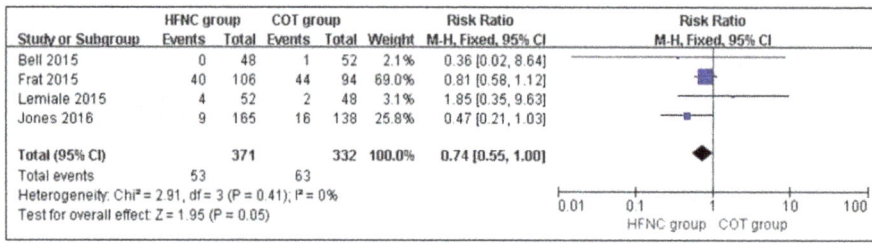

Fig. 5 Intubation rates in the HFNC and COT groups

included studies reported the rate of escalation of respiratory support. The strategies for the escalation of respiratory support in the 4 included studies were different (Table 3). There was significant heterogeneity between the studies (chi^2 = 6.85, df = 3, P = 0.08; I^2 = 56%). In the random-effects model, the HFNC group did not show a significant difference compared with the COT group (RR, 0.68; 95% CI, 0.37, 1.27; z = 1.20, P = 0.23, Fig. 3).

The subgroup analysis showed a significant 29% decrease in the escalation of respiratory support in the HFNC group when the patients were treated with HFNC therapy for ≥24 h compared with COT (RR, 0.71; 95% CI, 0.53, 0.97; z = 2.15, P = 0.03, Fig. 4). HFNC therapy did not demonstrate any benefit over COT in patients treated for less than 24 h (RR, 0.67; 95% CI, 0.08, 5.55; z = 0.38, P = 0.71, Fig. 4).

Intubation rate

All the included studies reported intubation rates. When the results of the 4 studies were analyzed, no significant heterogeneity was observed between the studies (chi^2 = 2.07, df = 3, P = 0.56; I^2 = 0%). The intubation rates of the COT group and the HFNC group were similar, with no significant difference between the two groups (RR, 0.74; 95% CI, 0.55, 1.00; z = 1.95, P = 0.05, Fig. 5).

The subgroup analysis also shown a significant decrease in the intubation rate in the HFNC group when patients were treated with HFNC therapy for ≥24 h compared with COT (RR, 0.71; 95% CI, 0.53, 0.97; z = 2.15, P = 0.03, Fig. 6). HFNC therapy did not demonstrate any benefit over COT in patients treated for less than 24 h (RR, 1.24; 95% CI, 0.31, 4.93; z = 0.30, P = 0.76, Fig. 6).

Mortality

Two of the four included studies reported mortality [22, 24]. There was significant heterogeneity between the studies (chi^2 = 4.49, df = 1, P = 0.03; I^2 = 78%). In addition, HFNC oxygen therapy did not decrease mortality compared with COT (RR, 0.82; 95% CI, 0.36, 1.88; z = 0.47, P = 0.64, Fig. 7).

Rate of transfer to the ICU

Two of the four studies were conducted in the emergency department and both reported the rate of admission to the ICU [2, 24]. No significant heterogeneity was observed between the two studies (chi^2 = 0.21, df = 1, P = 0.65; I^2 = 0%) and there was no significant difference in the rate of ICU transfer between the two groups (RR, 1.09; 95% CI, 0.57, 2.09; z = 0.26, P = 0.79, Fig. 8).

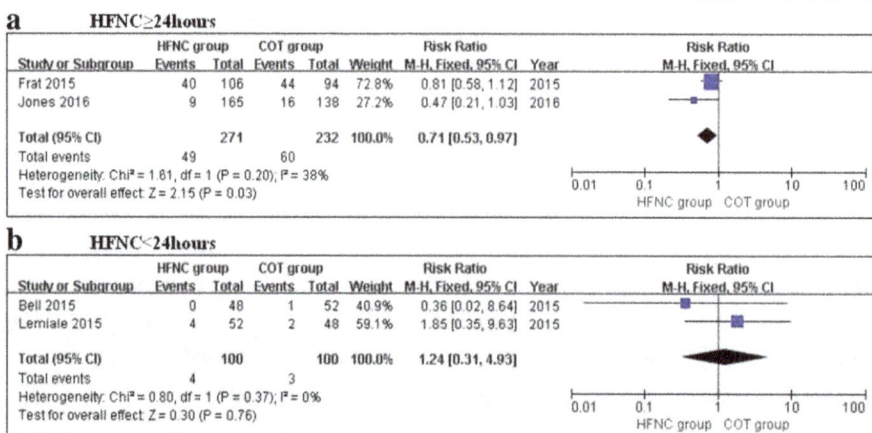

Fig. 6 Subgroup analysis of intubation rate in the HFNC and COT groups: (**a**) HFNC ≥ 24hours; (**b**) HFNC < 24hours

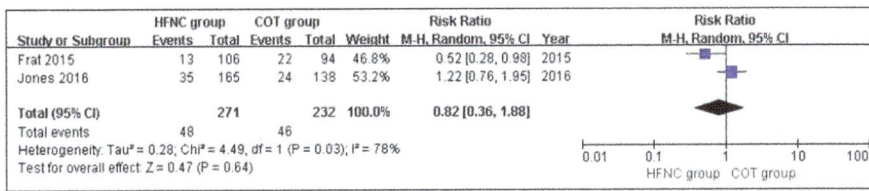

Fig. 7 Mortality between the HFNC and COT groups

Complications

Since the data on complications were insufficiently reported in the 4 included studies, we can only provide a description of their occurrence. In the studies by Bell et al. and Lemiale et al., no severe complications (i.e., nasal mucosa, skin trauma, infectious complications or hemodynamic instability due to HFNC) were reported. In the studies by Frat et al. and Jones et al., the overall incidence of serious adverse events was similar in the HFNC and COT groups (data not reported).

No publication bias was observed based on a visual inspection of the funnel plot (Fig. 9).

We had planned to analyze other variables, such as the lengths of stay in the ICU or hospital, patient comfort, the duration of HFNC therapy, maximal flow of the HFNC, and the costs of the two methods, but these variables were either not researched or were insufficiently reported in the included trials. Therefore, we could not perform any analyses with regard to these data.

Discussion

Recently, HFNC oxygen therapy has achieved widespread use in adult ARF patients in emergency departments and intensive care units [20, 31, 32]. However, the effect of HFNC therapy in adult ARF patients remains inconclusive. The present meta-analysis included 4 RCTs that studied 703 patients (371 HFNC and 332 COT patients) to examine whether there were differences between HFNC therapy and COT in the treatment of ARF. The overall estimates of this meta-analysis showed that there were no significant differences between the HFNC and COT groups in the rates of escalation of respiratory support (RR, 0.68; 95% CI, 0.37, 1.27; z = 1.20, $P = 0.23$), intubation (RR, 0.74; 95% CI, 0.55, 1.00; z = 1.95, $P = 0.05$), mortality (RR, 0.82; 95% CI, 0.36, 1.88; z = 0.47, P

$= 0.64$), or ICU transfer (RR, 1.09; 95% CI, 0.57, 2.09; z $= 0.26$, $P = 0.79$) in the treatment of ARF. Our results were similar to a previous study [26].

Although the present meta-analysis found no significant differences between HFNC therapy and COT for the treatment of adult ARF patients, it should be noted that there was significant heterogeneity between the RCTs included in the present study, which may have affected our conclusions. A series of factors may have led to this significant heterogeneity. First, as shown in Table 4, the criteria for ARF differed between the 4 studies (Table 4). The different criteria for inclusion led to different degrees of ARF among the patients in the four studies. In the study by Frat and colleagues, there was no significant difference in the intubation rate between the two groups, but when they conducted a post hoc analysis according to the ratio of PaO_2/FiO_2 at enrollment (≤ 200 mmHg versus >200 mmHg), they found that for the subgroup of patients with a $PaO_2/FiO_2 \leq 200$ mmHg, the intubation rate was significantly lower in the HFNC group than in the COT group [22]. Therefore, we consider the degree of ARF to be an important factor influencing the effectiveness of HFNC therapy. In addition, the differences in the degree of ARF experienced by the patients in the present meta-analysis may have eliminated the potential differences between the two groups. In fact, some therapies may only be useful in more critically ill patients.

Second, the starting flow of HFNC therapy may also affect results. The starting flows of HFNC therapy differed between the four studies (Table 2). In a study by Parke et al., researchers measured patients' nasopharyngeal pressure when HFNC therapy was performed with gas flows of 30, 40, and 50 L/min [14]. They found that during HFNC therapy, the mean nasopharyngeal airway pressures were 1.5 ± 0.6, 2.2 ± 0.8, and 3.1 ± 1.2 mmHg

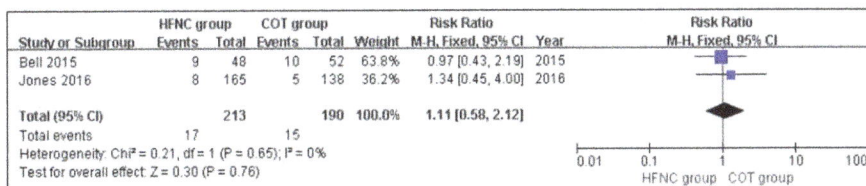

Fig. 8 Rate of transfers to the ICU between the HFNC and COT groups

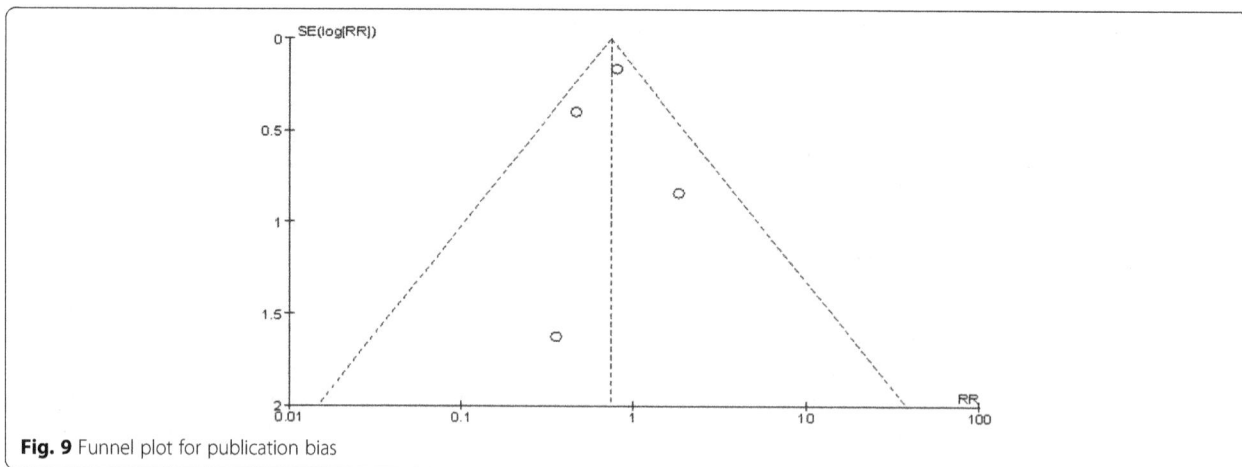

Fig. 9 Funnel plot for publication bias

at 30, 40, and 50 L/min, respectively. They demonstrated that the level of PEEP as a benefit of HFNC therapy was flow-dependent. The different starting flows may have led to different levels of PEEP and could have affected the results. Consistently, in two studies by Bell et al. and Frat et al., the starting flows were all 50 L/min and these studies showed more benefits in the HFNC group than in the COT group. [2, 22]

Third, as shown in Table 3, the criteria for the escalation of respiratory support differed between the 4 studies. In addition, the strategies for escalation also differed. The different criteria and strategies used for the escalation of respiratory support may have led to a bias. Furthermore, three of the studies included the option of escalating to NIV as a strategy for the escalation of respiratory support in the HFNC group. However, whether the patients who failed to improve with HFNC therapy could be recovered by escalating to NIV is currently unclear [8].

The subgroup analysis showed that HFNC therapy may decrease the rates of escalation of respiratory support (RR, 0.71; 95% CI, 0.53, 0.97; z = 2.15, $P = 0.03$) and intubation (RR, 0.71; 95% CI, 0.53, 0.97; z = 2.15, P = 0.03) when ARF patients are treated with HFNC therapy for ≥24 h compared with COT, which is not surprising. As we know, some therapies may only be useful with a sufficient duration. In the other two RCTs [2, 23], the durations of HFNC therapy were only 2 h, which may be too short to show its benefit. HFNCs have shown greater

benefits with longer durations in post-extubation patients. A previous randomized controlled study by Maggiore et al. compared HFNC therapy with COT in 105 patients after extubation [12]. The duration of HFNC therapy was at least 48 h. Notably, the results showed that the reintubation rate or any form of escalation of respiratory support was significantly lower in the HFNC group than in the COT group. The duration of HFNC therapy in their study was similar to that used in the study by Frat et al., which was included in this meta-analysis. In addition, in the study by Frat et al., HFNC oxygen therapy also showed a positive effect in decreasing 90-day mortality [22]. Conversely, when the duration of HFNC oxygen therapy was shorter, studies comparing HFNC therapy and COT often showed negative results, including the study by Lemiale et al. that was included in the present meta-analysis [23]. Therefore, it seems that the duration of HFNC therapy is associated with its efficacy, with longer durations of HFNC therapy potentially leading to better results. The optimal duration of HFNC therapy in patients with ARF is still unclear and the durations of HFNC therapy in the relevant studies varied greatly. Our present meta-analysis could provide useful information in this regard.

There are several limitations of our meta-analysis. First, there were few studies that compared HFNC therapy and COT in patients with ARF and the number of patients included in our meta-analysis was limited. According to the

Table 4 The criteria for ARF among the included studies

Bell 2016	Frat 2015	Lemiale 2015	Jones 2015
1. RRs >25 breaths /min 2. SpO₂ < 93%	1. RRs >25 breaths/min 2. PaO₂ / FiO₂ ≤ 300 mmHg when the patients breathed oxygen at a flow rate > 10 l/min over 15 min 3. PaCO₂ ≤ 45 mmHg 4. An absence of clinical history of underlying chronic respiratory failure	1. A need for oxygen greater than 6 L/min to maintain SpO₂ > 95% 2. Symptoms of respiratory distress*	1. SpO₂ ≤ 92% on air 2. RRs ≥22 breaths/min

RRs respiratory rates, *SpO₂* peripheral capillary oxygen saturation, *PaO₂* arterial partial pressure of oxygen, *FiO₂* fraction of the inspired oxygen, *PaCO₂* partial pressure of arterial carbon dioxide, *Min* minute; *: tachypnea >30/min, intercostal recession, labored breathing, and/or dyspnea at rest study by Frat et al., the intubation rate was 38% in the HFNC group and 47% in the COT group. Assuming an intubation rate of 45% in the COT group, to detect a 5-percentage point reduction in the intubation rate in the HFNC group with an α of 0.05 and a β of 0.20 would require each group to enroll approximately 1220 subjects. Therefore, further large-scale studies are needed to confirm our results. Second, the effects of HFNC therapy in hypoxic ARF may be different from those in hypercapnic ARF, however, we could not perform a subgroup analysis relative to this aspect due to a lack of raw data. Third, since only 4 studies were included in the present meta-analysis, a funnel plot could not provide sufficient power to reveal a publication bias. Fourth, it should be noted that the durations of HFNC therapy were different among the 4 studies, especially in the studies by Bell and Lemiale [2, 23] in which the durations of HFNC therapy were only 2 h. Our subgroup analysis showed that a longer duration of HFNC therapy (≥24 h) may benefit ARF patients, so the inclusion of studies with different durations of HFNC therapy might produce biases.

Conclusions

Our meta-analysis demonstrated that HFNC therapy was similar to COT in ARF patients. The subgroup analysis showed that HFNC therapy may decrease the rates of the escalation of respiratory support and intubation when ARF patients were treated with HFNC therapy for ≥24 h compared with COT. Further high-quality, large-scale studies are needed to confirm our results.

Abbreviations
ARF: Acute respiratory failure; CIs: Confidence intervals; COT: Conventional oxygen therapy; F: Female; FiO$_2$: Fraction of inspired oxygen; HFNC: High-flow nasal cannula; IMV: Invasive mechanical ventilation; M: Male; NIV: Noninvasive ventilation; RCTs: Randomized controlled trials, RRs: Risk ratios

Acknowledgements
We acknowledge all the people who helped us.

Funding
The authors received no specific funding for this work.

Authors' contributions
All authors conceived the study and contributed to the study design. HYY and RZ collected data and helped extract data. YFZ and JRW performed the analyses. YFZ and HYY performed the literature review. All authors contributed to the writing of the draft and approved the final manuscript.

Competing interests
The authors declare they have no competing interests.

Author details
[1]Department of Intensive Care Unit, Guangzhou Red Cross Hospital, Medical College, Jinan University, Tongfuzhong Road No. 396, Guangzhou, Guangdong province 510220, China. [2]Department of Cardiology, Guangzhou Red Cross Hospital, Medical College, Jinan University, Guangzhou, Guangdong province 510220, China.

References
1. Pandor A, Thokala P, Goodacre S, et al. Pre-hospital non-invasive ventilation for acute respiratory failure: a systematic review and cost-effectiveness evaluation. Health Technol Assess. 2015;19(42):1–102.
2. Bell N, Hutchinson CL, Green TC, Rogan E, Bein KJ, Dinh MM. Randomised control trial of humidified high flow nasal cannulae versus standard oxygen in the emergency department. Emerg Med Australas. 2015; 10.1111/1742-6723.12490. [Epub ahead of print]
3. Azevedo LC, Caruso P, Silva UV, et al. Outcomes for patients with cancer admitted to the ICU requiring ventilatory support: results from a prospective multicenter study. Chest. 2014;146(2):257–66.
4. Azoulay E, Mokart D, Pène F, et al. Outcomes of critically ill patients with hematologic malignancies: prospective multicenter data from France and Belgium—a Groupe de Recherche Respiratoire en reanimation Onco-Hématologique study. J Clin Oncol. 2013;31(22):2810–8.
5. Roca O, Riera J, Torres F, Masclans JR. High-flow oxygen therapy in acute respiratory failure. Respir Care. 2010;55(4):408–13.
6. Delclaux C, L'Her E, Alberti C, et al. Treatment of acute hypoxemic nonhyper-capnic respiratory insuff iciency with continuous positive airway pressure delivered by a face mask: a randomized controlled trial. JAMA. 2000;284(18):2352–60.
7. Martin TJ, Hovis JD, Costantino JP, et al. A randomized, prospective evaluation of noninvasive ventilation for acute respiratory failure. Am J Respir Crit Care Med. 2000;161(3):807–13.
8. Demoule A, Hill N, Navalesi P. Can we prevent intubation in patients with ARDS? Intensive Care Med. 2016;42(5):768–71.
9. Vignaux L, Vargas F, Roeseler J, et al. Patient-ventilator asynchrony during non-invasive ventilation for acute respiratory failure: a multicenter study. Intensive Care Med. 2009;35(5):840–6.
10. Antonelli M, Conti G, Esquinas A, et al. A multiple-center survey on the use in clinical practice of noninvasive ventilation as a first-line intervention for acute respiratory distress syndrome. Crit Care Med. 2007;35(1):18–25.
11. Nava S, Ceriana P. Causes of failure of non-invasive mechanical ventilation. Respir Care. 2004;49(3):295–303.
12. Corley A, Caruana LR, Barnett AG, Tronstad O, Fraser JF. Oxygen delivery through high-flow nasal cannulae increase end-expiratory lung volume and reduce respiratory rate in post-cardiac surgical patients. Br J Anaesth. 2011; 107(6):998–1004.
13. Parke R, McGuinness S, Eccleston M. Nasal high-flow therapy delivers low level positive airway pressure. Br J Anaesth. 2009;103(6):886–90.
14. Parke RL, McGuinness SP. Pressures delivered by nasal high flow oxygen during all phases of the respiratory cycle. Respir Care. 2013;58(10):1621–4.
15. Maggiore SM, Idone FA, Vaschetto R, et al. Nasal high-flow versus Venturi mask oxygen therapy after extubation. Effects on oxygenation, comfort, and clinical outcome. Am J Respir Crit Care Med. 2014;190(3): 282–8.
16. Rittayamai N, Tscheikuna J, Rujiwit P. High-flow nasal cannula versus conventional oxygen therapy after endotracheal extubation: a randomized crossover physiologic study. Respir Care. 2014;59(4): 485–90.
17. Sztrymf B, Messika J, Mayot T, Lenglet H, Dreyfuss D, Ricard JD. Impact of high-flow nasal cannula oxygen therapy on intensive care unit patients with acute respiratory failure: a prospective observational study. J Crit Care. 2012; 27(3):324.
18. Sztrymf B, Messika J, Bertrand F, et al. Beneficial effects of humidified high flow nasal oxygen in critical care patients: a prospective pilot study. Intensive Care Med. 2011;37(11):1780–6.
19. Schwabbauer N, Björn B, Gunnar B, Michael H, Jürgen H, Reimer R. Nasal high-flow oxygen therapy in patients with hypoxic respiratory failure: effect on functional and subjective respiratory parameters compared to conventional oxygen therapy and non-invasive ventilation (NIV). BMC Anesth. 2014;14(1):66.

20. Roca O, Gonzalo H, Salvador DL, et al. Current evidence for the effectiveness of heated and humidified high flow nasal cannula supportive therapy in adult patients with respiratory failure. Crit Care. 2016;20(1):109.

21. Kernick J, Magarey J. What is the evidence for the use of high flow nasal cannula oxygen in adult patients admitted to critical care units? A systematic review. Aust Crit Care. 2010;23(2):53–70.

22. Frat JP, Thille AW, Mercat A, et al. High-flow oxygen through nasal cannula in acute hypoxemic respiratory failure. N Engl J Med. 2015;372(23):2185–96.

23. Lemiale V, Djamel M, Julien M, et al. The effects of a 2-h trial of high-flow oxygen by nasal cannula versus Venturi mask in immunocompromised patients with hypoxemic acute respiratory failure: a multicenter randomized trial. Crit Care. 2015;19(1):380.

24. Jones PG, Kamona S, Doran O, Sawtell F, Wilsher M. Randomized controlled trial of humidified high-flow nasal oxygen for acute respiratory distress in the emergency department: the HOT-ER study. Respir Care. 2016;61(3):291–9.

25. Ni YN, Luo J, Yu H, Liu D, Zhong N, Cheng J, Liang BM, Liang ZA. Can high-flow nasal cannula reduce the rate of endotracheal intubation in adult patients with acute respiratory failure compared with conventional oxygen therapy and noninvasive positive pressure ventilation? A systematic review and meta-analysis. Chest. 2017;151(4):764–75. 10.1016/j.chest.2017.01.004.

26. Monro-Somerville T, Sim M, Ruddy J, Vilas M, Gillies MA. The effect of high-flow nasal cannula oxygen therapy on mortality and intubation rate in acute respiratory failure: a systematic review and meta-analysis. Crit Care Med. 2017;45(4):e449–56. 10.1097/CCM.0000000000002091.

27. Higgins J, Green S. Cochrane handbook for systematic reviews of interventions. Version 5.1.0 [updated March 2011]. The Cochrane Collaboration. 2011. (http://handbook.cochrane.org/).

28. Stéphan F, Barrucand B, Petit P, et al. High-flow nasal oxygen vs noninvasive positive airway pressure in hypoxemic patients after cardiothoracic surgery. JAMA. 2015;313(23):2331–9.

29. Vourc'h M, Asfar P, Volteau C, et al. High-flow nasal cannula oxygen during endotracheal intubation in hypoxemic patients: a randomized controlled clinical trial. Intensive Care Med. 2015;41(9):1538–48.

30. Hernández G, Vaquero C, González P, et al. Effect of Postextubation high-FlowNasal Cannula vs conventional oxygen therapy on Reintubation in low-risk patients. JAMA. 2016;315(3):1354–61.

31. Parke RL, Eastwood GM, McGuinness SP, the George Institute for Global Health and the Australian and New Zealand Intensive Care Society Clinical Trials Group. Oxygen therapy in non-intubated adult intensive care patients: a point prevalence study. Crit Care Resusc. 2013;15(4):287–93.

32. Sztrymf B, Messika J, Mayot T, Lenglet H, Dreyfuss D, Ricard JD. Impact of high-flow nasal cannula oxygen therapy on intensive care unit patients with acute respiratory failure: a prospective observational study. J Crit Care. 2012; 27(27):324. e9–324.e13

7

Implication of species change of Nontuberculous Mycobacteria during or after treatment

Jong Sik Lee[1], Jong Hyuk Lee[2], Soon Ho Yoon[2], Taek Soo Kim[3], Moon-Woo Seong[3], Sung Koo Han[1] and Jae-Joon Yim[1*]

Abstract

Background: Co-existence or subsequent isolation of multiple nontuberculous mycobacteria (NTM) species in same patient has been reported. However, clinical significance of these observations is unclear. The aim of this study was to determine clinical implications of changes of NTM species during or after treatment in patients with NTM lung disease.

Methods: Patients with NTM lung disease, who experienced changes of NTM species during treatment or within 2 years of treatment completion between January 1, 2009 and December 31, 2015, were included in the analysis. Demographic, clinical, microbiological, and radiographic data were reviewed and analyzed.

Results: During the study period, 473 patients were newly diagnosed with NTM lung disease. Treatment was started in 164 patients (34.6%). Among these 164 patients, 16 experienced changes of NTM species during or within 2 years of treatment completion. Seven showed changes from *M. avium* complex (MAC) to *M. abscessus* subspecies *abscessus* (MAA) and five patients displayed changes from *M. abscessus* subspecies *massiliense* (MAM) to MAC. With isolation of new NTM species, 6 out of 7 patients with change from MAC to MAA reported worsening of symptoms, whereas none of the five patients with change from MAM to MAC reported worsening of symptoms. All MAA isolated during or after treatment for MAC lung diseases showed inducible resistance to clarithromycin.

Conclusions: Change of NTM species may occur during or after treatment for NTM lung disease. Especially, changes from MAC to MAA is accompanied by symptomatic and radiographic worsening as well as inducible resistance to clarithromycin.

Keywords: Nontuberculous mycobacteria species change, *Mycobacterium avium* Complex, *Mycobacterium abscessus* subspecies *abscessus*, Clarithromcycin resistance

Background

Nontuberculous mycobacteria (NTM) are ubiquitous in environments including natural or treated water and soil. They have a relatively low pathogenicity but can cause lung disease in immunocompetent as well as immunocompromised hosts. [1, 2] Currently, approximately 150 NTM species have been identified. [3, 4] The incidence and prevalence of NTM lung disease are rising worldwide. [1, 5] The distribution of causative species of NTM lung disease varies according to country and region. In South Korea, *M. avium* complex (MAC) is the most common, comprising approximately 60%-70% of all cases, followed by *M. abscessus* complex, comprising approximately 20%-30%. [6–9].

Isolation of NTM different from initial NTM species in same patients has been reported. Co-culture of MAC was reported among 20% of patients with *M. abscessus* subspecies *abscessus* (MAA). [10] We also reported wide spectrum of NTM species changes including change of

* Correspondence: yimjj@snu.ac.kr
[1]Division of Pulmonary and Critical Care Medicine, Department of Internal Medicine, Seoul National University College of Medicine, 101, Daehak-ro, Jongno-gu, Seoul 03080, Republic of Korea

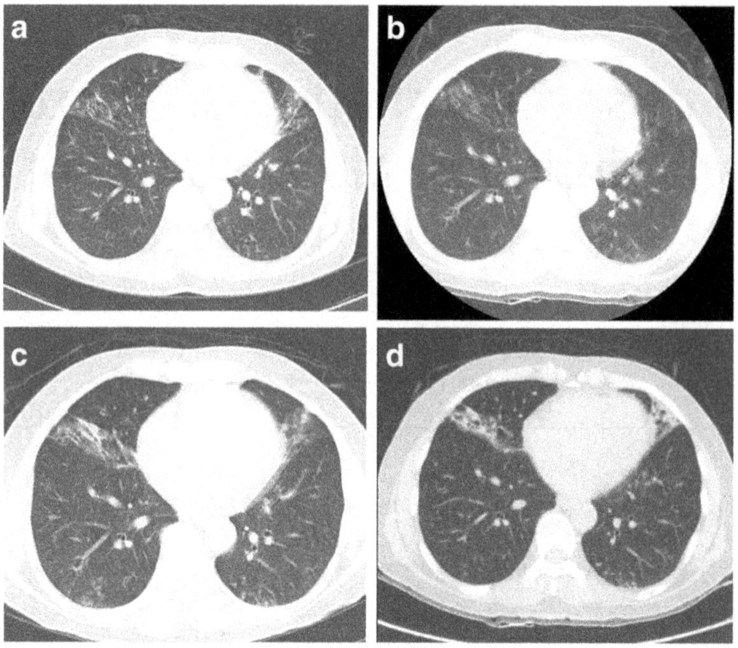

Fig. 1 a Chest CT scan of a patient with symptomatic *Mycobacterium intracellulare* lung disease before initiation of treatment. The scan shows bronchiectasis, nodules, and reticular densities in the right middle lobe and lingular segment. Treatment started 4 weeks after checking this CT scan. **b** Chest CT scan at 6 months after the initiation of treatment showing substantial improvement. **c** Chest CT scan at 12 months after the completion of 18-month treatment for *M. intracellulare* lung disease. Radiographic lesions and symptoms worsened; bloody sputum was also noted. Four weeks after this CT scan was taken, *M. abscessus* subspecies *abscessus*, instead of *M. intracellulare*, was isolated. **d** Chest CT scan at 6 months after initial isolation of *M. abscessus* subspecies *abscessus*. The patient's symptoms continued to worsen and sputum persistently tested positive for *M. abscessus* subspecies *abscessus*

species, alternative isolation of two or three species, or simultaneous isolation of multiple species in same patients [11].

We have experienced several patients with NTM lung diseases in whom changes of NTM species was identified during or after treatment. However, the clinical significance this of NTM change has not yet been reported. Therefore, the aim of this study was to determine the clinical implications of changes of NTM species during or after treatment completion in patients with NTM lung disease.

Methods

Study population

Among patients treated for NTM lung disease at Seoul National University Hospital between January 1, 2009 and December 31, 2015, patients with changes of NTM species during treatment or within 2 years of treatment completion were included in the analysis. Demographic, clinical, microbiological, and radiographic data of the included patients were reviewed. This study was conducted in accordance with the amended Declaration of Helsinki. The study protocol was approved by the institutional review board of Seoul National University Hospital (IRB No: 1608-046-784), and written informed consent was obtained from all patients.

Diagnosis of NTM lung disease and definition of newly isolated NTM species

Patients were diagnosed with NTM lung disease based on the diagnostic criteria of the American Thoracic Society (ATS)/Infectious Diseases Society of America (IDSA) guideline. [12] "Change of NTM species" were defined as disappearance of initially isolated NTM species and isolation of new species at least 2 times.

Follow up and treatment

Patients with NTM lung disease underwent follow-ups every 3 to 6 months and treatment was offered in cases of significant radiographic progression (i.e. new cavity formation) or worsening respiratory symptoms (i.e. development of hemoptysis). Once treatment was initiated, patients visited the clinic every 4 to 8 weeks for physical examination, mycobacterial cultures of sputum, and radiographic evaluations. Treatment regimen was selected based on the ATS/IDSA guideline. [12] After treatment completion, patients underwent follow-ups every 3–6 months.

Clinical and radiographic examination

Changes in respiratory symptoms were evaluated by the on-duty physician on every visit. If patients reported increased sputum production, worsened dyspnea, or development of hemoptysis, the symptoms were regarded as "worsened". Likewise, "no change" of symptoms and "improved" symptoms were defined based on patients' report.

Chest computed tomography (CT) was performed every 6 months during treatment and every 1–2 years after treatment completion. The severity of NTM lung diseases on CT was evaluated using a scoring system modified from a previously published one [13] by a board-certified radiologist (Fig. 1). The scoring system consists of severity, extent, and mucus plugging of bronchiectasis; severity and extent of cellular bronchiolitis; diameter, wall thickness, and extent of the cavity; nodules; and consolidation [13].

Microbiological examination

At every visit, patients were requested to submit sputum samples for mycobacterial culture. Sputum were decontaminated with same volume of 4% sodium hydroxide (NaOH), homogenized, and concentrated by centrifugation at 3000×g for 20 min. The processed sediments were stained using the Ziehl-Neelsen method. [12] Concentrated specimen were cultured in 3% Ogawa medium to minimize possibility of contamination and observed weekly for 9 weeks after inoculation. Once cultured, *M. tuberculosis* and NTM were differentiated using Gen-Probe® method (Gen-Probe; San diego, CA, USA). [14] Following isolation of a suspected mycobacterial species, NTM was confirmed by analyzing the sequences of three genes: *16S rRNA*, *rpoB*, and *tuf.*

Antimycobacterial drug susceptibility tests were conducted at the Korean Institute of Tuberculosis by using broth microdilution. Minimum inhibitory concentrations (MICs) of antibiotics (amikacin, cefoxitin, ciprofloxacin, clarithromycin, imipenem, moxifloxacin, rifampicin, ethambutol, linezolid for MAC; and amikacin, cefoxitin, ciprofloxacin, clarithromycin, imipenem, moxifloxacin, and linezolid for *M. abscessus* complex) were determined according to the CLSI guidelines. [15] For MAC, isolates were considered as resistant if the MIC of clarithromycin was ≥32 μg/ml and as susceptible if the MIC of clarithromycin was ≤8 μg/ml. For *M. abscessus* complex, isolates were considered as resistant if the MIC of clarithromycin was ≥8 μg/ml and as susceptible if the MIC of clarithromycin was ≤2 μg/ml. Inducible resistance was considered if the MIC of clarithromycin was ≤2 μg/ml for 3 days and ≥8 μg/ml for 14 days.

Statistical analysis

Data were summarized as medians with interquartile range (IQR) with non-normal distribution. We used repeated-measures data analysis with a Friedman model to test the significance of differences in CT scores. All statistical analyses were carried out using SPSS Statistics version 20 (IBM Corp, Chicago, IL, USA) and a P value < .05 was regarded as statistically significant.

Results
Characteristics of patients
During the study period, a total of 473 patients with NTM lung disease were diagnosed at Seoul National University Hospital. Of those, 164 patients started treatment for NTM lung disease. Among 164 patients with NTM lung disease, 54 patients (39 during treatment and 15 within 2 years of treatment completion) experienced isolation of another species of NTM. Among these 54 patients, 16 satisfied the definition of "change of NTM species", 12 patients during treatment and in 4 patients within 2 years of treatment completion. The median number of isolation of new NTM species was 5.5 (IQR 3-7). The median age of these 16 patients was 69 years (IQR 61.7-73.5) and 12 (75%) were female. The median body mass index was 20.8 (IQR 19.2-21.4) (Table 1).

Table 1 Baseline characteristics of 16 patients with nontuberculous mycobacteria lung disease included for the analysis

Patients, No.	$N = 16$
Age, years, median (IQR)	69 (61.7-73.5)
Sex, female	12 (75.0%)
BMI, kg/m², median (IQR)	20.8 (19.2-21.4)
Never smoker	14 (87.5%)
History of tuberculosis	6 (37.5%)
Underlying disease	
Connective tissue disease	4 (25.0%)
Diabetes	3 (18.7%)
Malignancy	1 (6.0%)
Respiratory symptoms	
Sputum	16 (100%)
Cough	13 (81.2%)
Dyspnea	4 (25.0%)
Hemoptysis	3 (18.7%)
General symptoms	
Weight loss	2 (12.5%)
Night sweating	1 (6.2%)
Laboratory findings, median (IQR)	
Leukocytes (×10³/μl)	6880 (5070-7542)
Hemoglobin (g/dl)	12.6 (11.9-13.3)
Cholesterol	168 (149-187.7)
Albumin	4 (3.8-4.4)
Creatinine	0.7 (0.6-0.9)

BMI body mass index, *IQR* interquartile range

Changes of NTM species during or after treatment for NTM lung disease

Of 16 patients who showed change of NTM species during or after initial NTM lung disease treatment, 7 patients (43.8%) showed changes from MAC to MAA, 4 during treatment and 3 after treatment for MAC. Five patients (31.2%) displayed changes from *M. abscessus* subspecies *massiliense* (MAM) to MAC during treatment for MAM. The other four patients exhibited change from and to other NTM species, 3 during treatment and 1 after treatment for initial NTM (Table 2). Among 12 patients with change of NTM species during treatment, the median interval from starting treatment for initial NTM lung disease to new species isolation was 7.3 months (IQR 4.2-17.4). The median interval from treatment completion for initial NTM lung disease to isolation of a new species was median 15.6 months (IQR 14.9-16.4) among the other four patients.

Changes of radiographic severities throughout treatment of initial NTM lung diseases and isolation of new NTM

Overall, the CT scores throughout the treatment course did not change. The median total CT scores at initiation of treatment for initial NTM, at 6–12 months after treatment, at isolation of a new NTM species, and at 6–12 months after isolation of a new NTM species was 13.2, 9.6, 12.9, and 13.0, respectively (P = .794) Likewise, CT scores before and after change of NTM species did not differ (median 12.9 vs 13.0, P = .763) (Table 3).

Table 2 Changes of NTM Species During and After Treatment

	N = 16
M. avium complex → M. abscessus subspecies abscessus	7 (43.8%)
M. intracellulare → M. abscessus subspecies abscessus	4
M. avium → M. abscessus subspecies abscessus	3
M. abscessus subspecies massiliense → M. avium complex	5 (31.2%)
M. abscessus subspecies massiliense → M. avium	3
M. abscessus subspecies massiliense → M. intracellulare	2
Others	
M. avium → M. fortuitum	1 (6.2%)
M. avium → M. intracellulare	1 (6.2%)
M. intracellulare → M. chimera	1 (6.2%)
M. abscessus subspecies massiliense → M. abscessus subspecies abscessus	1 (6.2%)

Table 3 Change of CT Scores Throughout Treatment of Initial NTM Lung Disease and Isolation of New NTM

	At initiation of treatment	At 6–12 months after treatment	At isolation of new NTM	At 6–12 months after isolation of new NTM	P Value
Bronchiectasis,					
Severity	1.7 (1-2)	1.8 (1.2-2)	2 (1.2-2)	1.7 (1.3-2)	.572
Extent	1 (1-2)	1 (1-2)	1 (1-2)	1 (1-2)	.733
Mucus plugging	1 (0-1)	0 (0-1)	1 (0-1)	1 (0-1)	.875
Cellular bronchiolitis					
Severity	1.8 (1.6-2.2)	1.7 (1.2-2)	2 (1.6-2)	1.8 (1.7-2)	.089
Extent	3 (1-3)	2.5 (1-3)	2 (1.5-3)	2 (1-3)	.112
Cavity					
Diameter (cm)	1 (0-2)	0 (0-1)	1 (0-1)	1 (0-2)	.245
Wall thickness (mm)	2 (0-2.5)	0 (0-2.1)	2 (0-2)	0.5 (0-2.4)	.978
Extent	1 (0-1)	0 (0-1)	1 (0-1)	1 (0-1)	1.000
Nodules	1 (0-1)	1 (0.8-1)	1 (1-1.5)	1 (0-1)	.572
Consolidation	0 (0-1)	0 (0-0.3)	0 (0-1)	1 (0-1)	.479
Total CT score	13.2 (7.2-17.6)	9.6 (6.4-14.4)	12.9 (9.0-14.8)	13 (8.0-14.6)	.794

Data are expressed as median (IQR). *CT* computed tomography, *NTM* nontuberculous mycobacteria

Changes of respiratory symptoms with isolation of new NTM species

Six out of seven patients with change from MAC to MAA reported worsening of symptoms with isolation of new species. Conversely, no patient with change from MAM to MAC complained of worsening symptoms (Table 4).

In vitro drug susceptibility to clarithromycin of newly isolated NTM species

All MAA isolated during or after the treatment for MAC lung diseases showed inducible resistance to clarithromycin. MAA isolated during treatment for MAM lung disease and *M. fortuitum* isolated during treatment for MAC lung diseases also showed inducible resistance to clarithromycin. One out of three MAC species isolated during or after treatment for MAM showed resistance to clarithromycin (Table 4). This patient refused to use intravenous drugs and took azithromycin only.

Treatment for newly isolated NTM species

Among 12 patients in whom another NTM species were isolated during treatment for initial NTM lung disease, the same treatment regimens were continued in 4 patients while the regimens were modified for the newly

Table 4 Symptomatic and Radiographic Changes, Clarithromycin Resistance, and Treatment for Newly Isolated NTM

No	NTM spices	Symptom changes at isolation of new NTM	Radiographic changes at isolation of new NTM	Clarithromycin resistance for initial NTM (MIC, μg/ml)	Clarithromycin resistance for new NTM(MIC, μg/ml)	Timing of new NTM isolation	Treatment for newly isolated NTM
M. avium complex → _M. abscessus_ subspecies _abscessus_							
1	_M. intracellulare_ → _M. abscessus_ subspecies _abscessus_	Worsening	Worsening	Susceptible (1)	Inducible resistance (1, 64)	After treatment for initial NTM	Not started
2	_M. intracellulare_ → _M. abscessus_ subspecies _abscessus_	Worsening	Unchanged	Susceptible (2)	Inducible resistance (2, 64)	During treatment for initial NTM	[a]Started
`3	_M. intracellulare_ → _M. abscessus_ subspecies _abscessus_	Worsening	Worsening	Susceptible (2)	Inducible resistance (2, 8)	After treatment for initial NTM	Not started
4	_M. intracellulare_ → _M. abscessus_ subspecies _abscessus_	Worsening	Worsening	Susceptible (2)	Inducible resistance (0.5, 64)	After treatment for initial NTM	Not started
5	_M. avium_ → _M. abscessus_ subspecies _abscessus_	Unchanged	Unchanged	Susceptible (4)	Inducible resistance (0.5, 64)	During treatment for initial NTM	Not started
6	_M. avium_ → _M. abscessus_ subspecies _abscessus_	Worsening	Worsening	Susceptible (1)	Inducible resistance (1, 64)	During treatment for initial NTM	Continued on-going treatment
7	_M. avium_ → _M. abscessus_ subspecies _abscessus_	Worsening	Unchanged	Susceptible (0.5)	Inducible resistance (1, 64)	During treatment for initial NTM	Modified regimen and continued treatment
M. abscessus subspecies _massiliense_ → _M. avium_ complex							
8	_M. abscessus_ subspecies _massiliense_ → _M. intracellulare_	Unchanged	Unchanged	Susceptible (0.5)	N/A	During treatment for initial NTM	Modified regimen and continued treatment
9	_M. abscessus_ subspecies _massiliense_ → _M. intracellulare_	Unchanged	Worsening	Susceptible (0.5)	Susceptible (1)	During treatment for initial NTM	Modified regimen and continued treatment
10	_M. abscessus_ subspecies _massiliense_ → _M. avium_	Unchanged	Unchanged	Susceptible (0.5)	Resistance (64)	During treatment for initial NTM	Continued on-going treatment
11	_M. abscessus_ subspecies _massiliense_ → _M. avium_	Unchanged	Improving	Susceptible (0.5)	Susceptible (2)	During treatment for initial NTM	Modified regimen and continued treatment
12	_M. abscessus_ subspecies _massiliense_ → _M. avium_	Unchanged	Unchanged	N/A	N/A	During treatment for initial NTM	[a]Started
Others							
13	_M. avium_ → _M. fortuitum_	Unchanged	Improving	Susceptible (0.5)	Inducible resistance (0.5, 16)	During treatment for initial NTM	Not started

Table 4 Symptomatic and Radiographic Changes, Clarithromycin Resistance, and Treatment for Newly Isolated NTM *(Continued)*

No	NTM spices	Symptom changes at isolation of new NTM	Radiographic changes at isolation of new NTM	Clarithromycin resistance for initial NTM (MIC, µg/ml)	Clarithromycin resistance for new NTM(MIC, µg/ml)	Timing of new NTM isolation	Treatment for newly isolated NTM
14	*M. avium → M. intracellulare*	Worsening	Worsening	N/A	Susceptible (1)	After treatment for initial NTM	Started
15	*M. intracellulare → M. chimerae*	Improving	Worsening	Susceptible (1)	Susceptible (2)	During treatment for initial NTM	Continued on-going treatment
16	*M. abscessus* subspecies *massiliense → M. abscessus* subspecies *abscessus*	Unchanged	Worsening	Susceptible (0.5)	Inducible resistance (1, 16)	During treatment for initial NTM	Continued on-going treatment

MIC minimal inhibitory concentration, *N/A* not available, *NTM* nontuberculous mycobacteria
[a]Treatment for initial NTM lung disease was completed. Then, treatment for newly isolated NTM was initiated

isolated NTM in 4 patients. Despite of isolation of new NTM species, the other 4 patients continued to receive and completed treatments for initial NTM lung disease and were observed for a while; in 2 out of these patients, treatments for newly isolated NTM were started eventually. (Table 4).

Among 4 patients in whom new NTM species were isolated after the completion of treatment for initial NTM lung disease, only one started to receive treatment for newly isolated NTM. (Table 4).

Discussion

In this study on patients with NTM lung diseases who received treatment, we identified several interesting findings. First, approximately 10% of patients with NTM lung disease exhibited changes to new NTM species during or within 2 years after treatment completion. Second, the most common pattern of NTM change species was from MAC to MAA. Third, change from MAC to MAA was associated with worsening of respiratory symptoms and radiographic lesions and most importantly with inducible resistance of clarithromycin.

Simultaneous or sequential isolation of several NTM species in the same patients has been reported. [10, 11, 16] In addition, repeated culture of different MAC strains in the same among patients with nodular bronchiectatic lung disease was also identified. [16] Through this study, we identified conversion of NTM species during or after treatment in 16 (9.8%) out of 164 patients treated for NTM lung diseases. The Majority of these patients (11 out of 16) experienced symptomatic and/or radiographic worsening with isolation of new NTM species. Similarly to the recent study [17], these could be regarded as development of new NTM lung disease.

In our study, conversion from lung disease by MAC to the caused by MAA, which is more difficult to treat, was most common than other conversion patterns.

Furthermore, all MAA isolated from patients who had been treated for MAC lung disease showed inducible resistance to clarithromycin. Inducible resistance to clarithromycin involves a functional erm(41) gene, related to a T/C polymorphism at the 28th nucleotide. [18, 19] The rate of inducible resistance among these patients was very high compared with our recent study, which showed 55.1% of MAA isolated from patients in our hospital. [20] It could be explained that MAA with C28 sequevar, which do not show inducible resistance, might be eradicated by previous treatment with regimen including macrolide.

Previous studies reported that patients with different MAC strains usually have nodular bronchiectatic features rather than cavitary disease. [16, 21] Different strains might reside in different ectatic bronchi or nodules in same patients. Likewise, in our study, all 16 patients with conversion of NTM species during or after treatment had nodular bronchiectatic features. We speculate that these patients already had two NTM species in different ectatic bronchi or nodules at initial diagnosis of NTM lung disease. The number of initially detected major NTM species might be minimized with treatment while minor NTM species prevailed. For patients with conversion from MAC lung disease to MAA lung disease, treatment with macrolide, ethambutol, and rifampicin might reduce the number of MAC as well as MAA which is sensitive to clarithromycin, but MAA with inducible resistance could resist treatment and turn into the major NTM species in those patients.

This study has several limitations. First, the number of patients included in the analysis was small, although all patients included were treated at an institution that routinely diagnoses and treats a large number patient with NTM lung disease. To confirm our observations, a large-scale study enrolling patients from multiple hospitals is needed. Secondly, this study was performed retrospectively. Time points of requesting mycobacterial culture of sputum or chest CT scans were not controlled strictly. Additionally, crucial data, such as drug susceptibility test for the secondary isolated NTM species, were missing in some patients.

Conclusions

NTM species changes could occur during or after treatment for NTM lung disease. Especially, changes from MAC to MAA were accompanied by symptomatic and radiographic worsening as well as inducible resistance to clarithromycin.

Abbreviations

CT: Chest computed tomography; IQR: Interquartile range; MAA: *M. abscessus* subspecies *abscessus*; MAC: *M. avium* complex; MAM: *M. abscessus* subspecies *massiliense*; MICs: Minimum inhibitory concentrations; NTM: nontuberculous mycobacteria

Funding

There was no funding for this study.

Authors' contributions

JSL contributed to the data acquisition, data interpretation, and writing of the manuscript. JHL, SHY, contributed to the collection and analysis of radiological data. TSK, HWS, SKH contributed substantially to the study design, data analysis and interpretation, and the writing of the manuscript. JJY is the guarantor of the entire manuscript and is responsible for the content of the manuscript, including the data collected and its analysis. All authors read and approved the final manuscript.

Competing interests

The authors declare that they have no competing interests.

Author details

[1]Division of Pulmonary and Critical Care Medicine, Department of Internal Medicine, Seoul National University College of Medicine, 101, Daehak-ro, Jongno-gu, Seoul 03080, Republic of Korea. [2]Department of Radiology, Seoul National University College of Medicine, 101, Daehak-ro, Jongno-gu, Seoul 03080, Republic of Korea. [3]Department of Laboratory Medicine, Seoul National University Hospital, 101, Daehak-ro, Jongno-gu, Seoul 03080, Republic of Korea.

References

1. Prevots DR, Marras TK. Epidemiology of human pulmonary infection with nontuberculous mycobacteria: a review. Clin Chest Med. 2015;36(1):13–34.
2. Falkinham JO. Environmental sources of nontuberculous mycobacteria. Clin Chest Med. 2015;36(1):35–41.
3. Tortoli E. Microbiological features and clinical relevance of new species of the genus mycobacterium. Clin Microbiol Rev. 2014;27(4):727–52.
4. Tortoli E. The new mycobacteria: an update. FEMS Immunology & Medical Microbiology. 2006;48(2):159–78.
5. Stout JE, Koh W-J, Yew WW. Update on pulmonary disease due to non-tuberculous mycobacteria. Int J Infect Dis. 2016;45:123–34.
6. Park Y, Lee C, Lee S, Yang S, Yoo C, Kim Y, Han S, Shim Y, Yim J. Rapid increase of non-tuberculous mycobacterial lung diseases at a tertiary referral hospital in South Korea [short communication]. The International Journal of Tuberculosis and Lung Disease. 2010;14(8):1069–71.
7. Lee SK, Lee EJ, Kim SK, Chang J, Jeong SH, Kang YA. Changing epidemiology of nontuberculous mycobacterial lung disease in South Korea. Scand J Infect Dis. 2012;44(10):733–8.
8. Koh W-J, Kwon OJ, Jeon K, Kim TS, Lee KS, Park YK, Bai GH. Clinical significance of nontuberculous mycobacteria isolated from respiratory specimens in Korea. CHEST Journal. 2006;129(2):341–8.
9. Jang M-A, Koh W-J, Huh HJ, Kim S-Y, Jeon K, Ki C-S, Lee NY. Distribution of nontuberculous mycobacteria by multigene sequence-based typing and clinical significance of isolated strains. J Clin Microbiol. 2014;52(4):1207–12.
10. Griffith DE, Girard WM, Wallace Jr RJ. Clinical features of pulmonary disease caused by rapidly growing mycobacteria: an analysis of 154 patients. Am Rev Respir Dis. 1993;147(5):1271–8.
11. Lim H-J, Park CM, Park YS, Lee J, Lee S-M, Yang S-C, Yoo C-G, Kim YW, Han SK, Yim J-J. Isolation of multiple nontuberculous mycobacteria species in the same patients. Int J Infect Dis. 2011;15(11):e795–8.
12. Griffith DE, Aksamit T, Brown-Elliott BA, Catanzaro A, Daley C, Gordin F, Holland SM, Horsburgh R, Huitt G, Iademarco MF. An official ATS/IDSA statement: diagnosis, treatment, and prevention of nontuberculous mycobacterial diseases. Am J Respir Crit Care Med. 2007;175(4):367–416.
13. Kim HS, Lee KS, Koh W-J, Jeon K, Lee EJ, Kang H, Ahn J. Serial CT findings of Mycobacterium Massiliense pulmonary disease compared with mycobacterium abscessus disease after treatment with antibiotic therapy. Radiology. 2012;263(1):260–70.
14. Bergmann JS, Yuoh G, Fish G, Woods GL. Clinical evaluation of the enhanced gen-probe amplified mycobacterium tuberculosis direct test for rapid diagnosis of tuberculosis in prison inmates. J Clin Microbiol. 1999; 37(5):1419–25.
15. CLSI: Susceptibility testing of Mycobacteria, Nocardiae, and other aerobic Actinomycetes. Approved standard-second edition CLSI document M24-A2 Wayne, PA: clinical and laboratory standards institute 2011.
16. Wallace Jr RJ, Zhang Y, Brown BA, Dawson D, Murphy DT, Wilson R, Griffith DE. Polyclonal Mycobacterium Avium Complex infections in patients with nodular bronchiectasis. Am J Respir Crit Care Med. 1998;158(4):1235–44.
17. Griffith DE, Philley JV, Brown-Elliott BA, Benwill JL, Shepherd S, York D, Wallace RJ. The significance of mycobacterium abscessus subspecies abscessus isolation during Mycobacterium Avium Complex lung disease therapy. CHEST Journal. 2015;147(5):1369–75.
18. Nash KA, Brown-Elliott BA, Wallace RJ. A novel gene, erm (41), confers inducible macrolide resistance to clinical isolates of mycobacterium abscessus but is absent from mycobacterium chelonae. Antimicrob Agents Chemother. 2009;53(4):1367–76.
19. Choi H, Kim S-Y, Kim DH, Huh HJ, Ki C-S, Lee NY, Lee S-H, Shin S, Shin SJ, Daley CL. Clinical characteristics and treatment outcomes of patients with acquired Macrolide-resistant mycobacterium abscessus lung disease. Antimicrob Agents Chemother. 2017;61(10):e01146–17.
20. Park J, Cho J, Lee CH, Han SK, Yim JJ. Progression and treatment outcomes of lung disease caused by mycobacterium abscessus and Mycobacterium Massiliense. Clin Infect Dis. 2017;64(3):301–8.
21. Mazurek GH, Hartman S, Zhang Y-s, Brown B, Hector J, Murphy D, Wallace R, Large DNA. Restriction fragment polymorphism in the Mycobacterium Avium-M. Intracellulare complex: a potential epidemiologic tool. J Clin Microbiol. 1993;31(2):390–4.

The use of an alternate side lying positioning strategy during inhalation therapy does not prolong nebulisation time in adults with Cystic Fibrosis

Ruth L. Dentice[1], Mark R. Elkins[2,3], Genevieve M. Dwyer[4]* ⓘ and Peter T. P. Bye[2,5]

Abstract

Background: Inhalation of nebulised medications is performed in upright sitting to maximise lung volumes. The pattern of deposition is poor for inhaled medications in people with Cystic Fibrosis. The pattern tends to be non-uniform and typically the upper lobes receive a reduced dose compared to the rest of the lung. One strategy that has been proposed as having the potential to improve homogeneity of deposition is to adopt an alternate side lying position for the inhalation procedure. This study sought to determine whether, among adults with Cystic Fibrosis, there is any disadvantage to delivery time of nebulised medications with a strategy of alternate side lying, compared to upright sitting.

Methods: A randomised crossover trial with concealed allocation, intention-to-treat analysis and blinded assessors was undertaken. The participants were 24 adults with stable Cystic Fibrosis. They inhaled 4 mL of normal saline via an LC Star™ nebuliser twice within 24 h. In random order, participants sat upright throughout nebulisation, or alternated between left and right side lying at each minute during the nebulisation period. The nebuliser was stopped and weighed each minute until the residual volume was reached. The primary outcome was the time required for 3.5 mL to be delivered. The secondary outcomes were: respiratory rate; ratio of the volume delivered on right and left sides; and calculation of how long the periods in side lying can be extended without causing greater than 20% discrepancy in dose delivered in the two positions.

Results: The delivery time did not significantly differ between sitting and side lying (mean difference 0.58 min, 95% confidence interval (CI) -1.40 to 0.24). There was no significant correlation between delivery time, lung function or subject height (all $R^2 < 0.4$). Increasing side lying duration from 1 to 2 min did not significantly impact the dose delivered on each side. Turning each 3 min however, significantly worsened the disparity (mean ratio 1.32, 95% CI 1.24 to 1.40).

Conclusion: Side lying during inhalation therapy does not prolong nebulisation time. 2-min periods should provide an equal dose in the two side lying positions.

Keywords: Cystic fibrosis, Body position, Nebuliser delivery rate

* Correspondence: g.dwyer@westernsydney.edu.au
[4]Physiotherapy Program, Western Sydney University, Sydney, Australia
Full list of author information is available at the end of the article

Background

Over the past few decades, research has established many nebulised therapies that improve the clinical status and quality of life of people with Cystic Fibrosis, including inhaled tobramycin [1] recombinant human deoxyribonuclease [2] and hypertonic saline [3]. However, these therapies, along with nebulised bronchodilators and other nebulised antibiotics, add considerably to the duration of a patient's treatment regimen. It is therefore not surprising that prolonged nebulisation times can adversely affect the acceptability of, or full compliance with, treatments for people with Cystic Fibrosis [4].

The distribution of ventilation (V), perfusion (Q), and V/Q matching in the lungs are primarily influenced by gravity [5, 6]. Ventilation is biased to the dependent lung regions regardless of body position. Thus in sitting, tidal ventilation is biased towards basal regions. In healthy subjects and in several patient populations, it has been demonstrated that drug deposition follows the distribution of tidal ventilation within the lungs [7–9]. Nebulised medications are traditionally recommended to be administered in upright sitting to: (a) maximise resting lung expansion in terms of total lung capacity, functional residual capacity, and residual volume [10–12]; (b) maximise ventilation; (c) minimise closing volume of dependent airways; (d) stimulate the sympathetic nervous system to increase alertness and concentration [13] and (e) minimise medication delivery to the oropharynx and gut. However, the disadvantage of the delivery of nebulised therapies in upright sitting is poor deposition of medication in the upper lobes. Poor deposition in the upper lobes has been identified in people with Cystic Fibrosis [7, 14–17], people with HIV [8, 18, 19], and other populations, including healthy people [9, 20, 21].

A strategy of alternate side lying has been proposed as a means to improve upper lobe deposition. In this strategy, patients alternate between right and left side lying at regular intervals during delivery of a single nebulised therapy. The rationale for this approach is that gravity will tend to increase ventilation in the most dependent region of the lungs. Adopting a sidelying position therefore will result in deposition of nebulised medication preferentially throughout the dependent lung, including its upper lobe. Importantly, regular turning is required to dose both sides (including both upper lobes) equally during a single nebulisation period. This is because the dose delivered by an LC Star nebuliser over time is initially rapid and then tapers after 8 to 10 min, rather than constant delivery. This has been demonstrated with its delivery of recombinant human deoxyribonuclease [22] and with its delivery of normal saline in our pilot data (see Additional file 1:. Pilot in-vitro data collected to establish the pattern of decay in the delivery rate of the LC Star nebuliser loaded with 4 mL of normal (0.9%) saline).

It remains unclear, however, whether this alternate sidelying strategy to improve homogeneity of deposition has an impact on nebulisation time. If the nebulisation time was significantly increased then any potential benefits in the pattern of drug deposition may be outweighed by poorer patient compliance in completing the drug administration regimen.

We assert that this is the first study to examine the alternate side lying strategy for nebulised delivery of medication. This assertion is reinforced by a Google Scholar search using the terms *nebuli-* AND *deliver-* AND (*body position* OR *side lying*), which identified no evidence about the side lying strategy.

Method

Aims

The aims of the study were to determine:

1. Among adults with Cystic Fibrosis, is there any disadvantage to delivery time of nebulised medications with a strategy of alternate side lying, compared to upright sitting?
2. How long can the periods in side lying be extended without causing greater than 20% discrepancy between the dose delivered in the two positions?

Design

A randomised, crossover trial with concealed allocation, blinding of assessors and intention-to-treat analysis was undertaken at Royal Prince Alfred Hospital, Sydney. Participants were recruited by personal approach by one of the investigators at the Cystic Fibrosis clinic at the hospital. Once enrolled in the trial, each participant was invited to attend the Department of Respiratory Medicine on two consecutive days. On both days, participants performed spirometry in standing in accordance with the most recent European Respiratory Society criteria [23]. Participants were then randomised, by flipping a coin, to one of two positioning regimens:

1. Upright sitting: maintained throughout the nebulisation period, or.
2. Alternate side lying: alternated between left and right at each minute during the nebulisation period. The starting side was also randomly allocated.

Participants were requested to adopt their allocated position and maintain a slightly deeper than normal tidal breathing pattern during the subsequent standard study inhalation. When participants returned for their second study day, they adopted the other positioning regimen.

All standard morning medications were inhaled on the study days, with the appointment scheduled at least 4 h after these medications, and not within 1 h of a meal. Participants were requested to keep their medication regimen constant during the two study days. After testing on each study day, participants were free to inhale medications and eat as usual.

Participants

Participants were required to meet the following criteria to be eligible for the study: aged at least 18 years; a diagnosis of Cystic Fibrosis confirmed with sweat testing or genotyping; and clinically stable with a forced expiratory volume in one second (FEV_1) within 10% of the best recorded value for the past 6 months. Potential participants were excluded if they: had received a lung transplant; were colonised with *Burkholderia cepacia* complex; were not clinically stable; had significant malignant, neurological or musculoskeletal co morbidities; had hepatomegaly, hepatosplenomegaly or current intestinal obstruction; or were pregnant. Research procedures were approved by the Ethics Committees of the Sydney Local Health District (RPAH Zone) (X08-0214, HREC/08/RPAH/358) and the University of Sydney. All participants provided written informed consent prior to participating in this study.

Intervention

Inhalation solution and body position

The standard study inhalation was 4 mL of normal saline (AstraZeneca, North Ryde, NSW), delivered by an LC Star nebuliser (Pari, Germany). The nebuliser and tubing were weighed before and after the 4 mL dose was loaded. The nebuliser was driven with 6 L/min of medical air via the hospital wall supply and a calibrated flow meter. This supply was interrupted after one minute of nebulisation time, as timed with an 870A electronic timer (Diamond Data, China). At this time, the nebuliser and tubing were weighed on a 1206MP Scale (Sartorius, UK). The nebulisation was then recommenced for another timed minute and then weighed again. This continued (with the patient swapping sides during the measurement time if randomised to the alternate side lying condition) until the weight indicated that 3.5 mL of the loaded dose had been delivered from the nebuliser. This approach assumed that the residual volume of 0.5 mL has been reached, in accordance with the manufacturer's specifications.

Blinding

Weighing of the nebuliser was performed by an investigator who was unaware of the position adopted by the participant. This 'blinding' was achieved by shielding the investigator from the patient by a curtain and blocking the sound of the participant changing position by padded headphones playing music. The investigator responsible for randomising and positioning the participant (RD)

passed the nebuliser and tubing around the curtain to the blinded investigator for weighing each minute. Each weight was recorded until the dead volume has been reached. An Excel file (Microsoft, USA) was used to store the data. The investigator responsible for randomising and positioning the participant recorded the respiratory rate of the participant, counted during the middle 30 s of each minute of nebulisation.

Outcome measures

The primary outcome was the time required for 3.5 mL of saline to be delivered by the nebuliser as determined by nebuliser weight. The secondary outcomes were respiratory rate, as an explanatory variable; ratio of the volume of saline delivered on the right and left sides; and calculation of how long the periods in side lying can be extended without causing greater than 20% discrepancy between the dose delivered in the two positions, i.e. the ratio exceeding 1:1.2.

Data analysis

For the primary outcome was nebulised medication delivery time, we were unable to find an estimate of the smallest effect on inhalation time that adults with Cystic Fibrosis would consider using a particular positioning regimen worthwhile. Clinical experience in our centre would indicate that time alone is not the only consideration used by patient for position selection when following a nebuliser regimen. Many patients prefer to nebulise in side lying due to comfort and convenience. Therefore we postulated that the increase in delivery time would need to be substantial to stop the use of this strategy in clinical practice. We considered that a minimum difference of 5 min in delivery time for the 3.5 mL dose would be large enough to contribute to clinical decision-making about which positioning regimen to use. Pilot data provided a standard deviation (SD) of 3.7 min for this change in delivery time among eight adults with Cystic Fibrosis who met the eligibility criteria. Assuming this SD, 20 participants would provide 80% power, at the 2-sided 5% significance level, to detect a 5-min difference in delivery time as statistically significant between two groups in the study. We increased participant recruitment to 24 to allow for possible drop outs.

As an explanatory variable, respiratory rates were compared between sitting and side lying, to see if this variable may have influenced the delivery rate due to breath activation. Respiratory rate in the two delivery positions was compared using a paired t-test. The alternate side lying data were further examined to assess whether the amount of saline delivered while in right side lying differed from that delivered while in left side lying, also using a paired t-test. As noted above, nebuliser delivery rates are not constant, with greater output initially tapering off to low output as the residual volume is approached [22]. To assess whether our strategy of alternating sides during the side lying positioning regimen was successful in balancing the amount of saline delivered in the two side lying positions, the ratio of the amount delivered while on each side was calculated, with a 95% confidence interval (CI). We extrapolated the data to estimate the effect of turning every two minutes, every three minutes, and so on, to identify at what point the amount delivered on each side became unbalanced by greater than 1:1.2.

Results

Flow of participants through the study
Twenty-four participants with Cystic Fibrosis were recruited and all completed the study (see Table 1). These participants had characteristics that were representative of the characteristics of patients attending the adult Cystic Fibrosis Clinic at Royal Prince Alfred Hospital in regards to age and lung function (FEV_1).

Delivery time
The delivery time did not significantly differ between the sitting regimen (mean $18.54 \pm SD$ 3.80 min) and the alternate side lying regimen (17.96 ± 3.53 min), a mean difference of 0.58 min (95% CI -1.40 to 0.24) (see Fig. 1).

Respiratory rate
Respiratory rate did not significantly differ between the sitting regimen (17.9 ± 3.7 breaths / min) and the alternate side lying regimen (17.1 ± 3.8 breaths / min), which was a mean difference of 0.8 breaths / min (95% CI -0.4 to 2.0).

Volume delivered in right and left side lying
There was no significant difference in the volume delivered in right (1.63 ± 0.14 mL) and left (1.60 ± 0.19 mL) side lying, which was a mean difference of 0.06 mL (95% CI -0.07 to 0.19). Based on extrapolation of the data, increasing side lying duration from 1 to 2 min would not significantly unbalance the dose delivered on each side (see Table 2). To limit the discrepancy between the dose delivered in the two side lying positions to less than 20%, the duration in a position could be extended to 2 min but not to 3 min.

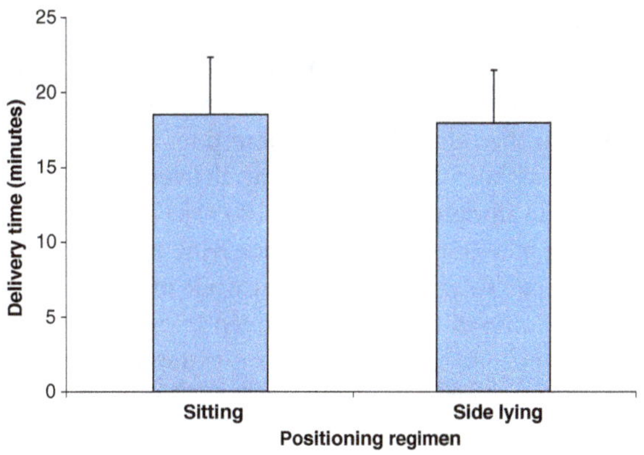

Mean and SD for each positioning regimen
MD: 0.58 min (95% CI -1.40 to 0.24)

Fig. 1 Delivery time in minutes for the two positioning regimens

Correlations
There was no significant correlation between delivery time and any of the following parameters in either position: FEV_1, FVC, FEV_1 % pred, FVC % pred, or participant height (all $R^2 < 0.4$).

Discussion
The delivery times in this study {sitting regimen (mean $18.54 \pm SD$ 3.80 min) and the alternate side lying regimen (17.96 ± 3.53 min)}are consistent with the anticipated delivery rates stated in the product information for an LC Star and observed in previous work in our centre. Clinicians may note that this is a longer duration than is often observed for the delivery of 4 mL of normal saline in clinical practice. We believe that this is because some patients only nebulise until the first sign of intermittent delivery, rather than continuing until the dead volume has been reached. The time burden of inhalation therapy supports the need to find strategies to improve convenience for individuals with cystic fibrosis.

Alternate side lying does not slow the delivery of nebulised medications substantially. The best estimate is that delivery of 3.5 mL of medication is just over half a minute faster, which would make up for the time spent turning, making it time neutral on average. This finding generates implications for further research. The time-

Table 1 Participant characteristics

	Mean ± SD	Range
Age (yr)	30 ± 9	18–47
Height (m)	1.69 ± 0.08	1.52–1.89
Gender (F: M)	13: 11	
FEV_1 (predicted %)	55 ± 34	14–108
FVC (predicted %)	76 ± 22	34–122

Mean, standard deviation (SD) and range of characteristics for the 24 participants who completed the study. Forced expiratory volume in 1 s (FEV_1), Forced vital capacity (FVC)

Table 2 Ratio of the dose delivered in the two side lying positions

Minute	Ratio	95% CI
1	1.05	0.97 to 1.13
2	1.14	1.09 to 1.19
3	1.32	1.24 to 1.40
4	1.41	1.34 to 1.48
5	1.51	1.40 to 1.61

neutral nature of the alternative side lying regimen indicates that it is suitable for further investigation of its effect on medication deposition pattern. This research could be pursued not just in people with Cystic Fibrosis but also in the other diseases where poor upper lobe deposition has been identified during delivery of nebulised therapies in upright sitting [8, 9, 18–21].

Turning between right and left side lying each minute delivered an equivalent dose by weight while in each side lying position. However, turning this frequently is likely to be impractical in clinical practice. Based on extrapolated data, increasing side lying duration from 1 to 2 min would not significantly unbalance the dose delivered on each side, but any further extension of time (≥ 3 min) would cause medication delivery imbalance. It is possible that patients with Cystic Fibrosis would choose to adopt a single side to nebulise for a therapy session and then lie on the other side for the next session. Alternatively, they may spend half the delivery side on one side and turn to the other side for the remainder, but alternate the starting side for subsequent doses. However, investigation of the side lying regimen's effect on the pattern of drug deposition is needed before it can be recommended in clinical practice. Therefore we do not recommend that the results of this study be used to generate any immediate clinical implications about positioning regimens during nebulised delivery of medications for people with Cystic Fibrosis. However, this study will be useful to inform the design of further studies about the effects of body position on nebulised drug delivery. Subsequent future work could then consider the impact of body position in relation to faster delivery systems and other inhaled therapies (dornase alfa, antibiotics) with differing viscosities.

Conclusions

The use of an alternate side lying positioning strategy during nebulised therapies does appear to be suitable, from the perspective of nebuliser delivery time, as an alternative to upright sitting. However while total nebuliser dosage delivered while in each side lying position does appear to be equitable if the side is changed at least every 2 min, further investigation of the side lying regimen's specific effect on the pattern of drug deposition is needed before this position can be recommended.

Abbreviations
CI: Confidence interval; FEV_1: Forced expiratory volume in one second; FVC: Forced vital capacity; Q: Perfusion; SD: Standard deviation; V: Ventilation

Acknowledgements
The authors are grateful to the participants at Royal Prince Alfred Hospital for their involvement.

Funding
This study was supported by the NHMRC CCRE in Respiratory & Sleep Medicine Postgraduate Research Scholarship and the US Cystic Fibrosis Foundation grant BYE04A0.

Authors' contributions
RD and ME wrote the first draft of the protocol. GD and PB reviewed the protocol for clinical issues, tolerability for participants, and relevance of the outcome measures to patients. RD and ME performed the data collection and analysis. All authors contributed to interpretation of the analysed data. All authors read and approved the final manuscript.

Competing interests
The authors declare that they have no competing interests.

Author details
[1]Physiotherapy Department, Royal Prince Alfred Hospital, Sydney, Australia. [2]Sydney Medical School, University of Sydney, Sydney, Australia. [3]Centre for Education & Workforce Development, Sydney Local Health District, Sydney, Australia. [4]Physiotherapy Program, Western Sydney University, Sydney, Australia. [5]Department of Respiratory & Sleep Medicine, Royal Prince Alfred Hospital, Sydney, Australia.

References
1. Ramsey BW, Pepe MS, Quan JM, Otto KL, Montgomery AB, Williams-Warren J, et al. Intermittent Administration of Inhaled Tobramycin in patients with cystic fibrosis. New Engl J Med. 1999;340(1):23–30.
2. Fuchs HJ, Borowitz DS, Christiansen DH, Morris EM, Nash ML, Ramsey BW, et al. Effect of aerosolized recombinant human DNase on exacerbations of respiratory symptoms and on pulmonary function in patients with cystic fibrosis. The Pulmozyme study group. New Engl J Med. 1994;331(10):637–42.
3. Elkins MR, Robinson M, Rose BR, Harbour C, Moriarty CP, Marks GB, et al. A controlled trial of long-term inhaled hypertonic saline in patients with cystic fibrosis. New Engl J Med. 2006;354(3):229–40.
4. Ballmann M, von der Hardt H. Hypertonic saline and recombinant human DNase: a randomised cross-over pilot study in patients with cystic fibrosis. J Cyst Fibros. 2002;1:35–7.
5. Amis T, Jones H, Hughes J. Effect of posture on inter-regional distribution of pulmonary perfusion and VA/Q ratios in man. Respir Physiol. 1984;56(2):169–82.
6. Lannefors L, editor Post-Conference Physiotherapy Workshop. Fifth Australian and New Zealand Cystic Fibrosis Conference; 2003; Melbourne.
7. Laube BL, Links JM, LaFrance ND, Wagner HNJ, Rosenstein BJ. Homogeneity of bronchopulmonary distribution of 99mTc aerosol in normal subjects and in cystic fibrosis patients. Chest. 1989;95(4):822–30.
8. O'Doherty MJ, Thomas SH, Page CJ, Bradbeer C, Nunan TO, Bateman NT. Does inhalation in the supine position increase deposition in the upper part of the lung? Chest. 1990;97:1343–8.
9. Regnis JA, Robinson M, Bailey DL, Cook P, Hooper P, Chan HK, et al. Mucociliary clearance in patients with cystic fibrosis and in normal subjects. Am J Respir Crit Care Med. 1994;150(1):66–71.
10. Porter-Jones G, Francis S, Benfield G. Running a nurse-led nebulizer clinic in a district general hospital. Brit J Nurs. 1999;8(16):1079–84.
11. Barnett M. Drug delivery: nebuliser therapy. J. Community Nurs. 2007;21(6):16.
12. Agostini E, et al. Statics of the Chest Wall. In: Macklem PT, editor. The thorax, part A. New York: Marcel Dekker, Inc; 1985.
13. Hahn-Winslow E. Cardiovascular consequences of bed rest. Heart Lung. 1985;14:236–46.
14. Laube BL, Jashnani R, Dalby RN, Zeitlin PL. Targeting aerosol deposition in patients with cystic fibrosis: effects of alterations in particle size and inspiratory flow rate. Chest. 2000;118(4):1069–76.
15. Robinson M, Hemming AL, Regnis JA, Wong AG, Bailey DL, Bautovich GJ, et al. Effect of increasing doses of hypertonic saline on mucociliary clearance in patients with cystic fibrosis. Thorax. 1997;52(10):900–3.
16. Robinson M, Regnis JA, Bailey DL, King M, Bautovich GJ, Bye PT. Effect of hypertonic saline, amiloride, and cough on mucociliary clearance in patients with cystic fibrosis. Am J Respir Crit Care Med. 1996;153(5):1503–9.

17. Wilson DM, Burniston E, Parkin MA, Smye S, Robinson P, Littlewood J. Improvement of nebulised antibiotic delivery in cystic fibrosis. Arch Dis Child. 1999;80(4):348–52.

18. Baskin M, Abd A, Ilowite J. Regional deposition of aerosolized pentamidine: effects of body position and breathing pattern. Ann Intern Med. 1990;113:677–83.

19. Ilowite J, Baskin MI, Sheetz MS, Abd AG. Delivered dose and regional distribution of aerosolized pentamidine using different delivery systems. Chest. 1991;99:1139–41.

20. Bendstrup KE, Chambers CB, Jensen JI, Newhouse MT. Lung deposition and clearance of inhaled 99mTc-heparin in healthy volunteers. Am J Respir Crit Care Med. 1999;160(5):1653–8.

21. Condos R, Hull FD, Schluger NW, Rom WN, Smaldone GC. Regional deposition of aerosolized interferon-gamma in pulmonary tuberculosis. Chest. 2004;125:2146–55.

22. Elkins M. Comparison of Pari LC-star and LC PLus nebulisers delivering 2.5mg of recombinant human deoxyribonuclease (rhDNase) [abstract]. J Cyst Fibros. 2006;5(Suppl 1):S42.

23. Miller MR, Hankinson JA, Brusasco V, Burgos F, Casaburi R, Coates A, et al. Standardisation of spirometry. Eur Respir J. 2005;26(2):319–38.

9

The relationship between high-dose corticosteroid treatment and mortality in acute respiratory distress syndrome: a retrospective and observational study using a nationwide administrative database in Japan

Takashi Kido[1,2*], Keiji Muramatsu[3], Takeshi Asakawa[4], Hiroki Otsubo[2], Takaaki Ogoshi[1], Keishi Oda[1], Tatsuhiko Kubo[3], Yoshihisa Fujino[3], Shinya Matsuda[3], Toshihiko Mayumi[2], Hiroshi Mukae[1,5] and Kazuhiro Yatera[1]

Abstract

Background: In the 1980s, randomized-controlled trials showed that high-dose corticosteroid treatment did not improve the mortality of acute respiratory distress syndrome (ARDS). However, while the diagnostic criteria for ARDS have since changed, and supportive therapies have been improved, no randomized-controlled trials have revisited this issue since 1987; thus, the effect of high-dose corticosteroid treatment may be different in this era. We evaluated the effect of high-dose corticosteroid treatment in patients with ARDS using a nationwide administrative database in Japan in a retrospective and observational study.

Methods: This study was performed with a large population using the 2012 Japanese nationwide administrative database (diagnostic procedure combination). We evaluated the mortality of ARDS patients receiving or not receiving high-dose corticosteroid treatment within 7 days of hospital admission. We employed propensity score weighting with a Cox proportional hazards model in order to minimize the bias associated with the retrospective collection of data on baseline characteristics and compared the mortality between the high-dose and non-high-dose corticosteroid groups.

Results: Data from 2707 patients were used; 927 patients were treated with high-dose corticosteroid and 1780 patients were treated without high-dose corticosteroid, within 7 days of admission. After adjusting for confounds, mortality rates within 3 months were significantly higher in the high-dose corticosteroid group compared to the non-high-dose corticosteroid group (weighted hazard ratio: 1.59; 95% CI: 1.37-1.84; $P < 0.001$).

Conclusions: Our results suggest that high-dose corticosteroid treatment does not improve the prognosis of patients with ARDS, even in this era. However, this study has limitations owing to its retrospective and observational design.

Keywords: Acute respiratory distress syndrome, Corticosteroid, Inverse probability of treatment weighting method, Nationwide administrative database, Propensity score

* Correspondence: t-kido@med.uoeh-u.ac.jp
[1]Department of Respiratory Medicine, University of Occupational and Environmental Health, 1-1 Iseigaoka, Yahatanishi-ku, Kitakyushu, Japan
[2]Department of Emergency Medicine, University of Occupational and Environmental Health, Kitakyushu, Japan
Full list of author information is available at the end of the article

Background

Acute respiratory distress syndrome (ARDS) is a critical respiratory syndrome. Recent advances in treatment strategies, such as protective mechanical ventilation techniques, have improved the mortality of patients with ARDS, according to many clinical trials [1–4]. However, no pharmacotherapies have yet been shown to be effective in improving the mortality rate; according to systematic reviews, mortalities due to ARDS were as high as 43 and 44% in 2008 and 2009, respectively, [2, 5].

A systemic inflammatory response is closely associated with the development of ARDS. Thus, anti-inflammatory corticosteroid treatment may be a logical choice for ARDS [6–8]. However, according to previous studies and meta-analyses, the efficacy of corticosteroids in ARDS is still controversial; while some reports have shown improvement in the mortality [9–13], others have not [14–16]. Furthermore, although meta-analyses have indicated the poor effectiveness of corticosteroids, they also highlight the difficulties in confirming the role of corticosteroids due to the heterogeneity of ARDS studies [8, 17]. The dosage of corticosteroids for the treatment of ARDS is also controversial. In the 1980s, a few randomized-controlled trials (RCTs) showed that high-dose corticosteroids did not improve mortality, and subsequently, for almost three decades, no RCTs have revisited this topic due to the results of these reports [14, 18]. However, the ARDS diagnostic criteria, supportive methods, and treatments for underlying diseases have changed over the years. In 1994, the American-European Consensus Conference (AECC) resulted in the development of new diagnostic criteria for ARDS [19], which were subsequently modified (Berlin definition [20]). We therefore speculated that the effectiveness of high-dose corticosteroid treatment might be different in the present era. In this retrospective and observational study, we investigated the effectiveness of high-dose corticosteroid treatment using the Japanese nationwide administrative database: the diagnostic procedure combination (DPC). To minimize the bias associated with the retrospective collection of data (i.e. the baseline characteristics in the high-dose and non-high-dose corticosteroid groups), we employed propensity score weighting with a Cox proportional hazards model [21–25].

Methods

Data source

The DPC is a case-mix patient classification system that was introduced by the Japanese government in 2002 and is linked with a lump-sum payment system [26]. It covers approximately 40% of all acute-care hospitalizations in Japan and has been actively utilized for the evaluation of treatments [27–29]. The database contains the following information: disease name, treatment costs, comorbid illnesses at admission and during hospitalization (coded by the *International Classification of Diseases, 10th revision*; ICD-10), patients' age, sex, length of stay, medical procedures, intensive-care unit (ICU) admission, interventional procedures (including mechanical ventilation and hemodialysis), medications, state of consciousness according to the Japan Coma Scale (JCS) on admission, and discharge status (including in-hospital deaths) [26, 29].

Any patient identifiable information was removed from the data. This study was conducted according to guidelines laid down in the Declaration of Helsinki and was approved by Ethics Committee of Medical Research, University of Occupational and Environmental Health, Japan. Informed consent was waived because of the retrospective study design.

Patient selection

Patients who were diagnosed with ARDS, ICD-10 code J80 or pneumonia at admission (and subsequently diagnosed with ARDS as the predominant reason for hospitalization as indicated by the cost during hospitalization) and discharged within 2012 were included. Patients who were discharged and died within 7 days of hospitalization or who did not receive mechanical ventilation were excluded, as we believed that if the duration of administration was too short, the effect of high-dose corticosteroid on ARDS could not be analyzed properly, and the use of mechanical ventilation is necessary for the diagnosis according to the criteria of ARDS [19, 20].

Variables

Patients' sex and age (years), hospital volume (number of patients with ARDS treated in 2012), emergency transport, diagnoses of sepsis, cancer, pneumonia, pancreatitis, lung or abdominal trauma, liver dysfunction (diagnosed as liver failure, hepatitis, or liver cirrhosis) at admission, hemodialysis performed within 7 days of admission, neurological dysfunction (JCS at admission of ≥ 100 indicating coma) [29], shock (use of a vasopressor within 7 days of admission), medication use (insulin, antithrombin III, recombinant human soluble thrombomodulin, heparin, synthetic protease inhibitors, or sivelestat within 7 days from admission), transfusion of platelets and red cells within 7 days of admission, administration of albumin and immunoglobulin within 7 days of admission, mechanical ventilation, and ICU transfer within 7 days of admission were used as variables.

Statistical analyses

The high-dose corticosteroid group was defined as the patients who received treatment with methylprednisolone at doses of > 500 mg/day for > 1 day within 7 days of admission. The definition of high-dose corticosteroid was taken from previous meta-analyses [8], and infusion of 500 mg of methylprednisolone every 12 h for < 72 h is the most common regimen of high-dose corticosteroid therapy in Japan.

The primary outcome was mortality; the secondary endpoints were the duration (in days) for which mechanical ventilation was used and the duration of ICU stay within the 28 days after admission. We employed propensity score weighting with a Cox proportional hazards model, as described previously [8, 25, 29, 30]. The propensity score was calculated using a logistic model with baseline variables that potentially influenced the use of high-dose corticosteroid, including patients' sex and age, hospital volume, sepsis, cancer, pneumonia, pancreatitis, lung and abdominal trauma, liver dysfunction, hemodialysis, neurological dysfunction, shock, use of antithrombin III, recombinant human soluble thrombomodulin, heparin, synthetic protease inhibitors and sivelestat, platelet and red cell transfusions, albumin and immunoglobulin administration, and mechanical ventilation status.

The C-statistic was used to evaluate goodness of fit. To check the balance of the measured covariates, χ^2 or Fisher's exact tests were used for categorical data, and unpaired t-tests or Mann-Whitney U tests were used for continuous variables to evaluate the between-group (high-dose vs. non-high-dose corticosteroid group) differences before and after adjusting for confounders using propensity score weighting. The adjusted Kaplan-Meier curves were depicted, and the adjusted hazard ratio

(HR) and robust 95% confidence interval (CI) were estimated in a Cox regression model [8, 25, 30, 31]. This method was performed using the IBM SPSS 22.0 (Armonk, NY, USA) and STATA/IC 14.0 (StataCorp, College Station, TX, USA) software programs. Differences of $P < 0.05$ were considered statistically significant in all tests.

Results

Among the data of 4982 patients diagnosed with ARDS in the DPC database (as described in the Methods), the data of 706 patients were excluded because the patients were discharged within 7 days of admission. The data of 1569 patients were also excluded because the patients did not receive mechanical ventilation within 7 days of admission. Of the remaining 2707 patients, 927 received high-dose corticosteroid treatment, and 1780 received non-high-dose corticosteroid treatment within 7 days of admission (Fig. 1).

To minimize the bias associated with the retrospective collection of data in the high-dose and non-high-dose corticosteroid groups, we employed propensity score weighting with a Cox proportional hazards model. The C-statistic (area under the receiver operating characteristic curve) of the propensity score was 0.72. Patient baseline characteristics, before and after adjusting for confounders, are shown in Table 1. Before adjustment, the baseline variables of patient age, hospital volume, emergency transport, sepsis, cancer, pneumonia, pancreatitis, lung and abdominal trauma, hemodialysis,

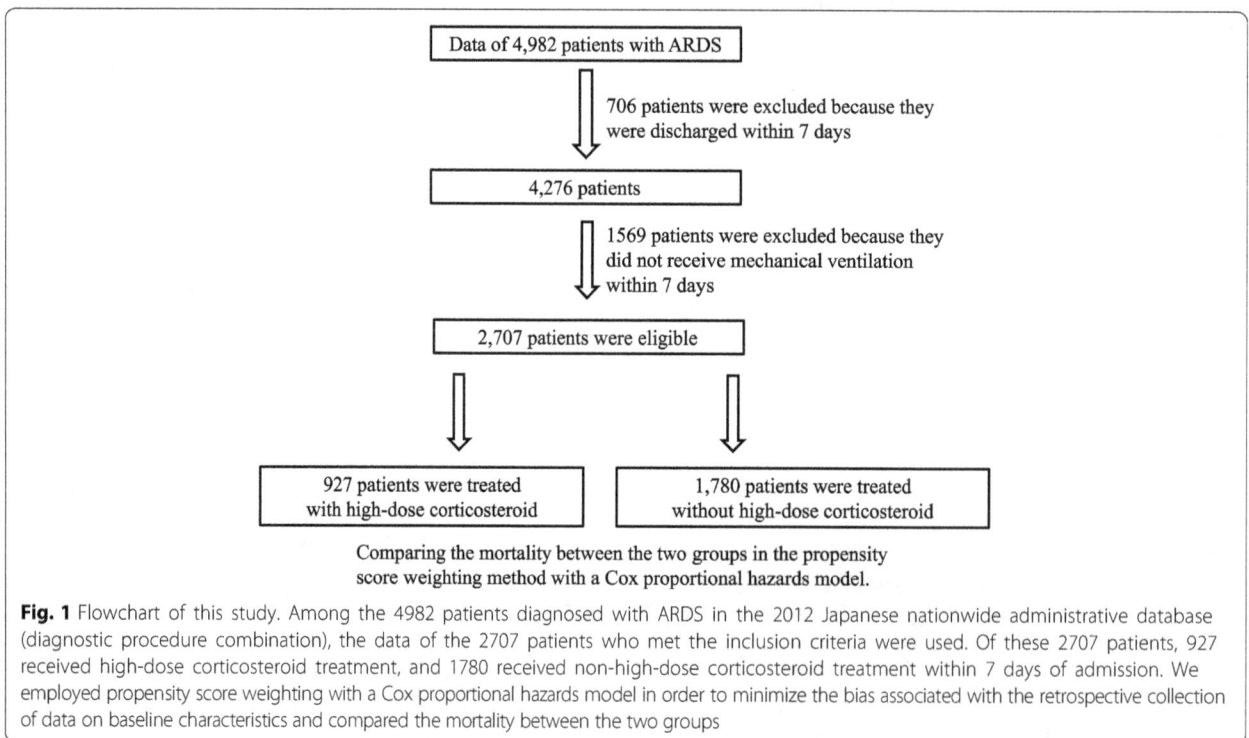

Fig. 1 Flowchart of this study. Among the 4982 patients diagnosed with ARDS in the 2012 Japanese nationwide administrative database (diagnostic procedure combination), the data of the 2707 patients who met the inclusion criteria were used. Of these 2707 patients, 927 received high-dose corticosteroid treatment, and 1780 received non-high-dose corticosteroid treatment within 7 days of admission. We employed propensity score weighting with a Cox proportional hazards model in order to minimize the bias associated with the retrospective collection of data on baseline characteristics and compared the mortality between the two groups

Table 1 Baseline characteristics of the patients treated with or without high-dose corticosteroid before and after group adjustment

	Before adjustment			After adjustment		
	High-dose corticosteroid (n = 927)	Non-high-dose corticosteroid (n = 1780)	p-value	High-dose corticosteroid (n = 927)	Non-high-dose corticosteroid (n = 1780)	p-value
Sex	68.1	66.9	0.562	68.1	67.8	0.771
Age (years)	71.6 ± 0.5	67.9 ± 0.5	< 0.001	67.7 ± 1.0	69.3 ± 0.4	0.05
Hospital volume per year	10.3 ± 0.3	13.0 ± 0.3	< 0.001	12.2 ± 0.6	12.1 ± 0.2	0.806
Sepsis	12.1	22.1	< 0.001	19.9	19	0.373
Cancer	12.3	8.3	0.001	10.2	9.7	0.487
Pneumonia	52.6	62.4	< 0.001	63.6	60.3	< 0.001
Pancreatitis	0.3	1.1	0.041	0.4	0.8	0.001
Lung and abdominal trauma	0.1	0.7	0.043	0.2	0.4	0.009
Liver dysfunction	2.1	2.2	0.88	3.0	2.2	0.392
Hemodialysis	10.1	13.1	0.023	14.0	12.4	0.085
Neurological dysfunction	10.6	22.5	< 0.001	21.8	18.8	0.034
Shock	44.2	48.1	0.053	47.4	47.2	0.848
Insulin	61.7	45.9	< 0.001	48.7	51.2	0.016
Antithrombin III	9.0	15.4	< 0.001	13.9	13.2	0.537
rhTM	10.0	14.1	0.002	14.6	12.9	0.159
Heparin	58.2	61.5	0.094	62.8	61.7	0.088
Protease inhibitors	17.8	19.4	0.318	20.1	19.2	0.331
Sivelestat	72.9	56.2	< 0.001	59.7	61.8	0.074
Platelet transfusion	8.0	10.2	0.045	9.7	9.7	0.938
Red blood cell transfusion	16.4	26.5	< 0.001	24.8	23.3	0.241
Albumin administration	31.7	41.6	< 0.001	38.9	38.5	0.706
Immunoglobulin administration	18.1	23.5	0.001	22.2	21.8	0.637
Intensive-care unit	33.3	32.9	0.852	33.7	33.4	0.754

Data are presented as the % or mean ± standard error, unless otherwise stated. Groups were adjusted using the inverse probability of treatment weighting method
rhTM recombinant human soluble thrombomodulin

neurological dysfunction, shock, insulin, antithrombin III, recombinant human soluble thrombomodulin, platelet and red cell transfusions, albumin administration, immunoglobulin administration, and ICU transfer were significantly different between the high-dose and non-high-dose corticosteroid groups. After adjusting for confounders using the IPTW method, patient baseline characteristics between the two groups were similar across these variables, although pneumonia, pancreatitis, lung and abdominal trauma, neurological dysfunction, and insulin were still significantly different between the groups. In the propensity score-weighted Cox proportional hazards model, the mortality was significantly lower in the high-dose corticosteroid group than in the non-high-dose corticosteroid group (weighted HR: 1.59; 95% CI: 1.37-1.84; $P < 0.001$; Fig. 2). There were no significant differences between the two groups with regard to the duration for which mechanical ventilation was

used (3.5 ± 0.2 versus 3.3 ± 0.1 days, $P = 0.323$), and the duration of the ICU stay (13.2 ± 0.3 versus 12.8 ± 0.2 days, $P = 0.330$) within the 28 days after admission (Table 2).

Discussion
To date, no pharmacotherapies have demonstrated robust, beneficial effects on the outcomes of patients with ARDS. In the present study, we observed the effects of high-dose corticosteroid treatment in a large number of Japanese patients with ARDS using a Japanese nationwide administrative database (DPC) by propensity score weighting with a Cox proportional hazards model. After adjusting for baseline characteristics, the mortality was found to be significantly worse in patients who received high-dose corticosteroid treatment than in those who received non-high-dose corticosteroid treatment.

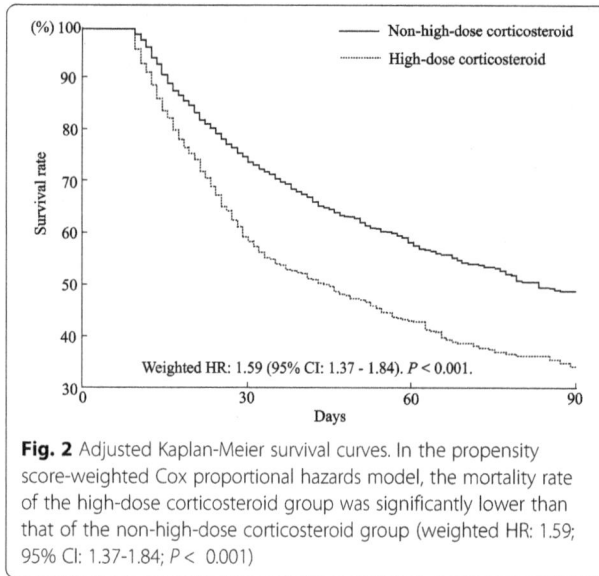

Fig. 2 Adjusted Kaplan-Meier survival curves. In the propensity score-weighted Cox proportional hazards model, the mortality rate of the high-dose corticosteroid group was significantly lower than that of the non-high-dose corticosteroid group (weighted HR: 1.59; 95% CI: 1.37-1.84; $P <$ 0.001)

The efficacy of corticosteroids is still controversial; some reports have shown improvements in mortality [9–13], while others have not [14–16]. Our results showed a higher mortality following high-dose corticosteroid use than without the use of such agents. Previous reports of the high-dose corticosteroid treatment showed that high-dose corticosteroid did not improve the mortality [7, 8, 13, 14, 16, 17, 32]. Among these, Bernard et al. showed that 30 mg/kg of body weight of methylprednisolone every 6 h for 24 h did not improve the mortality of patients with ARDS [14]. Very recently, a meta-analysis showed that high-dose corticosteroid treatment did not improve the mortality [13], and a recent retrospective propensity-matched study also showed that high-dose corticosteroid treatment increased the mortality compared to low-dose corticosteroid treatment [32]. However, the reasons for this are unclear. Weigelt et al. showed that high-dose corticosteroid treatment (30 mg/kg of body weight every 6 h for 48 h) did not prevent patients with respiratory failure from developing ARDS but did increase the risk of infectious complications [33]. In our patients, approximately 60 and 20% of patients were diagnosed with pneumonia

and sepsis, respectively, at the time of admission. Thus, high-dose corticosteroids may have exacerbated infectious diseases or increased infectious complications in the present study, similar to a recent study by Takaki et al. [32]. Other than mortality, we have also shown the effects of corticosteroids on the duration for which mechanical ventilation is used and the duration of the ICU stay within the 28 days after admission, which did not differ between the groups to a statistically significant extent. On the other hand, several studies that have investigated lower dosages of corticosteroids and different protocols have shown the effects on shortening the duration of mechanical ventilation usage and ICU stay [12, 15]. Further studies might be needed to investigate the effects of high-dose corticosteroids on these secondary outcomes.

Propensity score weighting has recently been used in observational studies to assess the effect of treatment after adjusting for baseline characteristics in order to minimize the drawbacks associated with the propensity score matching method, such as sampling biases and loss of sample numbers. ARDS is relatively rare and clinically severe; therefore, it may be not easy to perform new and large RCTs, especially for the reevaluation of clinically used medications that have the potential to be clinically effective in different scenarios from previous studies. Even in retrospective studies, we speculate that propensity score weighting with a Cox proportional hazards model and a large subject population is suitable for evaluating the clinical effect of certain medications, such as high-dose corticosteroid, in patients with ARDS.

There are several limitations associated with this study, similar to previous studies using the DPC database [27–29, 34]. First, this study was observational and retrospective; however, our application of propensity score weighting with a Cox proportional hazards model reduced the effects of this limitation. Second, even after adjustment, there were still significant differences in the characteristics of the high-dose and non-high-dose corticosteroid groups, such as in the rates of pneumonia, pancreatitis, lung and abdominal trauma, neurological dysfunction and insulin. However, after adjusting for confounders, the differences between the two groups

Table 2 Secondary endpoints of the patients treated with or without high-dose corticosteroids before and after group adjustment.

	Before adjustment			After adjustment		
	High-dose corticosteroid (n = 927)	Non-high-dose corticosteroid (n = 1780)	p-value	High-dose corticosteroid (n = 927)	Non-high-dose corticosteroid (n = 1780)	p-value
Duration of mechanical ventilation use within 28 days (days)	13.3 ± 0.2	12.9 ± 0.2	0.108	13.2 ± 0.3	12.8 ± 0.2	0.330
Duration of intensive-care unit stay within 28 days (days)	3.4 ± 0.2	3.3 ± 0.1	0.863	3.5 ± 0.2	3.3 ± 0.1	0.323

Data are presented as the mean ± standard error. Groups were adjusted using the inverse probability of treatment weighting method were small. For example, the frequency of neurological dysfunction in the high-dose corticosteroid and non-high-dose corticosteroid groups were 10.6% versus 22.5%, respectively, before adjustment, and 21.8% versus 18.8% after adjustment. While this remains one of the limitations of the present study, we consider these differences to be relatively small. Third, we were unable to include several clinical data, such as the peripheral blood laboratory findings, radiological findings, physiological data, including vital signs, and mechanical ventilation settings, which could also influence the mortality in patients with ARDS. Fourth, the ARDS diagnostic criteria have changed over the years [19, 20], so it was unclear which criteria had been used to diagnose ARDS in each patient in this retrospective study.

Despite these limitations, the major advantages of this study were the inclusion of a large number of patients and evaluation of the effect of high-dose corticosteroid treatment in this era. To our knowledge, this is the largest study of high-dose corticosteroid treatment for ARDS, even compared to previous meta-analyses [7, 8, 13, 17].

Conclusions

We observed a higher mortality with the administration of high-dose corticosteroids within 7 days of hospital admission in patients with ARDS than without the administration of such agents. We used a nationwide administrative database, making this the largest study to observe high-dose corticosteroid treatment for ARDS, to our knowledge. However, this study has some limitations owing to its retrospective and observational design.

Abbreviations
AECC: American-European Consensus Conference; ARDS: Acute respiratory distress syndrome; CI: Confidence interval; DPC: Diagnostic procedure combination; HR: Hazard ratio; ICD-10: International Classification of Diseases, 10th revision; ICU: Intensive-care unit; IPTW: Inverse probability of treatment weighting; JCS: Japan Coma Scale; RCT: Randomized controlled trial

Acknowledgements
Not applicable.

Funding
This research was partially supported by the Practical Research Project for Rare Intractable Diseases from the Japan Agency for Medical Research and Development (AMED), and a grant from the Ministry of Health, Labour, and Welfare of Japan, which was awarded to the study group for Diffuse Pulmonary Disorders, Scientific Research/Research on Intractable Diseases.

Authors' contributions
TK had full access to all study data and takes responsibility for the integrity of the data and accuracy of the data analysis. KM, TA, TK, YF, and SM contributed to the study design, and data collection, analysis, and interpretation. HO, TO, KO, TM, HM, and KY contributed to the study design and drafting the important intellectual content of the manuscript. All authors read and approved the final manuscript.

Competing interests
The authors declare that they have no competing interests.

Author details
[1]Department of Respiratory Medicine, University of Occupational and Environmental Health, 1-1 Iseigaoka, Yahatanishi-ku, Kitakyushu, Japan. [2]Department of Emergency Medicine, University of Occupational and Environmental Health, Kitakyushu, Japan. [3]Department of Preventive Medicine and Community Health, University of Occupational and Environmental Health, Kitakyushu, Japan. [4]Department of Information Systems Center, University of Occupational and Environmental Health, Kitakyushu, Japan. [5]Second Department of Internal Medicine, Nagasaki University Hospital, Nagasaki, Japan.

References
1. The Acute Respiratory Distress Syndrome Network. Ventilation with lower tidal volumes as compared with traditional tidal volumes for acute lung injury and the acute respiratory distress syndrome. N Engl J Med. 2000; 342(18):1301–8.
2. Zambon M, Vincent JL. Mortality rates for patients with acute lung injury/ ARDS have decreased over time. Chest. 2008;133(5):1120–7.
3. Briel M, Meade M, Mercat A, Brower RG, Talmor D, Walter SD, Slutsky AS, Pullenayegum E, Zhou Q, Cook D, et al. Higher vs lower positive end-expiratory pressure in patients with acute lung injury and acute respiratory distress syndrome: systematic review and meta-analysis. JAMA. 2010;303(9):865–73.
4. Guerin C, Reignier J, Richard JC, Beuret P, Gacouin A, Boulain T, Mercier E, Badet M, Mercat A, Baudin O, et al. Prone positioning in severe acute respiratory distress syndrome. N Engl J Med. 2013;368(23):2159–68.
5. Phua J, Badia JR, Adhikari NK, Friedrich JO, Fowler RA, Singh JM, Scales DC, Stather DR, Li A, Jones A, et al. Has mortality from acute respiratory distress syndrome decreased over time?: a systematic review. Am J Respir Crit Care Med. 2009;179(3):220–7.
6. Ware LB, Matthay MA. The acute respiratory distress syndrome. N Engl J Med. 2000;342(18):1334–49.
7. Peter JV, John P, Graham PL, Moran JL, George IA, Bersten A. Corticosteroids in the prevention and treatment of acute respiratory distress syndrome (ARDS) in adults: meta-analysis. BMJ. 2008;336(7651):1006–9.
8. Horita N, Hashimoto S, Miyazawa N, Fujita H, Kojima R, Inoue M, Ueda A, Ishigatsubo Y, Kaneko T. Impact of corticosteroids on mortality in patients with acute respiratory distress syndrome: a systematic review and meta-analysis. Intern Med. 2015;54(14):1473–9.
9. Meduri GU, Headley AS, Golden E, Carson SJ, Umberger RA, Kelso T, Tolley EA. Effect of prolonged methylprednisolone therapy in unresolving acute respiratory distress syndrome: a randomized controlled trial. JAMA. 1998; 280(2):159–65.
10. Keel JB, Hauser M, Stocker R, Baumann PC, Speich R. Established acute respiratory distress syndrome: benefit of corticosteroid rescue therapy. Respiration. 1998;65(4):258–64.
11. Lee HS, Lee JM, Kim MS, Kim HY, Hwangbo B, Zo JI. Low-dose steroid therapy at an early phase of postoperative acute respiratory distress syndrome. Ann Thorac Surg. 2005;79(2):405–10.
12. Meduri GU, Golden E, Freire AX, Taylor E, Zaman M, Carson SJ, Gibson M, Umberger R. Methylprednisolone infusion in early severe ARDS: results of a randomized controlled trial. Chest. 2007;131(4):954–63.
13. Yang ZG, Lei XL, Li XL. Early application of low-dose glucocorticoid improves acute respiratory distress syndrome: a meta-analysis of randomized controlled trials. Exp Ther Med. 2017;13(4):1215–24.
14. Bernard GR, Luce JM, Sprung CL, Rinaldo JE, Tate RM, Sibbald WJ, Kariman K, Higgins S, Bradley R, Metz CA, et al. High-dose corticosteroids in patients with the adult respiratory distress syndrome. N Engl J Med. 1987;317(25):1565–70.

15. Steinberg KP, Hudson LD, Goodman RB, Hough CL, Lanken PN, Hyzy R, Thompson BT, Ancukiewicz M. Efficacy and safety of corticosteroids for persistent acute respiratory distress syndrome. N Engl J Med. 2006;354(16):1671–84.

16. Zhang Z, Chen L, Ni H. The effectiveness of corticosteroids on mortality in patients with acute respiratory distress syndrome or acute lung injury: a secondary analysis. Sci Rep. 2015;5:17654.

17. Agarwal R, Nath A, Aggarwal AN, Gupta D. Do glucocorticoids decrease mortality in acute respiratory distress syndrome? A meta-analysis. Respirology. 2007;12(4):585–90.

18. Laggner AN, Lenz K, Base W, Druml W, Schneeweiss B, Grimm G, Sommer G, Kleinberger G. Effect of high-dose prednisolone on lung fluid in patients with non-cardiogenic lung edema. Wien Klin Wochenschr. 1987;99(7):245–9.

19. Bernard GR, Artigas A, Brigham KL, Carlet J, Falke K, Hudson L, Lamy M, Legall JR, Morris A, Spragg R. The American-European consensus conference on ARDS. Definitions, mechanisms, relevant outcomes, and clinical trial coordination. Am J Respir Crit Care Med. 1994;149(3 Pt 1):818–24.

20. Ranieri VM, Rubenfeld GD, Thompson BT, Ferguson ND, Caldwell E, Fan E, Camporota L, Slutsky AS. Acute respiratory distress syndrome: the Berlin definition. JAMA. 2012;307(23):2526–33.

21. Robins JM, Hernan MA, Brumback B. Marginal structural models and causal inference in epidemiology. Epidemiology. 2000;11(5):550–60.

22. Kurita T, Yasuda S, Oba K, Odani T, Kono M, Otomo K, Fujieda Y, Oku K, Bohgaki T, Amengual O, et al. The efficacy of tacrolimus in patients with interstitial lung diseases complicated with polymyositis or dermatomyositis. Rheumatology (Oxford). 2015;54(8):1536.

23. Lunceford JK, Davidian M. Stratification and weighting via the propensity score in estimation of causal treatment effects: a comparative study. Stat Med. 2004;23(19):2937–60.

24. Morshed S, Knops S, Jurkovich GJ, Wang J, MacKenzie E, Rivara FP. The impact of trauma-center care on mortality and function following pelvic ring and acetabular injuries. J Bone Joint Surg Am. 2015;97(4):265–72.

25. Kido T, Muramatsu K, Yatera K, Asakawa T, Otsubo H, Kubo T, Fujino Y, Matsuda S, Mayumi T, Mukae H. Efficacy of early sivelestat administration on acute lung injury and acute respiratory distress syndrome. Respirology (Carlton, Vic). 2017;22(4):708–13.

26. Matsuda S, Ishikawa KB, Kuwabara K, Fujimori K, Fushimi K, Hashimoto H. Development and use of the Japanese case-mix system. Eur Secur. 2008; 14(3):25–30.

27. Yasunaga H, Hashimoto H, Horiguchi H, Miyata H, Matsuda S. Variation in cancer surgical outcomes associated with physician and nurse staffing: a retrospective observational study using the Japanese diagnosis procedure combination database. BMC Health Serv Res. 2012;12:129.

28. Chikuda H, Yasunaga H, Takeshita K, Horiguchi H, Kawaguchi H, Ohe K, Fushimi K, Tanaka S. Mortality and morbidity after high-dose methylprednisolone treatment in patients with acute cervical spinal cord injury: a propensity-matched analysis using a nationwide administrative database. Emerg Med J. 2014;31(3):201–6.

29. Iwagami M, Yasunaga H, Doi K, Horiguchi H, Fushimi K, Matsubara T, Yahagi N, Noiri E. Postoperative polymyxin B hemoperfusion and mortality in patients with abdominal septic shock: a propensity-matched analysis. Crit Care Med. 2014;42(5):1187–93.

30. Guo S, Fraser MW. Propensity score analysis: statistical methods and applications. 2nd ed. Thousand Oaks: Sage; 2015.

31. Cole SR, Hernan MA. Adjusted survival curves with inverse probability weights. Comput Methods Prog Biomed. 2004;75(1):45–9.

32. Takaki M, Ichikado K, Kawamura K, Gushima Y, Suga M. The negative effect of initial high-dose methylprednisolone and tapering regimen for acute respiratory distress syndrome: a retrospective propensity matched cohort study. Critical Care (London, England). 2017;21(1):135.

33. Weigelt JA, Norcross JF, Borman KR, Snyder WH 3rd. Early steroid therapy for respiratory failure. Arch Surg. 1985;120(5):536–40.

34. Hamada T, Yasunaga H, Nakai Y, Isayama H, Horiguchi H, Matsuda S, Fushimi K, Koike K. Continuous regional arterial infusion for acute pancreatitis: a propensity score analysis using a nationwide administrative database. Critical Care (London, England). 2013;17(5):R214.

Eplerenone attenuates pathological pulmonary vascular rather than right ventricular remodeling in pulmonary arterial hypertension

Mario Boehm[1], Nadine Arnold[2], Adam Braithwaite[2], Josephine Pickworth[2], Changwu Lu[1], Tatyana Novoyatleva[1], David G. Kiely[3], Friedrich Grimminger[1], Hossein A. Ghofrani[1], Norbert Weissmann[1], Werner Seeger[1], Allan Lawrie[2], Ralph T. Schermuly[1]* and Baktybek Kojonazarov[1]

Abstract

Background: Aldosterone is a mineralocorticoid hormone critically involved in arterial blood pressure regulation. Although pharmacological aldosterone antagonism reduces mortality and morbidity among patients with severe left-sided heart failure, the contribution of aldosterone to the pathobiology of pulmonary arterial hypertension (PAH) and right ventricular (RV) heart failure is not fully understood.

Methods: The effects of Eplerenone (0.1% Inspra® mixed in chow) on pulmonary vascular and RV remodeling were evaluated in mice with pulmonary hypertension (PH) caused by Sugen5416 injection with concomitant chronic hypoxia (SuHx) and in a second animal model with established RV dysfunction independent from lung remodeling through surgical pulmonary artery banding.

Results: Preventive Eplerenone administration attenuated the development of PH and pathological remodeling of pulmonary arterioles. Therapeutic aldosterone antagonism – starting when RV dysfunction was established - normalized mineralocorticoid receptor gene expression in the right ventricle without direct effects on either RV structure (Cardiomyocyte hypertrophy, Fibrosis) or function (assessed by non-invasive echocardiography along with intra-cardiac pressure volume measurements), but significantly lowered systemic blood pressure.

Conclusions: Our data indicate that aldosterone antagonism with Eplerenone attenuates pulmonary vascular rather than RV remodeling in PAH.

Keywords: PAH, Eplerenone, Right ventricle

Background

Pulmonary arterial hypertension (PAH) is a devastating disorder characterized by aberrant remodeling of pulmonary arteries that results in sustained pulmonary vasoconstriction, progressively increases pulmonary vascular resistance (PVR) and right ventricular (RV) afterload [1–3]. The persistent increase in afterload maintains high shear stress on the RV myocardium and leads to structural RV remodeling. Current interventions approved for PAH therapy consist of vasodilators that relieve the pulmonary vasoconstrictive component of the disease while the underlying pathological lung and heart remodeling progresses. Therefore, future treatment strategies need to go beyond vasodilation by targeting maladaptive remodeling processes in both, pulmonary vasculature and RV myocardium.

An accumulating body of evidence suggests that dysregulation of the Renin-Angiotensin-Aldosterone-System (RAAS) contributes to the pathogenesis of PAH [4–7]. In particular, the potential contribution of aldosterone – a mineralocorticoid hormone critically involved in

* Correspondence: Ralph.Schermuly@innere.med.uni-giessen.de
[1]Universities of Giessen and Marburg Lung Center (UGMLC), Excellence Cluster Cardio-Pulmonary System (ECCPS), Member of the German Center for Lung Research (DZL), Aulweg 130, 35392, Giessen, Germany

systemic blood pressure regulation – to PAH pathogenesis has recently drawn attention. Elevated levels of circulating aldosterone were found in PH patients and correlate with key cardio-pulmonary indices [8]. In line, PH rat models demonstrate increased plasma and lung tissue aldosterone concentrations that correlate with cardio-pulmonary hemodynamics as well as pulmonary vascular remodeling [8, 9] pointing towards a causative role for aldosterone signaling in mediating adverse lung remodeling as seen in PAH development. Pharmacological aldosterone antagonism by the FDA approved drugs Spironolactone or Eplerenone, respectively, directly reduced the pathologic pulmonary vascular remodeling in PAH animal models [10].

On a cellular level, it was demonstrated that aldosterone induces oxidative stress, endothelial dysfunction, inflammation and fibrosis within the pulmonary vasculature. In pulmonary artery smooth muscle cells (PASMCs), aldosterone promotes proliferation, viability and apoptosis resistance [10, 11]. In pulmonary artery endothelial cells (PAECs), aldosterone activates oxidant stress signaling pathways that decrease the bioavailability of the vasodilator nitric oxide, increases inflammation, promotes fibrosis and increases cell proliferation and migration [9, 12, 13]. In PAH, both PASMCs and PAECs are considered key cell types, whose aberrant activation is thought to drive maladaptive remodeling of the pulmonary vasculature.

Aldosterone activation is also associated with decreased diuresis which elevates blood volume and thereby blood pressure. Thus, by closely monitoring electrolytes (sodium/fluid retention and potassium/magnesium wasting), diuretics in combination with aldosterone antagonists effectively reduce blood volume, thereby cardiac load and thus decrease RV wall stress in patients with severe left heart failure [14]. Retrospectively, Spironolactone and Eplerenone therapy have shown direct beneficial effects on the RV in patients with PAH [15]. However, in an experimental rat model of RV failure independent from afterload, RAAS inhibition with Losartan (angiotensin II receptor blocker) and Eplerenone had no direct effects on either RV structure or function [16].

Eplerenone itself is a small molecule suggested to selectively compete with aldosterone for mineralocorticoid receptor binding and as compared with the nonselective mineralocorticoid receptor antagonist Spironolactone has lower affinity for progesterone and androgen receptor binding which is associated with drug-induced gynecomastia, breast pain and impotence [17]. Eplerenone is clinically FDA approved for the treatment of left-sided heart failure and systemic hypertension [18].

Taken together, clinical and experimental data suggest that increased circulating aldosterone levels contribute to the pathogenesis of PAH. To test this hypothesis, we investigated whether pharmacological aldosterone antagonism with Eplerenone attenuates pathological remodeling of the lung and the RV in experimental mouse models. In order to differentiate afterload-dependent from direct myocardial effects, we utilized the SuHx and a pulmonary artery banding (PAB) mouse model.

Methods

All experiments were performed according to the institutional guidelines that comply with national and international regulations (EU directive 2010/63). The local authorities for animal research approved the study protocol (Regierungspräsidium Giessen, Germany, Gi 32/2013 and The UK Home Office under PPL 40/3517).

Animal models

Adult male C57BL/6 J mice were purchased from Charles River Laboratories (Sulzfeld, Germany and United Kingdom) and housed under controlled conditions with free access to rodent chow and tap water.

Mice were kept for three weeks under normobaric hypoxia ($\sim$ 10% O_2) and were concomitantly given an injection of sugen5416 (20 mg/kg dissolved in MCC, Tocris) once per week subcutaneously. All animals were randomly assigned for either placebo (standard diet, hereafter referred to as SuHx) or Eplerenone therapy (hereafter referred to as Epl) starting on day one for additional three weeks. Effective dosing was estimated according to prior reports demonstrating efficacy of 200 mg/kg Eplerenone administration [19, 20], wherefore 50 mg Inspra® tablets were homogenized and mixed into standard rodent chow (Altromin, Lage, Germany) to receive a final concentration of 0.1% Eplerenone mixed in chow. Based on prior uptake data, this concentration was estimated to result in $\sim$ 200 mg/kg/d Eplerenone. Control animals were kept under normobaric conditions without sugen5416 injections and were fed standard diet for the entire study period (hereafter referred to as cntrl). Maintained pressure overload was surgically induced by pulmonary artery banding (PAB) as described before [21–23]. PAB-challenged animals were randomly assigned for either placebo (hereafter referred to as PAB) or Eplerenone (0.1% mixed in chow, hereafter referred to as Epl) therapy starting one week after disease commencement for additional two weeks. Control animals underwent the identical surgical procedure without pulmonary artery clipping and were fed control diet for the entire study period (hereafter referred to as sham).

Heart function assessment

All animals underwent non-invasive transthoracic imaging under continuous isoflurane anesthesia (1.5–2%)

to measure RV cardiac output (CO), RV internal diameter (RVID), tricuspid annular plane systolic excursion (TAPSE) and myocardial performance index (MPI) in a blinded manner as described before [24, 25]. Total pulmonary resistance index (TPRi) was calculated as RV systolic pressure divided by echocardiographically determined CI. Subsequently, intra-cardiac catheterization was performed in all animals as previously reported [21, 26]. Terminally, all mice were euthanized by exsanguination and the RVs dissected for tissue weight measurements.

Histomorphology

Formalin fixed tissue samples were dehydrated, paraffin embedded, sectioned (5 μm) and stained for Alcian Blue Elastic van Gieson (ABVEG), alpha smooth muscle actin (αSMA) and von Willebrand factor (vWF) or picrosirius red and wheat germ agglutinin (WGA) as described before [22, 26, 27].

Gene expression analysis

Total mRNA was extracted from frozen mouse RV tissues, subsequently transcribed into cDNA and qPCR was performed. Intron-spanning mouse-specific primers for mineralocorticoid receptor (5'-CCGAGATCGTG TATGCAGGC-3' and 5'-CGCACGAACTGAAGGCT GAT-3'), Collagen 1A1 (Col1A1; 5'-CCGGCTCCTGC TCCTCTTAG-3' and 5'-CCTCGGGTTTCCACGTC TCA-3'), Collagen 3A1 (Col3A1; 5'-CCAGGAGCCA GTGGCCATAA-3' and 5'-GGGGCACCAGGAGAAC CATT-3') and porphobilinogen deaminase (PBGD; 5'-GGGAA CCAGCTCTCTGAGGA-3' and 5'-GAATTCC TGCAGCTCATCCA-3') were designed using sequence information from the NCBI database and were purchased from Metabion (Martinsried, Germany). Target gene Ct values were normalized to the housekeeping gene PBGD and expression was calculated as percentage of sham controls.

Data analysis

All data are presented as mean ± SD analyzed with one-way ANOVA followed by Newman-Keuls multiple comparison post-hoc test. Differences were considered statistically significant for $p < 0.05$.

Results

Eplerenone attenuates SuHx-induced PH and pulmonary vascular remodeling

Oral Eplerenone administration (0.1% mixed in chow) for three consecutive weeks significantly attenuated the development of PH in the SuHx mouse model (Sugen-5416 injection followed by chronic hypoxia) demonstrated by reduced RV hypertrophy (1.2 ± 0.1 vs. 1.4 ± 0.1, $p < 0.05$) (RV/BW, Fig. 1a) and reduced RV systolic

pressure (33.8 ± 4.3 vs. 39.5 ± 4.0 mmHg, $p < 0.05$) (RVSP, Fig. 1b) as compared with controls. Total pulmonary resistance index tended to decrease upon Eplerenone administration (48.6 ± 13.0 vs. 51.4 ± 7.2 mmHg·ml^{-1}·min^{-1}·g^{-1}, $p > 0.05$) (TPRi, Fig. 1c) without affecting systemic blood pressure (82.8 ± 10.0 vs. 79.7 ± 8.8 mmHg, $p > 0.05$) (systemic BP, Fig. 1d) indicating a selective direct effect on the diseased pulmonary circulation. Reduced remodeling of pulmonary arteries was demonstrated by histomorphology (Fig. 1e) and quantified as medial hypertrophy (0.47 ± 0.08 vs. 0.64 ± 0.05, $p < 0.05$) (media/cross sectional vessel area, Fig. 1f) and percentage of muscularized pulmonary arterioles (Fig. 1g).

Eplerenone therapy reduces systemic blood pressure upon chronic RV pressure overload without direct effects on RV structure or function

Therapeutic efficacy of Eplerenone – starting after one week when animals in both PAB groups showed comparable signs of established RV dysfunction (data not shown) – normalized mineralocorticoid receptor gene expression in the RV (92 ± 12% vs. 118 ± 8%, $p < 0.05$) (Fig. 2a) without affecting RV hypertrophy (1.3 ± 0.4 vs. 1.1 ± 0.2, $p > 0.05$) (RV/BW, Fig. 2b), RV systolic blood pressure (54.0 ± 13.7 vs. 55.7 ± 8.7 mmHg, $p > 0.05$) (RVSP, Fig. 2c) or cardiac output (9.8 ± 2.2 vs. 10.3 ± 1.8 ml·min^{-1}, $p > 0.05$) (Fig. 2d) as compared with placebo controls, demonstrating no direct cardioprotective effects of Eplerenone on the RV. Importantly, systemic blood pressure dropped down (52.0 ± 11.3 vs. 69.8 ± 6.5 mmHg, $p < 0.05$) (Fig. 2e) indicating effective dosing and a significant systemic impact of Eplerenone on the stressed heart. Pressure-volume analysis (Fig. 2f) demonstrated unchanged contractility by RV end-systolic elastance (1.04 ± 0.08 vs. 1.02 ± 0.11 mmHg·μl^{-1}, $p > 0.05$) (Ees, Fig. 2g). In addition, echocardiography revealed no change in RV dilatation (unchanged RV internal diameter (2.4 ± 0.1 vs. 2.1 ± 0.3 mm, $p > 0.05$) (RVID, Fig. 2h)) and tricuspid annular plane systolic excursion (1.0 ± 0.1 vs. 1.0 ± 0.1 mm, $p > 0.05$) (TAPSE, Fig. 2i) upon Eplerenone therapy as compared with placebo controls.

Furthermore, chronic pressure overload-induced structural RV adaptation remained unaltered by Eplerenone therapy as total RV collagen content (8.6 ± 1.4 vs. 8.5 ± 0.4%, $p > 0.05$) (Fig. 3a), Col1A1 (147 ± 7 vs. 159 ± 14%, $p > 0.05$) (Fig. 3b) and Col3A1 (196 ± 25 vs. 227 ± 23%, $p > 0.05$) (Fig. 3c) gene expression were not affected. Also, pharmacological aldosterone antagonism had no effect on cardiomyocyte hypertrophy (23.9 ± 0.6 vs. 20.9 ± 0.8 μm, $p > 0.05$) (CM diameter, Fig. 3d) and heart failure marker gene expression (221 ± 6 vs. 220 ± 16%, $p > 0.05$ for ANP, Fig. 3e and 167 ± 10 vs. 154 ± 4%, $p > 0.05$ for BNP, Fig. 3f).

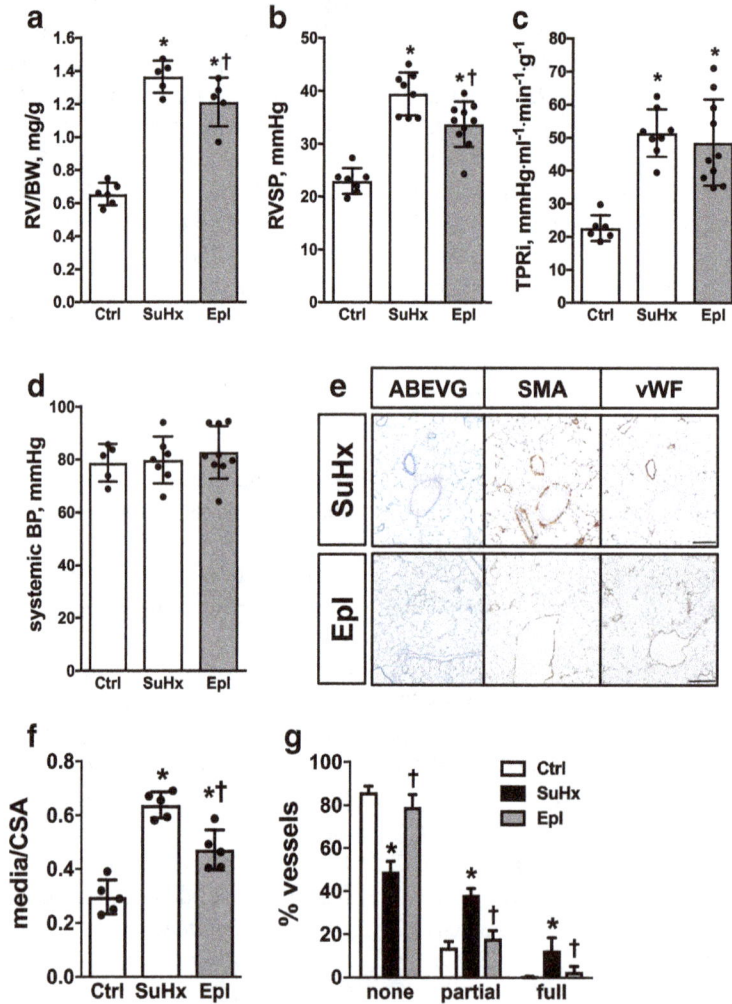

Fig. 1 Eplerenone attenuates SuHx-induced PH and pulmonary vascular remodeling. Preventive Eplerenone administration (Inspra®, 0.1% mixed in chow) to mice attenuated the development of SuHx-induced RV hypertrophy (RV/BW, mg/g; **a**) and increased RV systolic pressure (RVSP, mmHg; **b**). Total pulmonary resistance index (TPRi, $ml^{-1} \cdot min^{-1} \cdot g^{-1}$; **c**) and systemic blood pressure (systemic BP, mmHg; **d**) remained unaltered by Eplerenone administration. Representative lung sections stained for Alcian Blue Elastic van Gieson (ABEVG), smooth muscle actin (SMA) and von Willebrand factor (vWF) are shown in **e**. Medial hypertrophy is presented as ratio of media to cross sectional area [CSA] (**f**). Remodeling of pulmonary blood vessels is demonstrated by muscularization (percentage of vessels). $n = 5–10$ mice per group; *: $p < 0.05$ vs. cntrl; †: $p < 0.05$ vs. SuHx

Discussion

The current study demonstrates that oral administration of an aldosterone receptor antagonist attenuates maladaptive remodeling of the pulmonary vasculature without direct effects on RV structure and function in rodent models. Eplerenone decreased SuHx-induced remodeling of small pulmonary arteries without affecting the systemic circulation. In a PAB mouse model, Eplerenone induced systemic hypotension in animals with established RV dysfunction - most likely due to cardiac unloading - while RV structure and function remained unaffected, demonstrating no direct cardioprotective effects independent from afterload. Taken together, these data suggest that aldosterone plays a pathological role in maladaptive remodeling of the pulmonary vasculature

rather than the RV. The therapeutic effect of Eplerenone on the diseased pulmonary circulation, however, remains to be characterized (including the effects of Eplerenone on PASMCs and PAECs).

The development of PH in mice following vascular endothelial growth factor receptor (VEGFR) blockade and chronic hypoxia (SuHx model) was effectively attenuated by concomitant treatment with the oral available aldosterone antagonist Eplerenone (Inspra®, 0.1% mixed in standard chow) through reduced remodeling of small pulmonary arteries. Eplerenone was oral available and efficacious by decreasing RV systolic pressure and hypertrophy without affecting the systemic circulation - showing a direct effect on the pulmonary circulation. We estimated 0.1% Eplerenone mixed in chow to result in ~

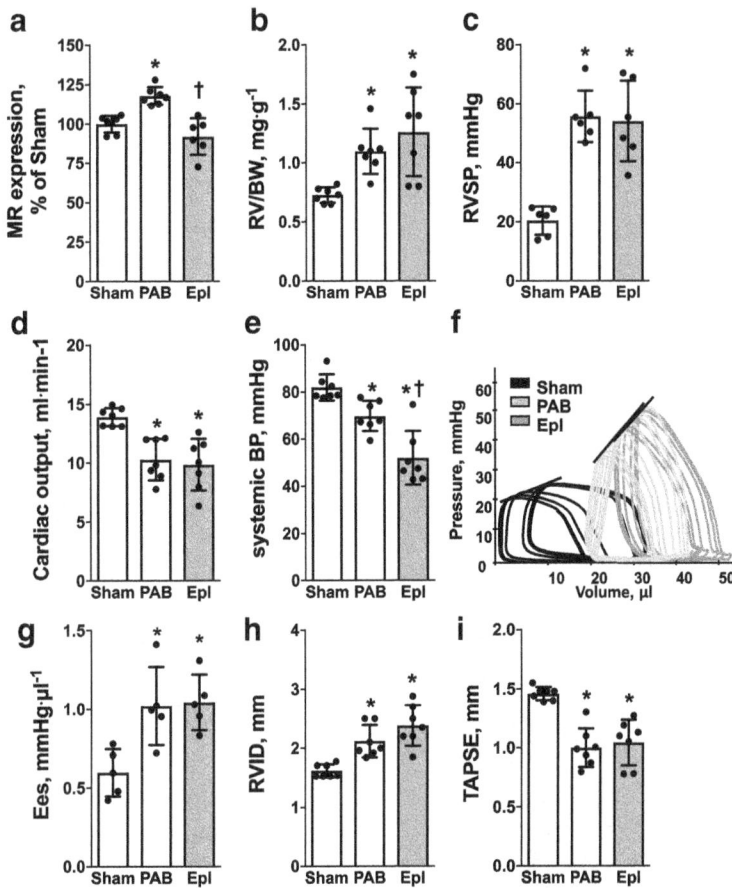

Fig. 2 Eplerenone reduces systemic blood pressure without direct effects on RV structure and function upon PAB. Eplerenone therapy normalizes RV mineralocorticoid receptor gene expression (MR expression, percentage of sham; **a** without affecting RV hypertrophy (RV/BW, mg/g; **b** RV systolic pressure (RVSP, mmHg; **c** or cardiac output (ml·min^{-1}, **d** while systemic blood pressure (systemic BP, mmHg; **e** dropped down significantly. Representative pressure-volume loops with lined end-systolic elastances (**f**). Quantification of end-systolic elastance (Ees, mmHg·µl; **g**), echocardiography-derived RV internal diameter (RVID, mm; **h**) and Tricuspid annular plane systolic excursion (TAPSE, mm; **i**) reveal no difference between PAB and Eplerenone treated mice. $n = 5–7$ mice per group; *: $p < 0.05$ vs. cntrl; †: $p < 0.05$ vs. PAB

200 mg/kg/d effective dosing, confirmed by PH attenuation in the SuHx model, while an exact free plasma concentration for Eplerenone is not available, may vary between animals and is a clear limitation to this study. Though, a pathological role for aldosterone in maladaptive remodeling of pulmonary arteries has previously been described in PH rat models. In monocrotaline-induced PH, pharmacological aldosterone antagonism with either Spironolactone or Eplerenone decreased vascular hyperplasia and vessel thickening [10, 11]. Also, aldosterone antagonism has been shown to reduce neointimal hyperplasia in rats with SuHx-induced PH [10]. These data are consistent with the decreased pulmonary vascular remodeling observed in the current study, which show that preventive Eplerenone administration reduced vascular thickening. On a cellular level, previous studies have demonstrated that aldosterone activates an Akt/mTOR/Raptor axis that promotes pulmonary artery smooth muscle cell (PASMC)

proliferation, cell migration, viability and apoptosis resistance [10, 11]. It was shown that chronic hypoxia itself selectively induces aldosterone synthesis autonomously in pulmonary artery endothelial cells (PAECs) by upregulation of the steroidogenic acute regulator protein (StAR). Elevated aldosterone levels were linked to vasoconstriction by PAEC-derived endothelin 1 release, reactive oxidant signaling, reduced nitric oxide bioavailability and fibrosis [9, 12, 13]. In PAH, both PASMCs and PAECs are considered key cell types whose aberrant activation leads to pulmonary vascular remodeling that results in a sustainably increased RV afterload.

Therapeutic strategies for the treatment of PAH aim to halt or even reverse maladaptive lung remodeling thereby reducing RV afterload, wall stress, myocardial oxygen consumption, and ischemia to improve the contractile state of the heart. Currently, RV afterload and wall stress reduction in PAH is achieved through

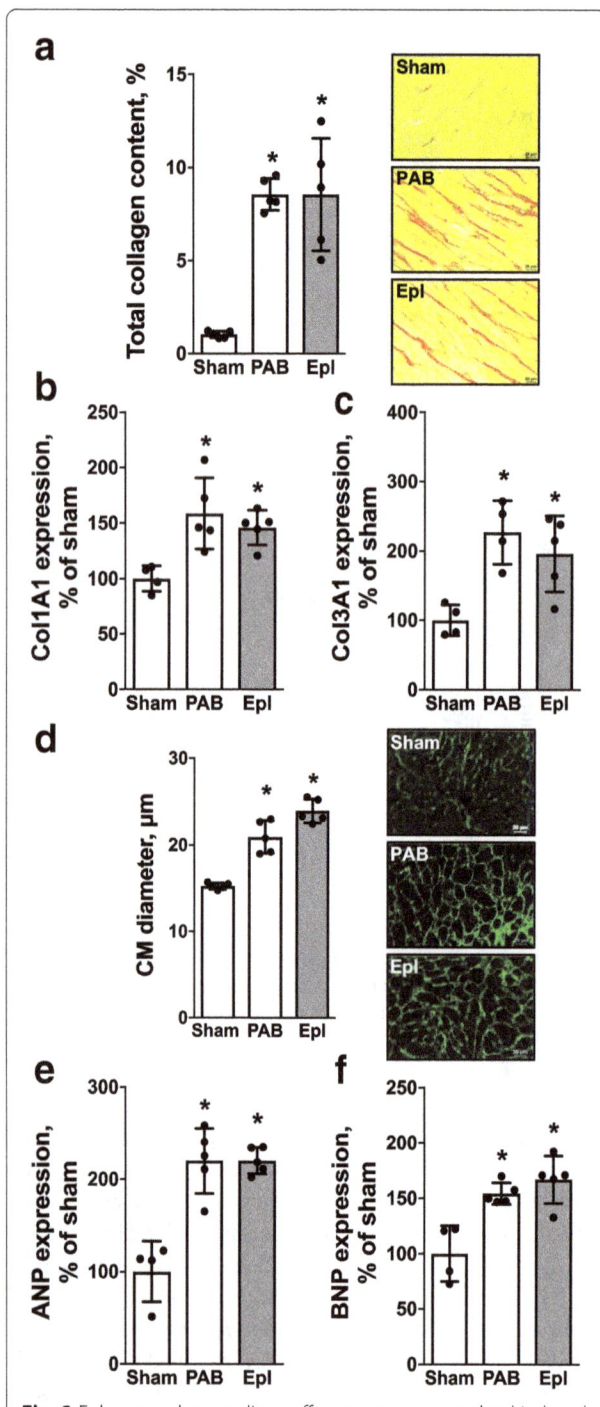

Fig. 3 Eplerenone has no direct effect on pressure overload-induced structural RV remodeling. Pharmacological aldosterone antagonism with Eplerenone had no effect on RV total collagen content assessed by picrosirius red stains (percentage of the total RV; **a**), *Col1A1* (percentage of sham; **b**) and *Col3A1* gene expression (percentage of sham; **c**). Eplerenone did not affect cardiomyocyte hypertrophy (CM diameter, μm; **d**), ANP (**e**) or BNP gene expression (percentage of sham; **f**). $n = 4$–5 mice per group; *: $p < 0.05$ vs. cntrl

pulmonary vasodilation [28]. Extensive work from the field of left-sided heart failure has already revealed that in addition to vasodilation, cardiac unloading through blood volume reduction via RAAS inhibition beneficially affects cardiac structure and function [14, 17]. In line, several reports link dysfunctional RAAS activation to PAH pathogenesis [4, 5, 7]. However, experimental and clinical data demonstrate that RAAS blockade has no or only minor direct beneficial effects on the RV myocardium despite systemic unloading, suggesting that the response to RAAS therapy might be critically different between the LV and the RV [16, 29, 30]. The current study extends these observations into oral administration of Eplerenone in mice with isolated RV pressure overload independent from afterload in a dosage that has proven efficacy in attenuating pathologic pulmonary vascular remodeling. Beneficial effects observed in PH animal models might be secondary due to afterload reductions. Here, Eplerenone therapy starting when RV dysfunction was established had no direct effect on the RV myocardium while systemic blood pressure dropped down. Interestingly, Eplerenone lowered the systemic blood pressure only when administered to animals with established RV dysfunction but not in the preventive SuHx model, pointing towards a differential role in the stressed RV which might be more vulnerable to aldosterone antagonism. Similar observations were made in a study addressing the effects of RAAS inhibition on the RV in a chronic pressure overload rat model [16].

A clinical role for Eplerenone has been described in cardiovascular protection, was confirmed in several clinical trials in patients with left-sided heart failure (RALES, EPHESUS, ENPHASIS-HF) and has been extensively characterized in models of LV remodeling [14, 31, 32]. However, the molecular mechanisms are not fully understood. A growing body of evidence suggests that Eplerenone mediates its effects in part through competing with aldosterone for mineralocorticoid receptor binding – however, the mechanistic insights how Eplerenone might affect mineralocorticoid receptor expression, as it was observed in this study, are still elusive. In heart failure mouse models, genetic inactivation of the mineralocorticoid receptor signaling pathway improved LV function [33]. Specifically, cardiomyocyte but not fibroblast restricted mineralocorticoid receptor deficiency improved LV function and reduced LV dilation upon trans-aortic constriction pointing towards a key role for cardiomyocyte mineralocorticoid receptor signaling in the pathogenesis of left heart failure [34]. In line, Eplerenone therapy in wildtype animals with heart failure improved LV function and reduced LV dilation [35]. Whether elevated cardiac mineralocorticoid receptor signaling is a disease consequence or drives heart failure progression is not clear. In the current study, we report increased mineralocorticoid receptor gene expression directly in the hypertrophied RV – suggesting increased mineralocorticoid receptor signaling - which was normalized by Eplerenone therapy without functional or structural RV improvements. These data show that increased mineralocorticoid receptor activation is rather a disease consequence than a driver of RV heart failure pathogenesis.

Conclusions

In summary, this study reports a benefit of pharmacological aldosterone antagonism with Eplerenone in PAH by directly targeting the pulmonary vasculature while further studies are warranted to fully characterize the therapeutic benefit of Eplerenone on the diseased pulmonary vasculature and dissect the mechanistic role of aldosterone in PAH pathophysiology. The clinical relevance of aldosterone antagonism as a therapeutic approach for PAH is currently being evaluated in clinical trials. Patients are recruited for a Phase 2, dose-ranging, randomized, placebo controlled study (→→→→ClinicalTrials.gov identifier: NCT01712620) that is designed to compare the effectiveness of Spironolactone in treating PAH versus placebo. By targeting the maladaptive pulmonary vascular remodeling processes, that current PAH therapies do not, aldosterone antagonism with Spironolactone is expected to improve exercise capacity and endothelial dysfunction in PAH. To find out whether an enhanced cardiopulmonary fitness (exercise capacity and RV function) improves the quality of life, Spironolactone in combination with an endothelin receptor type A blocker will be administered to PAH patients with a LV ejection fraction > 50% in a prospective, double blind, placebo-controlled phase 4 study (ClinicalTrials.gov identifier: NCT02253394).

Acknowledgements
We thank Christina Vroom and Elena Jenike for technical assistance.

Funding
This work was supported by the Universities of Giessen and Marburg Lung Center (UGMLC), Excellence Cluster Cardio-Pulmonary System (ECCPS), German Center for Lung Research (DZL), Collaborative Research Center (CRC) 1213, British Heart Foundation Senior Basic Science Research Fellowship (FS/13/48/30453), British Heart Foundation Project Grant (PG/06/125/21633), National Institute for Health Research, Sheffield Clinical Research Facility.

Authors' contributions
MB, AL, RTS and BK designed and performed experiments, analyzed and interpreted data. MB wrote the manuscript. NA, AB, JP, CL and TN performed experiments, analyzed and interpreted data. DGK, FG, HAG, NW and WS analyzed and interpreted data. All authors were involved in critically revising the manuscript.

Competing interests
The authors declare that they have no competing interests.

Author details
[1]Universities of Giessen and Marburg Lung Center (UGMLC), Excellence Cluster Cardio-Pulmonary System (ECCPS), Member of the German Center for Lung Research (DZL), Aulweg 130, 35392, Giessen, Germany. [2]Department of Infection, Immunity and Cardiovascular Disease, University of Sheffield, Sheffield, UK. [3]Sheffield Pulmonary Vascular Disease Unit, Royal Hallamshire Hospital, Sheffield, UK.

References
1. Schermuly RT, Ghofrani HA, Wilkins MR, Grimminger F. Mechanisms of disease: pulmonary arterial hypertension. Nat Rev Cardiol. 2011;8(8):443–55.
2. Rabinovitch M. Molecular pathogenesis of pulmonary arterial hypertension. J Clin Invest. 2008;118(7):2372–9.
3. Leopold JA, Maron BA. Molecular mechanisms of pulmonary vascular remodeling in pulmonary arterial hypertension. Int J Mol Sci. 2016;17(5)
4. Morrell NW, Danilov SM, Satyan KB, Morris KG, Stenmark KR. Right ventricular angiotensin converting enzyme activity and expression is increased during hypoxic pulmonary hypertension. Cardiovasc Res. 1997; 34(2):393–403.
5. de Man FS, Tu L, Handoko ML, Rain S, Ruiter G, Francois C, Schalij I, Dorfmuller P, Simonneau G, Fadel E, et al. Dysregulated renin-angiotensin-aldosterone system contributes to pulmonary arterial hypertension. Am J Respir Crit Care Med. 2012;186(8):780–9.
6. Maron BA, Leopold JA. Emerging concepts in the molecular basis of pulmonary arterial hypertension: part II: Neurohormonal signaling contributes to the pulmonary vascular and right ventricular Pathophenotype of pulmonary arterial hypertension. Circulation. 2015; 131(23):2079–91.
7. Orte C, Polak JM, Haworth SG, Yacoub MH, Morrell NW. Expression of pulmonary vascular angiotensin-converting enzyme in primary and secondary plexiform pulmonary hypertension. J Pathol. 2000;192(3):379–84.
8. Maron BA, Opotowsky AR, Landzberg MJ, Loscalzo J, Waxman AB, Leopold JA. Plasma aldosterone levels are elevated in patients with pulmonary arterial hypertension in the absence of left ventricular heart failure: a pilot study. Eur J Heart Fail. 2013;15(3):277–83.
9. Maron BA, Zhang YY, White K, Chan SY, Handy DE, Mahoney CE, Loscalzo J, Leopold JA. Aldosterone inactivates the endothelin-B receptor via a cysteinyl thiol redox switch to decrease pulmonary endothelial nitric oxide levels and modulate pulmonary arterial hypertension. Circulation. 2012; 126(8):963–74.
10. Aghamohammadzadeh R, Zhang YY, Stephens TE, Arons E, Zaman P, Polach KJ, Matar M, Yung LM, Yu PB, Bowman FP, et al. Up-regulation of the mammalian target of rapamycin complex 1 subunit raptor by aldosterone induces abnormal pulmonary artery smooth muscle cell survival patterns to promote pulmonary arterial hypertension. FASEB J. 2016;30(7):2511–27.
11. Preston IR, Sagliani KD, Warburton RR, Hill NS, Fanburg BL, Jaffe IZ. Mineralocorticoid receptor antagonism attenuates experimental pulmonary hypertension. Am J Physiol Lung Cell Mol Physiol. 2013;304(10):L678–88.
12. Leopold JA, Dam A, Maron BA, Scribner AW, Liao R, Handy DE, Stanton RC, Pitt B, Loscalzo J. Aldosterone impairs vascular reactivity by decreasing glucose-6-phosphate dehydrogenase activity. Nat Med. 2007;13(2):189–97.
13. Maron BA, Oldham WM, Chan SY, Vargas SO, Arons E, Zhang YY, Loscalzo J, Leopold JA. Upregulation of steroidogenic acute regulatory protein by hypoxia stimulates aldosterone synthesis in pulmonary artery endothelial cells to promote pulmonary vascular fibrosis. Circulation. 2014;130(2):168–79.
14. Pitt B, Zannad F, Remme WJ, Cody R, Castaigne A, Perez A, Palensky J, Wittes J. The effect of spironolactone on morbidity and mortality in patients with severe heart failure. Randomized Aldactone evaluation study investigators. N Engl J Med. 1999;341(10):709–17.
15. Brown NJ. Aldosterone and end-organ damage. Curr Opin Nephrol Hypertens. 2005;14(3):235–41.
16. Borgdorff MA, Bartelds B, Dickinson MG, Steendijk P, Berger RM. A cornerstone of heart failure treatment is not effective in experimental right ventricular failure. Int J Cardiol. 2013;169(3):183–9.
17. Nappi JM, Sieg A. Aldosterone and aldosterone receptor antagonists in patients with chronic heart failure. Vasc Health Risk Manag. 2011;7:353–63.
18. Craft J. Eplerenone (Inspra), a new aldosterone antagonist for the treatment of systemic hypertension and heart failure. Proc (Baylor Univ Med Cent). 2004;17(2):217–20.

19. Keidar S, Hayek T, Kaplan M, Pavlotzky E, Hamoud S, Coleman R, Aviram M. Effect of eplerenone, a selective aldosterone blocker, on blood pressure, serum and macrophage oxidative stress, and atherosclerosis in apolipoprotein E-deficient mice. J Cardiovasc Pharmacol. 2003;41(6):955–63.

20. Keidar S, Kaplan M, Pavlotzky E, Coleman R, Hayek T, Hamoud S, Aviram M. Aldosterone administration to mice stimulates macrophage NADPH oxidase and increases atherosclerosis development: a possible role for angiotensin-converting enzyme and the receptors for angiotensin II and aldosterone. Circulation. 2004;109(18):2213–20.

21. Boehm M, Lawrie A, Wilhelm J, Ghofrani HA, Grimminger F, Weissmann N, Seeger W, Schermuly RT, Kojonazarov B. Maintained right ventricular pressure overload induces ventricular-arterial decoupling in mice. Exp Physiol. 2017;102(2):180–9.

22. Janssen W, Schymura Y, Novoyatleva T, Kojonazarov B, Boehm M, Wietelmann A, Luitel H, Murmann K, Krompiec DR, Tretyn A, et al. 5-HT2B receptor antagonists inhibit fibrosis and protect from RV heart failure. Biomed Res Int. 2015;2015:438403.

23. Shi L, Kojonazarov B, Elgheznawy A, Popp R, Dahal BK, Bohm M, Pullamsetti SS, Ghofrani HA, Godecke A, Jungmann A, et al. miR-223-IGF-IR signalling in hypoxia- and load-induced right-ventricular failure: a novel therapeutic approach. Cardiovasc Res. 2016;111(3):184–93.

24. Savai R, Al-Tamari HM, Sedding D, Kojonazarov B, Muecke C, Teske R, Capecchi MR, Weissmann N, Grimminger F, Seeger W, et al. Pro-proliferative and inflammatory signaling converge on FoxO1 transcription factor in pulmonary hypertension. Nat Med. 2014;20(11):1289–300.

25. Budas GR, Boehm M, Kojonazarov B, Viswanathan G, Tian X, Veeroju S, Novoyatleva T, Grimminger F, Hinojosa-Kirschenbaum F, Ghofrani HA, et al. ASK1 inhibition halts disease progression in preclinical models of pulmonary arterial hypertension. Am J Respir Crit Care Med. 2017

26. Hameed AG, Arnold ND, Chamberlain J, Pickworth JA, Paiva C, Dawson S, Cross S, Long L, Zhao L, Morrell NW, et al. Inhibition of tumor necrosis factor-related apoptosis-inducing ligand (TRAIL) reverses experimental pulmonary hypertension. J Exp Med. 2012;209(11):1919–35.

27. Lawrie A, Hameed AG, Chamberlain J, Arnold N, Kennerley A, Hopkinson K, Pickworth J, Kiely DG, Crossman DC, Francis SE. Paigen diet-fed apolipoprotein E knockout mice develop severe pulmonary hypertension in an interleukin-1-dependent manner. Am J Pathol. 2011;179(4):1693–705.

28. Hoeper MM, McLaughlin VV, Dalaan AM, Satoh T, Galie N. Treatment of pulmonary hypertension. Lancet Respir Med. 2016;4(4):323–36.

29. Therrien J, Provost Y, Harrison J, Connelly M, Kaemmerer H, Webb GD. Effect of angiotensin receptor blockade on systemic right ventricular function and size: a small, randomized, placebo-controlled study. Int J Cardiol. 2008;129(2):187–92.

30. van der Bom T, Winter MM, Bouma BJ, Groenink M, Vliegen HW, Pieper PG, van Dijk AP, Sieswerda GT, Roos-Hesselink JW, Zwinderman AH, et al. Effect of valsartan on systemic right ventricular function: a double-blind, randomized, placebo-controlled pilot trial. Circulation. 2013;127(3):322–30.

31. Pitt B, Remme W, Zannad F, Neaton J, Martinez F, Roniker B, Bittman R, Hurley S, Kleiman J, Gatlin M. Eplerenone, a selective aldosterone blocker, in patients with left ventricular dysfunction after myocardial infarction. N Engl J Med. 2003;348(14):1309–21.

32. Zannad F, McMurray JJ, Krum H, van Veldhuisen DJ, Swedberg K, Shi H, Vincent J, Pocock SJ, Pitt B. Eplerenone in patients with systolic heart failure and mild symptoms. N Engl J Med. 2011;364(1):11–21.

33. Montes-Cobos E, Li X, Fischer HJ, Sasse A, Kugler S, Didie M, Toischer K, Fassnacht M, Dressel R, Reichardt HM. Inducible knock-down of the mineralocorticoid receptor in mice disturbs regulation of the renin-angiotensin-aldosterone system and attenuates heart failure induced by pressure overload. PLoS One. 2015;10(11):e0143954.

34. Lother A, Berger S, Gilsbach R, Rosner S, Ecke A, Barreto F, Bauersachs J, Schutz G, Hein L. Ablation of mineralocorticoid receptors in myocytes but not in fibroblasts preserves cardiac function. Hypertension. 2011;57(4):746–54.

35. Kuster GM, Kotlyar E, Rude MK, Siwik DA, Liao R, Colucci WS, Sam F. Mineralocorticoid receptor inhibition ameliorates the transition to myocardial failure and decreases oxidative stress and inflammation in mice with chronic pressure overload. Circulation. 2005;111(4):420–7.

Comparative bench study evaluation of different infant interfaces for non-invasive ventilation

Giorgio Conti[1], Giorgia Spinazzola[1], Cesare Gregoretti[2], Giuliano Ferrone[1], Andrea Cortegiani[2]* ⓘ, Olimpia Festa[1], Marco Piastra[1], Luca Tortorolo[1] and Roberta Costa[1]

Abstract

Background: To compare, in terms of patient-ventilator interaction and performance, a new nasal mask (Respireo, AirLiquide, FR) with the Endotracheal tube (ET) and a commonly used nasal mask (FPM, Fisher and Paykel, NZ) for delivering Pressure Support Ventilation (PSV) in an infant model of Acute Respiratory Failure (ARF).

Methods: An active test lung (ASL 5000) connected to an infant mannequin through 3 different interfaces (Respireo, ET and FPM), was ventilated with a standard ICU ventilator set in PSV. The test lung was set to simulate a 5.5 kg infant with ARF, breathing at 50 and 60 breaths/min). Non-invasive ventilation (NIV) mode was not used and the leaks were nearly zero.

Results: The ET showed the shortest inspiratory trigger delay and pressurization time compared to FPM and Respireo ($p < 0.01$). At each respiratory rate tested, the FPM showed the shortest Expiratory trigger delay compared to ET and Respireo ($p < 0.01$). The Respireo presented a lower value of Inspiratory pressure–time product and trigger pressure drop than ET ($p < 0.01$), while no significant difference was found in terms of pressure-time product at 300 and 500 ms. During all tests, compared with the FPM, ET showed a significantly higher tidal volume (V_T) delivered ($p < 0.01$), while Respireo showed a trend toward an increase of tidal volume delivered compared with FPM.

Conclusions: The ET showed a better patient-ventilator interaction and performance compared to both the nasal masks. Despite the higher internal volume, Respireo showed a trend toward an increase of the delivered tidal volume; globally, its efficiency in terms of patient-ventilator interaction was comparable to the FPM, which is the infant NIV mask characterized by the smaller internal volume among the (few) models on the market.

Keywords: Non invasive ventilation, Bench test, Infant mask, Patient-ventilator interaction, Mechanical ventilation, Acute respiratory failure

Background

The role of Non-Invasive Ventilation (NIV) in children with acute respiratory failure (ARF) treated in the Pediatric Intensive Care Unit (PICU) is well established [1–7].

During NIV, ventilator modes, settings and interfaces may deeply affect patient-ventilator interaction. Pressure Support Ventilation (PSV) still remains the mode most commonly used in PICU during NIV, although Neurally Adjusted Ventilatory Assist (NAVA) has been recently proposed to improve patient-ventilator synchrony in infants [8, 9]. Nevertheless, NAVA requires the placement of an indwelling catheter making its use more invasive and expensive [8–10]. As a matter of fact, the use of a comfortable and well-fitted interface, as well as an appropriate ventilator mode and setting are both important factors to optimize patient-ventilator interaction and increase patient's compliance during NIV [6, 11].

NIV is usually delivered with different interfaces, such as face and nasal masks or helmets. However, only few pediatric interfaces are present on the market and, more

* Correspondence: cortegiania@gmail.com
[2]Department of Biopathology and Medical Biotechnologies (DIBIMED), Section of Anesthesia, Analgesia, Intensive Care and Emergency. Policlinico Paolo Giaccone, University of Palermo, Via del vespro 129, 90127 Palermo, Italy

often than never, their sub-optimal design can deeply affect patient-ventilator synchrony, compared to the benchmark, represented by the endotracheal tube. In a recent study on a pediatric model breathing at high respiratory rates, the helmet demonstrated the worst patient-ventilator interaction, suggesting that the face mask should be considered the first choice for delivering NIV in babies [6].

Nevertheless, considering that infants are usually nose breathers, the nasal mask is largely employed in this patient population [12]. So far, no study has investigated the role of different nasal interfaces on patient-ventilator interaction in infants, even though nasal masks may have different internal volumes and may behave differently in various clinical settings.

We hypothesized that, compared to the ET, considered as the benchmark, different nasal masks with specific features in terms of internal volume and dead space could perform differently in terms of patient- ventilator synchrony. In order to test this hypothesis, a comparative bench study using an active lung simulator connected to a mannequin was designed to determine whether different interfaces and ventilator settings might influence patient-ventilator interaction in an infant model of restrictive respiratory failure.

Methods

This study was performed at the Respiratory Mechanics Laboratory (Ventil@b) of the Catholic University of Rome, Italy. A Laerdal Resusci Baby mannequin (Laerdal Medical, Stavanger, Norway) has been chosen for this study, being the most widely used resuscitation mannequin and the most realistic for the purposes of our bench study [13–16].

We connected the artificial airway of the mannequin with an active test lung (ASL 5000, Ingmar Medical, Pittsburgh, Pennsylvania) in order to test three different interfaces: the endotracheal tube (ET, size ID 4 mm, Covidien, Mansfield, Massachusetts), a new infant nasal mask (Respireo, extrasmall size, AirLiquide, FR) and a commonly used infant nasal mask (FPM, Infant Nasal Mask, large size, Fisher and Paykel, NZ) [17–19]. The two masks differ for shape and design characteristic, FPM presenting two parallel connections with a complete separation between inspiratory and expiratory limbs, while Respireo is characterized by a single limb connected to the Y piece with a flexible tube able to rotate at 360°.

A standard intensive care unit (ICU) ventilator wad used to ventilate the Resusci Baby mannequin (Servo I, Maquet, Sweden) [20, 21] in neonatal PSV mode, without using the air leak compensation software, since air leaks were eliminated during NIV by sealing the masks to the mannequin's face. The ET and the masks were

connected to the ventilator using a standard double limbs neonatal circuit. The mouth of the mannequin was filled and closed to reduce the dead space. Pressure Support (PS) and Positive End Expiratory Pressure (PEEP) were set at13cmH$_2$O and 5 cmH$_2$O, respectively. The inspiratory flow trigger was set at 1.5 L/min and optimized to the lowest level, to avoid auto-trigger.

Inspiratory trigger, pressurization time (Time$_{press}$) and expiratory trigger threshold (Tr$_{exp}$) were set to optimize patient-ventilator interaction and maintained constant throughout the trials. The test lung was set to simulate a 5.5 Kg BW infant, with a restrictive condition simulating a mild Acute Respiratory Distress Syndrome (ARDS). Compliance was set at 0.8 ml/cmH$_2$O/kg, respiratory system resistances at 25 cmH$_2$O/L/s and inspiratory muscle pressure (Pmus) at 12 cmH$_2$O. Respiratory Rate (RR) was set at 50 and 60 breaths/min. Each test condition lasted 20 min, and the last 5 min of each trial were recorded for analysis.

Data acquisition and analysis

Air flow (V′) was measured with a pneumotachograph (Fleish No.1, Metabo, Epalinges, Switzerland), while airway pressure (P$_{aw}$) was measured by a pressure transducer with a differential pressure of ±100 cmH$_2$O (Digima Clic-1, ICULab system; KleisTek Engineering, Bari, Italy), placed distally from the pneumotachograph. When the mannequin was ventilated through the ET or the Respireo, the pneumotachograph and the pressure transducer were positioned at the Y-connection of the ventilator circuit (Fig. 1). In the FPM, Flow and P$_{aw}$ were not measured because of the mask design, which determines a complete separation of inspiratory and expiratory limbs, not allowing the correct positioning of an external pneumotachograph. All the signals were acquired, amplified, filtered, and digitized at 100 Hz, then recorded on a dedicated personal computer and analyzed through specific software (ICULab 2.7; KleisTek). Ventilator inspiratory and expiratory time (mechanical T$_I$ and mechanical T$_E$, respectively), and ventilator rate of cycling were all determined on the flow tracing. The inspiratory duty cycle (mechanical T$_I$/T$_{tot}$) was calculated as the ratio between mechanical T$_I$ and the total mechanical breath duration (T$_{tot}$). Airflow (V′) and tidal volume (V$_T$) delivered to the simulator, airway opening pressure (Paw), and inspiratory muscles effort were displayed online on the computer screen. The signals obtained with the ASL were transmitted to a PC host via 10/100MBit Ethernet, sampled and processed in real time by means of specific software (Lab View, Ingmar Medical). The signals obtained with the ASL were integrated with the signals from the ICULab system by using a specific application of the ICULab (ICULab 2.7, KleisTek). The numerical integration of flow over time

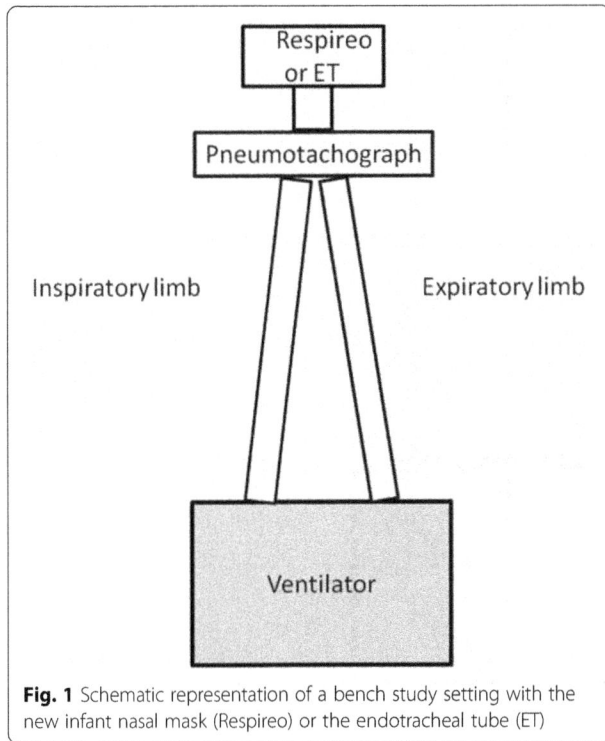

Fig. 1 Schematic representation of a bench study setting with the new infant nasal mask (Respireo) or the endotracheal tube (ET)

determined the mechanical tidal volume (mechanical V_T). The amount of tidal volume delivered to the simulator during its active inspiration (ie, the neural tidal volume, V_T) was calculated as the volume generated from the onset of inspiratory muscle effort negative deflection to its nadir. Interfaces performance was evaluated using the following parameters [20–22]:

1) Trigger pressure drop ($Swing_{trigger}$), defined as the pressure swing generated by the simulator inspiratory effort in the airway during the triggering phase;
2) Inspiratory pressure–time product ($PTP_{trigger}$), defined as the area under the Paw curve relative to the time between the onset of inspiratory effort and the start of mechanical assistance;
3) Pressure-time product at 300 ms (PTP_{300}) defined as the integration of Paw over time during the first 300 msec and representing the speediness of the ventilator in reaching the preset level of pressure support;
4) Pressure-time product at 500 ms (PTP_{500}), defined as the integral Paw area over insufflation time from the simulated effort onset, representing the ventilator capability of maintaining pressurization;
5) PTP_{500} index, expressed as a percentage of the ideal PTP, which is unattainable because it would imply a trigger pressure drop and an instantaneous pressurization of the ventilator.

Patient–ventilator interaction (Fig. 2) was evaluated by determining:

1) Pressurization time ($Time_{press}$), defined as the time necessary to achieve the pre-set level of pressure support from the baseline value;
2) Inspiratory trigger delay ($Delay_{trinsp}$), calculated as the time lag between the onset of inspiratory muscle effort negative swing and the start of the ventilator support (i.e., P_{aw} positive deflection);
3) Expiratory trigger delay ($Delay_{trexp}$), assessed as the delay between the end of the inspiratory effort and the end of the mechanical insufflations (i.e., flow deflection);
4) Time of synchrony ($Time_{sync}$), defined as the time during which inspiratory muscle effort and Paw are in phase (ideally 100%);
5) Simulator V_T/mechanical V_T, intended as the percentage of V_T delivered during inspiratory muscle effort negative deflection;
6) Wasted efforts, defined as ineffective inspiratory efforts, not assisted by the ventilator;
7) Auto-triggering, namely a mechanical insufflation in absence of inspiratory effort.

Statistical analysis

All data are expressed as mean ± SD. All variables were compared with each interface used. All variables were compared by using a non-parametric Kruskal-Wallis test for analysis of variance (ANOVA) on ranks. Pairwise comparisons were done with the Dunn's multiple comparison test. The Mantel-Haenszel extended chi-square test was used. P value < 0.05 was considered statistically significant.

Results

During all study conditions, the V_T delivered to the mannequin was significantly higher with the ET than with the FPM ($p < 0.01$). No significant differences were found in terms of V_T during Respireo NIV compared to the other two settings, although this mask showed a not trend toward an increase of the delivered V_T compared to the FPM (Fig. 3).

At RR 50 the ET showed significantly shorter $Delay_{trinsp}$ and $Time_{press}$ compared to the Respireo ($p < 0.05$), while no significant differences were observed between the two masks. At RR 60 no difference was observed in terms of $Delay_{trinsp}$ between the three interfaces.

At both RR tested, the FPM showed a significantly shorter $Delay_{trexp}$ compared both to the ET and the Respireo ($p < 0.01$) (Fig. 4).

At RR60 Time of Synchrony ($Time_{sync}$) did not show significant differences between all the interfaces, while at RR50 the Respireo, but not the FPM, showed a

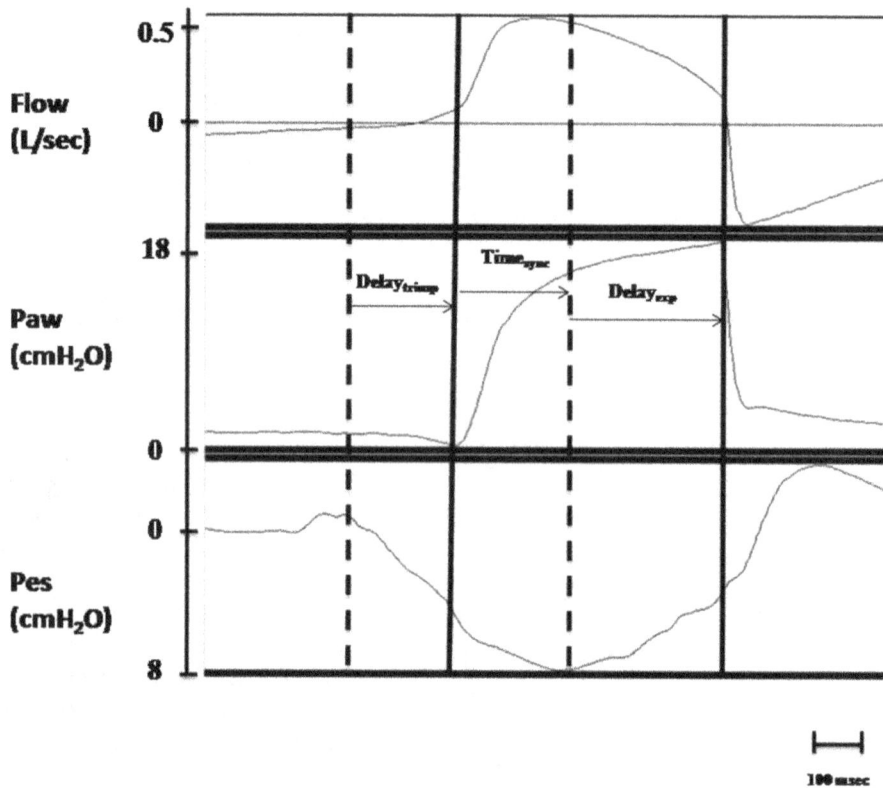

Fig. 2 Example from a real patient tracing (from our database) of patient-ventilator interaction measurements during NIV. From the top to the bottom: Flow (V'), Airway pressure (Paw) and Esophageal pressure (Pes). $Delay_{trinsp}$: between the first dotted line and the first black line is the delay between the onset of patient inspiration and the start of the mechanical assistance. $Delay_{trexp}$: between the second dotted line and the second black line is the delay between the end of patient inspiration and the end of the mechanical insufflation. $Time_{sync}$: between the first black line and the second dotted line is the time during which the patient and the ventilator are in phase

significantly shorter $Time_{sync}$ compared to the ET ($p < 0.01$) (Fig. 5).

The performance analysis was conducted only between the ET and the Respireo, as the FPM design did not allow positioning an external pneumotacograph. At both RR, the Respireo showed a significantly shorter $Swing_{trigger}$ and $PTP_{trigger}$ compared to the ET ($p < 0.01$). No significant difference was found between the Respireo and the ET in terms of PTP_{300} at both RR tested. Finally, at RR 60 the Respireo showed a better PTP_{500}index compared to the ET ($p < 0.05$) (Table 1).

Discussion

To the best of our knowledge, this is the first study aimed at evaluating different NIV interfaces in a simulated infant restrictive model. The main results of this bench study can be summarized as follows:

1) At RR 50 the ET showed a better patient-ventilator interaction in terms of $Delay_{trinsp}$ and $Time_{press}$ compared to the nasal masks tested. At RR 60, no difference was observed in terms of $Delay_{trinsp}$ between the three interfaces. The Respireo showed

better $Swing_{trigger}$ and $PTP_{trigger}$ compared to the ET at both RR.

2) The V_T delivered to the mannequin was between 6 and 8 ml/Kg, although, during ET, V_T showed a trend toward an increase compared during Respireo NIV and it was significantly higher than during FPM NIV. No differences were found between ET and Respireo and between Respireo and FPM.

3) No significant differences were observed in terms of PTP_{300} and PTP_{500} between the Respireo and the ET. Nevertheless, at RR 60 the Respireo showed a significantly better performance in terms of PTP_{500}index compared to the ET.

Despite the ET represents the standard of care for the treatment of ARF in infants, there is an increasing evidence of physicians trying to avoid intubation or extubate their patients and continue the ventilator assistance on NIV [23].

In the last years, many efforts have been made to improve the interfaces. This has involved interface physical characteristics, materials and design. Neonates and infants are preferentially nose breathers and the choice

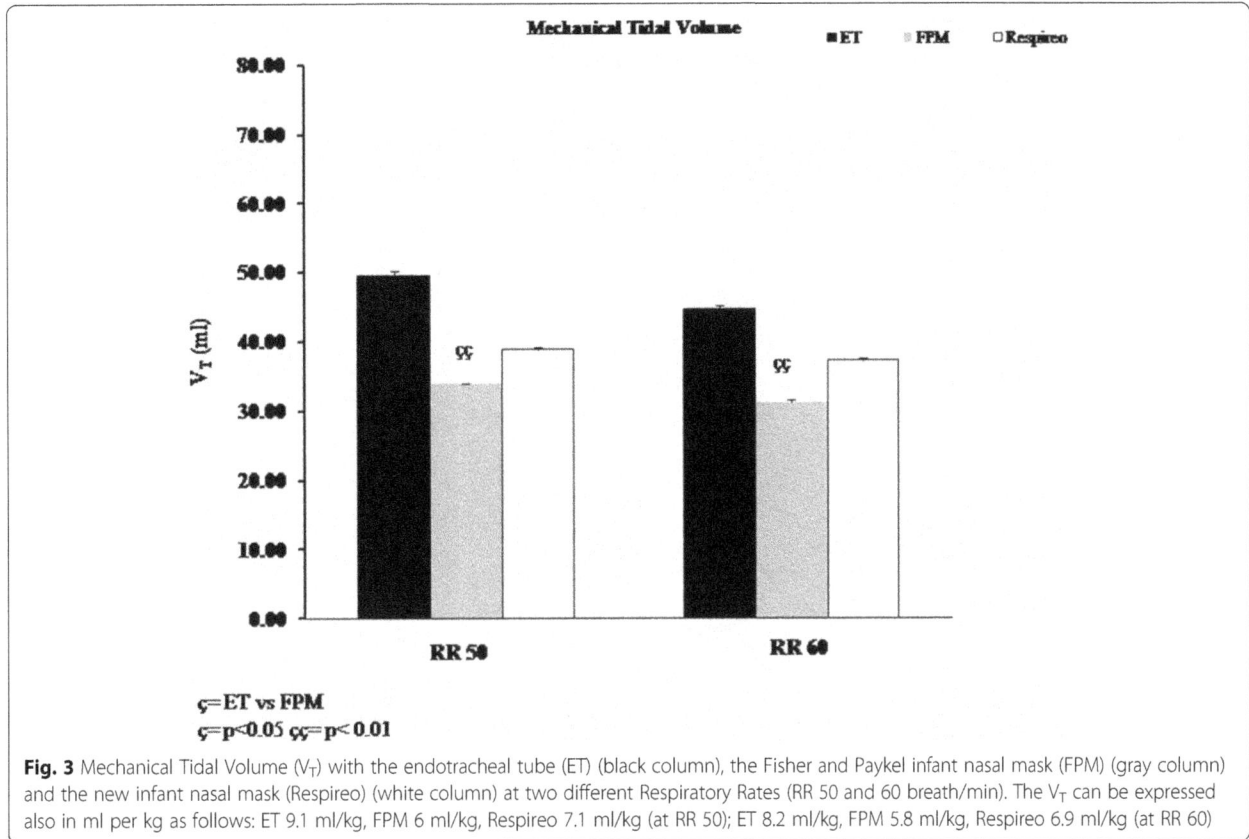

Fig. 3 Mechanical Tidal Volume (V_T) with the endotracheal tube (ET) (black column), the Fisher and Paykel infant nasal mask (FPM) (gray column) and the new infant nasal mask (Respireo) (white column) at two different Respiratory Rates (RR 50 and 60 breath/min). The V_T can be expressed also in ml per kg as follows: ET 9.1 ml/kg, FPM 6 ml/kg, Respireo 7.1 ml/kg (at RR 50); ET 8.2 ml/kg, FPM 5.8 ml/kg, Respireo 6.9 ml/kg (at RR 60)

of the interface is determined both by the age and by the type of ventilator support. During NIV the likelihood of leaks, with subsequent patient-ventilator asynchrony is higher than during nasal Continuous Positive Airway Pressure (CPAP) [24].

In order to understand this issue, it is important to note that in PICU, CPAP is delivered through "leaking systems", where intentional air leaks are an intrinsic feature of the CPAP system. In the same way, NIV can be administered using intentional leaks ventilators, namely ventilators that are coupled with masks provided with embedded "exhalation holes", also named as vented masks. Conversely, in our bench study, NIV was delivered by an high pressure ICU ventilator with active valves adopting a double circuit, without any intentional leak. For these reasons we used a non-vented mask.

We chose to use PSV to compare nasal masks with the ET, where mechanical ventilation is provided with high pressure ICU ventilator. We used an infant mannequin [25] and developed a system that allowed to avoid air leaks during both mask and ET ventilation, although we are aware that non intentional leaks are routinely observed both during invasive and non-invasive ventilation in infants [26, 27]. In this study we wanted to have an accurate estimation of flow and pressure curves as well as of the delivered V_T during simulated positive pressure ventilation.

In addition, other studies where leaks were allowed tested the efficiency of face masks in the resuscitation of newborn infants [26, 28], measuring the expired tidal volumes during bag and mask ventilation or NIV similar to our setting with a flow sensor (pneumotachograph) placed between the Y connection of the circuit and the interface [29–31]. Our results demonstrated that the ET, as expected, showed an overall better patient-ventilator interaction compared to the nasal masks at both RR tested. Interestingly, the Respireo showed a better Swing$_{trigger}$ and PTP$_{trigger}$ compared to the ET at both RR. This result can be explained considering the higher inspiratory resistance generated by the ET compared to the Respireo mask, that determines a deeper Swing trigger and thus, an higher PTP trigger.

In addition, compared to the FPM, the Respireo showed a trend toward an increase of the delivered V_T at both RR. This result may be explained considering, on one side, that Respireo has a double internal volume than FPM and on the other that FPM, for its specific design, generates a complete separation of the inspiratory and expiratory limbs, thus increasing inspiratory resistances with consequent generation of lower V_T for a comparable level of transpulmonary pressure. It can also be speculated that the Respireo lower resistance, compared to the ET, was responsible of a better performance in terms of PTP$_{500}$ index at RR 60.

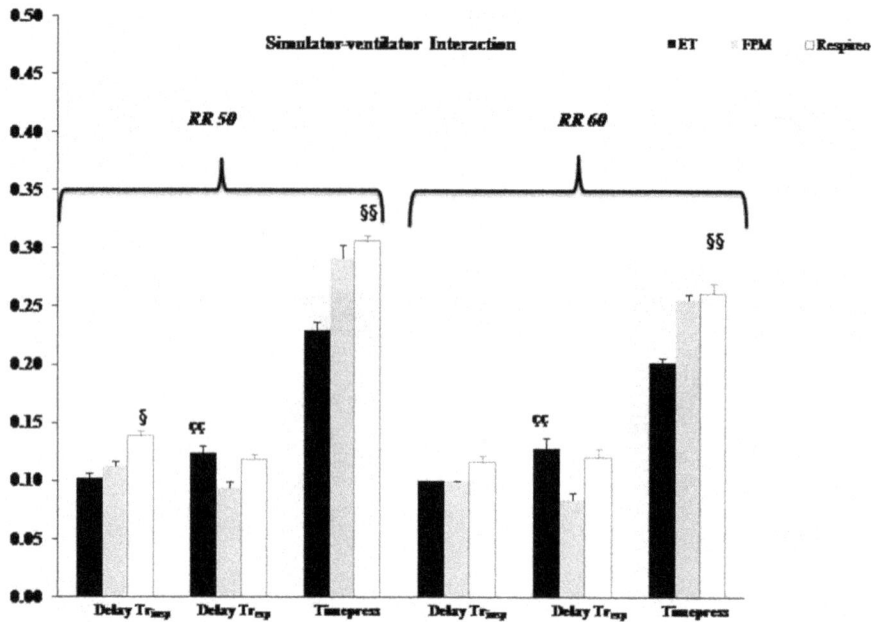

ç= ET vs FPM
§= ET vs Respireo
#= FPM vs Respireo
ç, §, #= p< 0,05, çç, §§, ##= p< 0,01

Fig. 4 Inspiratory trigger delay (Delay$_{trinsp}$), Pressurization Time (Time$_{press}$) and Expiratory Trigger delay (Dealy$_{trexp}$) with the endotracheal tube (ET) (black column), the Fisher and Paykel infant nasal mask (FPM) (gray column) and the new infant nasal mask (Respireo) (white column) at two different Respiratory Rates (RR 50 and 60 breath/min)

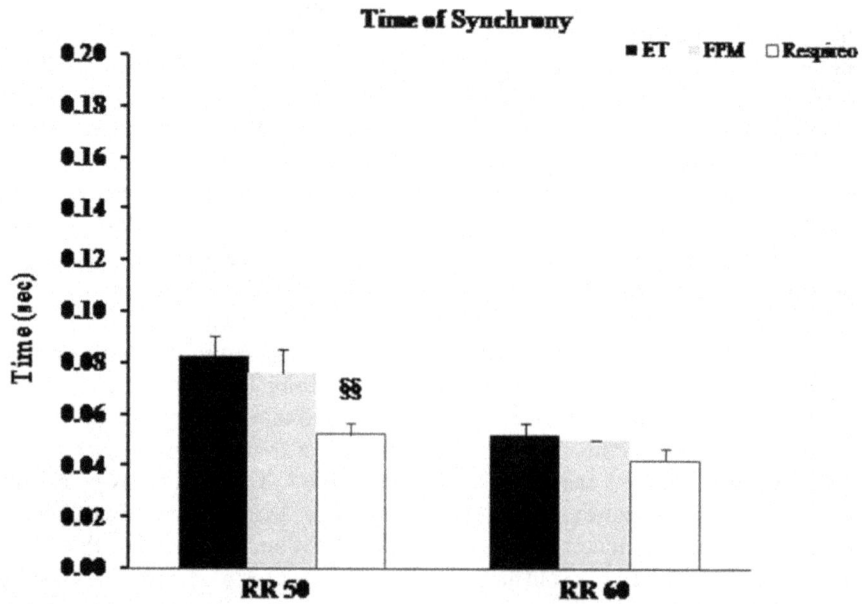

§= ET vs Respireo
§=p<0.05; §§=p<0.01

Fig. 5 Time of synchrony with the endotracheal tube (ET) (black column), the Fisher and Paykel infant nasal mask (FPM) (gray column) and the new infant nasal mask (Respireo) (white column) at two different Respiratory Rates (RR 50 and 60 breath/min)

Table 1 Interfaces performance

RR 50	ET	Respireo	P	RR 60	ET	Respireo	p
$Swing_{trigger}$ (cmH2O)	1.82 ± 0.1	0.83 ± 0.08	< 0.001		2.75 ± 0.12	0.78 ± 0.09	< 0.001
$PTP_{trigger}$ (cmH2O/s)	0.09 ± 0.01	0.06 ± 0.01	< 0.001		0.14 ± 0.01	0.05 ± 0.02	< 0.001
PTP_{300} (cmH2O/s)	1.8 ± 0.11	1.61 ± 0.19	NS		1.7 ± 0.1	1.7 ± 0.18	NS
PTP_{500}index (%)	55%	56%	NS		48%	50%	< 0.05

Performance evaluation of the endotracheal tube (ET) and the new infant nasal mask (Respireo) in terms of Trigger pressure drop ($Swing_{trigger}$), Inspiratory pressure–time product ($PTP_{trigger}$), Pressure-Time Product at 300(PTP_{300}), and PTP_{500} index at two respiratory rates (RR 50 and RR 60 breaths/min)
Values are mean ± SD

Our study has several limitations that need to be discussed. The major limitation is that it is a bench study conducted on an active lung simulator breathing with a repetitive respiratory rhythm that does not fully represent the clinical behavior of an infant receiving NIV. Moreover, during a bench study, the interfaces are evaluated in "optimal" conditions (i.e. without air leaks or secretions) to obtain a pure performance evaluation. For all these reasons, our results need to be confirmed by clinical studies assessing the effectiveness of the masks in ventilating infants in different conditions and evaluating their performance in response to the variability of a real clinical scenario.

Unfortunately, it is technically and ethically impossible to perform a direct comparison between different interfaces, especially when an ET is included in the same (pediatric) patient. Moreover, despite the mannequin used is considered one of the best devices for simulation, the anatomy of the upper airways is not perfectly representative of the human infant ones. In details, the nostrils are probably more resistive than the "in vivo" nostrils and the rhino- and oro-pharynx are larger than the "in vivo" ones. These differences increase both the resistive work (nostrils), and the dead space, making the "in vitro" study setting adopted in this evaluation a worst scenario than the "in vivo" conditions.

Conclusions

We have developed an active model for assessing the delivery of invasive and non-invasive ventilation in infants. With this model, the ET showed a better patient-ventilator interaction and performance compared to the nasal masks. Respireo was superior to the FPM in terms of delivered V_T at both RR; at the higher RR both masks showed similar results, despite the double internal volume of Respireo. Respireo showed a better $Swing_{trigger}$ and $PTP_{trigger}$ compared to the ET, while in terms of pressurization and PTP_{300} and PTP_{500} the results were similar. Globally, the Respireo performance was comparable and sometime superior to the FPM, which is the infant NIV mask characterized by the smaller internal volume among the (few) models on the market.

Abbreviations

ARDS: Acute respiratory distress syndrome; ARF: Acute respiratory failure; $Delay_{trexp}$: Expiratory trigger delay; $Delay_{trinsp}$: Inspiratory trigger delay; ET: Endotracheal tube; ICU: Intensive care unit; NAVA: Neurally Adjusted Ventilatory Assist; NIV: Noninvasive ventilation; P_{aw}: Airway pressure; PEEP: Positive end expiratory pressure; Pmus: Inspiratory muscle pressure; PS: Pressure support; PSV: Pressure support ventilation; PTP_{500}: Pressure-time product at 500 ms; $PTP_{trigger}$: Inspiratory pressure–time product; RR: Respiratory Rate; $Swing_{trigger}$: Trigger pressure drop; T_E: Expiratory time; T_I: Inspiratory time; T_I/T_{tot}: Inspiratory duty cycle; $Time_{press}$: Pressurization ramp; $Time_{sync}$: Time of synchrony; T_{rexp}: Expiratory trigger threshold; T_{tot}: Total mechanical breath duration; V': Air flow

Acknowledgements
None

Funding
None

Authors' contributions

GC, GS, CG, GF, AC, OF, MP. LT, RC participated in study design, data acquisition, writing the manuscript. All authors read and approved the manuscript.

Competing interests

All authors declare that they have no competing interests.

Author details

[1]Intensive Care and Anaesthesia Department and Ventilab, Catholic University of Rome, Policlinico A. Gemelli, Largo Agostino Gemelli 8, 00168 Rome, Italy. [2]Department of Biopathology and Medical Biotechnologies (DIBIMED), Section of Anesthesia, Analgesia, Intensive Care and Emergency. Policlinico Paolo Giaccone, University of Palermo, Via del vespro 129, 90127 Palermo, Italy.

References

1. Yanez LJ, Yunge M, Emilfork M, Lapadula M, Alcantara A, Fernandez C, Lozano J, Contreras M, Conto L, Arevalo C, Gayan A, Hernandez F, Pedraza M, Feddersen M, Bejares M, Morales M, Mallea F, Glasinovic M, Cavada G. A prospective, randomized, controlled trial of noninvasive ventilation in pediatric acute respiratory failure. Pediatr Crit Care Med. 2008;9:484–9.
2. Gregoretti C, Pisani L, Cortegiani A, Ranieri VM. Noninvasive ventilation in critically ill patients. Crit Care Clin. 2015;31:435–57.
3. Bimkrant DJ, Pope JF, Eiben RM. Topical review: pediatric noninvasive nasal ventilation. J Child Neurol. 2016;12:231–6.
4. Fortenberry JD, Del Toro J, Jefferson LS, Evey L, Haase D. Management of Pediatric Acute Hypoxemic Respiratory Insufficiency with Bilevel Positive Pressure (BiPAP) nasal mask ventilation. Chest. 1995;108:1059–64.

5. Padman R, Lawless S, Nessen Von S. Use of BiPAP by nasal mask in the treatment of respiratory insufficiency in pediatric patients: preliminary investigation. Pediatr Pulmonol. 1994;17:119–23.

6. Conti G, Gregoretti C, Spinazzola G, Festa O, Ferrone G, Cipriani F, Rossi M, Piastra M, Costa R. Influence of different interfaces on synchrony during pressure support ventilation in a pediatric setting: a bench study. Respir Care. 2015;60:498–507.

7. Teague WG. Noninvasive ventilation in the pediatric intensive care unit for children with acute respiratory failure. Pediatr Pulmonol. 2003;35:418–26.

8. Bordessoule A, Emeriaud G, Morneau S, Jouvet P, Beck J. Neurally adjusted ventilatory assist improves patient-ventilator interaction in infants as compared with conventional ventilation. Pediatr Res. 2012;72:194–202.

9. Conti G, Costa R. Technological development in mechanical ventilation. Curr Opin Crit Care. 2010;16:26–33.

10. Longhini F, Ferrero F, De Luca D, Cosi G, Alemani M, Colombo D, Cammarota G, Berni P, Conti G, Bona G, Corte Della F, Navalesi P. Neurally adjusted ventilatory assist in preterm neonates with acute respiratory failure. Neonatology. 2015;107:60–7.

11. Costa R, Navalesi P, Spinazzola G, Ferrone G, Pellegrini A, Cavaliere F, Proietti R, Antonelli M, Conti G. Influence of ventilator settings on patient-ventilator synchrony during pressure support ventilation with different interfaces. Intensive Care Med. 2010;36:1363–70.

12. Shott SR, Myer CM, Willis R, Cotton RT. Nasal obstruction in the neonate. Rhinology. 1989;27:91–6.

13. De Luca D, Costa R, Visconti F, Piastra M, Conti G. Oscillation transmission and volume delivery during face mask-delivered HFOV in infants: bench and in vivo study. Pediatr Pulmonol. 2016;51:705–12.

14. Howells R, Madar J. Newborn resuscitation training–which manikin. Resuscitation. 2002;54:175–81.

15. Campbell DM, Barozzino T, Farrugia M, Sgro M. High-fidelity simulation in neonatal resuscitation. Paediatr Child Health. 2009;14:19–23.

16. Udassi JP, Udassi S, Theriaque DW, Shuster JJ, Zaritsky AL, Haque IU. Effect of alternative chest compression techniques in infant and child on rescuer performance. Pediatr Crit Care Med. 2009;10:328–33.

17. Neuzeret P-C, Morin L. Impact of different nasal masks on CPAP therapy for obstructive sleep apnea: a randomized comparative trial. Clin Respir J. 2016; 11:990–98.

18. Goel S, Mondkar J, Panchal H, Hegde D, Utture A, Manerkar S. Nasal mask versus nasal prongs for delivering nasal continuous positive airway pressure in preterm infants with respiratory distress: a randomized controlled trial. Indian Pediatr. 2015;52:1035–40.

19. Ramanathan R. Nasal respiratory support through the nares: its time has come. J Perinatol. 2010;30(Supp 1):S67–72.

20. Vignaux L, Vargas F, Roeseler J, Tassaux D, Thille AW, Kossowsky MP, Brochard L, Jolliet P. Patient–ventilator asynchrony during non-invasive ventilation for acute respiratory failure: a multicenter study. Intensive Care Med. 2009;35:840.

21. Vignaux L, Piquilloud L, Tourneux P, Jolliet P, Rimensberger PC. Neonatal and adult ICU ventilators to provide ventilation in neonates, infants, and children: a bench model study. Respir Care. 2014;59:1463–75.

22. Olivieri C, Costa R, Spinazzola G, Ferrone G, Longhini F, Cammarota G, Conti G, Navalesi P. Bench comparative evaluation of a new generation and standard helmet for delivering non-invasive ventilation. Intensive Care Med. 2013;39:734–8.

23. Yoder BA, Stoddard RA, Li M, King J, Dirnberger DR, Abbasi S. Heated, humidified high-flow nasal cannula versus nasal CPAP for respiratory support in neonates. Pediatrics. 2013;131:e1482–90.

24. Essouri S, Nicot F, Clement A, Garabedian E-N, Roger G, Lofaso F, Fauroux B. Noninvasive positive pressure ventilation in infants with upper airway obstruction: comparison of continuous and bilevel positive pressure. Intensive Care Med. 2005;31:574–80.

25. O'Donnell C, Kamlin C, Davis P, Morley C. Neonatal resuscitation 1: a model to measure inspired and expired tidal volumes and assess leakage at the face mask. Arch Dis Child Fetal Neonatal Ed. 2005;90:F388–91.

26. Beck J, Reilly M, Grasselli G, Mirabella L, Slutsky AS, Dunn MS, Sinderby C. Patient-ventilator interaction during neurally adjusted ventilatory assist in low birth weight infants. Pediatr Res. 2009;65:663–8.

27. Shaffer TH, Alapati D, Greenspan JS, Wolfson MR. Neonatal non-invasive respiratory support: physiological implications. Pediatr Pulmonol. 2012;47:837 47.

28. Palme C, Nystrom B, Tunell R. An evaluation of the efficiency of face masks in the resuscitation of newborn infants. Lancet. 1985;1:207–10.

29. Milner AD, Vyas H, Hopkin IE. Efficacy of facemask resuscitation at birth. Br Med J. 1984;289:1563–5.

30. Field D, Milner AD, Hopkin IE. Efficiency of manual resuscitators at birth. Arch Dis Child. 1986;61:300–2.

31. Hoskyns EW, Milner AD, Hopkin IE. A simple method of face mask resuscitation at birth. Arch Dis Child. 1987;62:376–8.

Anti-fibrotic effects of pirfenidone and rapamycin in primary IPF fibroblasts and human alveolar epithelial cells

M. Molina-Molina[1,2,3], C. Machahua-Huamani[2], V. Vicens-Zygmunt[1,2], R. Llatjós[4], I. Escobar[5], E. Sala-Llinas[3,7], P. Luburich-Hernaiz[6], J. Dorca[1,2,3] and A. Montes-Worboys[1,2,3,8*]

Abstract

Background: Pirfenidone, a pleiotropic anti-fibrotic treatment, has been shown to slow down disease progression of idiopathic pulmonary fibrosis (IPF), a fatal and devastating lung disease. Rapamycin, an inhibitor of fibroblast proliferation could be a potential anti-fibrotic drug to improve the effects of pirfenidone.

Methods: Primary lung fibroblasts from IPF patients and human alveolar epithelial cells (A549) were treated in vitro with pirfenidone and rapamycin in the presence or absence of transforming growth factor β1 (TGF−β). Extracellular matrix protein and gene expression of markers involved in lung fibrosis (tenascin-c, fibronectin, collagen I [COL1A1], collagen III [COL3A1] and α-smooth muscle actin [α-SMA]) were analyzed. A cell migration assay in pirfenidone, rapamycin and TGF−β-containing media was performed.

Results: Gene and protein expression of tenascin-c and fibronectin of fibrotic fibroblasts were reduced by pirfenidone or rapamycin treatment. Pirfenidone-rapamycin treatment did not revert the epithelial to mesenchymal transition pathway activated by TGF−β. However, the drug combination significantly abrogated fibroblast to myofibroblast transition. The inhibitory effect of pirfenidone on fibroblast migration in the scratch-wound assay was potentiated by rapamycin combination.

Conclusions: These findings indicate that the combination of pirfenidone and rapamycin widen the inhibition range of fibrogenic markers and prevents fibroblast migration. These results would open a new line of research for an anti-fibrotic combination therapeutic approach.

Keywords: Pirfenidone, Rapamycin, Idiopathic pulmonary fibrosis, Pulmonary fibrosis, Cell migration, Extracellular matrix proteins, Epithelial-mesenchymal transition

Background

Idiopathic pulmonary fibrosis (IPF) is the most common and deadly form of idiopathic interstitial pneumonia. The mortality from diagnosis is estimated between 3 and 5 years, and onset of the disease usually occurs in elderly adults [1]. The pathogenic mechanisms are still unclear; however, recent studies agree that the disease is the result of abnormal wound healing in response to micro-injuries of the alveolar epithelium. The activated alveolar epithelial cells cause the migration, proliferation, and activation of mesenchymal cells with the formation of myofibroblast foci [2]. The myofibroblasts secrete excessive amounts of extracellular matrix (ECM) proteins, including tenascin-c, fibronectin and collagens, with the subsequent distortion of lung homoeostasis and architecture [1, 3]. These changes in the ECM composition besides an increase in cytokines and growth factors, such as transforming growth factor (TGF)−β, contribute to IPF progression [2].

Over the past decade, growing evidence has demonstrated the clinical benefits of anti-fibrotic treatment in IPF, and two anti-fibrotic drugs are now recommended in patients in the mild-moderate stage of the disease [4].

* Correspondence: amontesw@idibell.cat
[1]Department of Pneumology, Bellvitge University Hospital, Barcelona, Spain
[2]Pneumology Research Group, IDIBELL, University of Barcelona, Barcelona, Spain

In particular, pirfenidone (5-methyl-1-phenyl-2-[1H]-pyri-done) has been shown to slow down the decline in FVC. [5, 6]. Pirfenidone is a pleiotropic molecule that inhibits TGF–β, collagen synthesis, and fibroblast proliferation, and mediates tissue repair [7–12]. The anti-fibrotic activity and safety of this novel agent has been established in lung, liver and kidney tissue [13]. Several molecular mechanisms responsible for the anti-fibrotic action of pirfenidone are still under study. The current clinical objective in IPF treatment is to inhibit disease progression with anti-fibrotic therapy [14], and the current research objective is to find an anti-fibrotic capable of completely halting or abrogate fibrosis. In this context, the in vitro anti-fibrotic effect of drug combinations, together with the safety profile of this therapeutic approach, should be explored in future clinical trials.

Rapamycin, an inhibitor of mammalian target of rapamycin (mTOR)-mediated and a potent anti-proliferative drug, was initially introduced into clinical practice to prevent transplant rejection and later to treat mTOR diseases such as lymphangioleiomiomatosis (LAM) [15, 16]. Rapamycin presents some metabolic and bioavailability differences with other analogs such as everolimus [17]. All the rapalogs are structurally similar to rapamycin differing mainly at a single position of the lactone ring (C-40) [17]. Although everolimus exhibits greater polarity than rapamycin, the bioavailability is only slightly improved and is still relatively low. There are differences in the half-life, potentially affecting the optimal dosing schedules [17]. More recently, the potent anti-fibrogenic action of rapamycin has been demonstrated in animal models of hepatic [18], renal [19], and pulmonary fibrosis [20]. The anti-fibrotic effects of rapamycin in human lung fibroblasts are mediated by a decrease in collagen synthesis (COL1A1, COL1A2, and COL3A1) [20, 21]. Thus, it has been suggested as a new anti-fibrotic pathway to explore in pulmonary fibrosis [22] and is being tested in clinical trials.

Currently, the efforts of the scientific community are focused on the search for anti-fibrotic strategies that stop the abnormal repair process that leads to fibrosis and dysfunction of the lung tissue in order to avoid the progression of this devastating disease. Within this framework, it is essential to find novel agents or combinations of anti-fibrotic therapies. In this study, we aim to elucidate the role of pirfenidone and rapamycin as a new therapeutic approach for the treatment of lung fibrosis by analyzing first their anti-fibrotic potential in vitro as a primary step.

Methods

Isolation of human lung fibroblasts

Adult human lung fibroblasts were obtained from lung biopsies of six different IPF patients who underwent surgical biopsy for the diagnosis of the disease (histologically confirmed usual interstitial pneumonia). The harvested lung tissue samples were maintained in DMEM high Glucose with L-Glutamine (Gibco Life Technologies) medium with HEPES (Sigma-Aldrich, St Louis, MO, USA) and insulin human transferrin and sodium selenite (ITS) (Sigma-Aldrich) until processing. Then cut into small pieces, and placed into 6 well plates (Nunc Thermo Scientific, Waltham, MA, USA) with growth medium; DMEM supplemented with 10% fetal bovine serum (FBS, Gibco Life Technologies), penicillin (100 U/ml)/streptomycin (100 μg/ml) solution (Gibco Life Technologies) and 25 μg/ml amphotericin B (Sigma-Aldrich). Cells were cultured at 37 °C in a humidified atmosphere of 5% CO_2. Spindle-like primary fibroblasts started to grow separately from tissue samples on day 2 to 3. Outgrowth of fibroblasts took 1 to 2 weeks. Tissue samples were then removed by aspiration, and cells were allowed to reach confluence. Fibroblasts at confluence were expanded by trypsinization and passaged every 4 to 5 days at 1:4 ratio. Pulmonary fibroblasts were identified by the typical spindle morphology and immunohistochemistry; vimentin and α-smooth muscle actin (α-SMA) positive, and factor VIII and surfactant C-negative staining. Cells between passage numbers 4 and 7 were used in this study.

Cell line culture

Bronchial-alveolar epithelial human cells (A549) were purchased from the American Type Culture Collection (ATCC CRM-CCL-185, Manassas, VA, USA) and cultured in F12 K (Gibco Life Technologies, Grand Island, NY, USA) medium supplemented with 10% FBS (Gibco Life Technologies) and penicillin (100 U/ml) / streptomycin (100 μg/ml) solution (Gibco Life Technologies) according to the manufacturer's recommendations. Cells were maintained at 37 °C in a humidified 5% CO_2 atmosphere.

Cell viability assay

Cell viability was evaluated using a commercial colorimetric assay (Quick Cell Proliferation Assay Kit II. MBL, International Corporation, Woburn, MA, USA) according to the recommended protocol. Briefly, cells (5×10^4/well) were cultured in a 96-well microtiter plate (Nunc Thermo Scientific) and treated with pirfenidone (Hoffmann-La Roche) (1 mg/ml), and rapamycin (Sigma-Aldrich) (1 μg/ml), and the combination of both agents in the presence of TGF–β (5 ng/ml) in a final volume of 100 μl/well of 2% FBS culture medium in triplicates for 72 h. Then, 10 μl/well of WST reagent was added and plates were incubated for 2 h at 37 °C in standard culture conditions. After shaking the plates for 1 min, the absorbance was computed at a wavelength of 450 nm in each well using a microplate reader (Thermo Scientific) with 650 nm of reference wavelength. The amount of the dye generated by activity of dehydrogenase is directly proportional to the number of living cells.

Cell culture stimulation

Human lung primary fibroblasts and A549 cell line were cultured in 6 well plates (Nunc Thermo Scientific) in the appropriated medium with 10% FBS; when cells reached 80% confluence the medium was changed at 2% FBS. Cells were stimulated with activated TGF–β (5 ng/ml) (R&D Systems Minneapolis, MN, USA), in the presence of pirfenidone (1 mg/ml) and rapamycin (1 μg/ml) during 72 h. Besides, we stimulated cells with a combination of rapamycin and pirfenidone without TGF–β, rapamycin with TGF–β, pirfenidone with TGF–β and rapamycin, pirfenidone and TGF–β. After the incubation period, cells and supernatants were collected, separated by centrifugation and frozen for further analysis. Doses of pirfenidone and rapamycin were chosen based on previous reported studies [7, 9, 23–27] and our results from the cell viability assay.

Western blot assay

Cells were grown in 6-well plates (Nunc) and incubated with TGF–β (5 ng/ml), pirfenidone (1 mg/ml) and rapamycin (1 μg/ml) for 72 h at 37 °C. Cells were then lysed in Radio-Immunoprecipitation Assay (RIPA) Buffer (25 mM Tris-HCl, 150 mM NaCl, 1% NP-40, 0.1% sodium deoxycholate SDS) containing 1:100 phenylmethylsulfonyl fluoride and phosphatase inhibitors (Sigma-Aldrich). The final protein concentrations were determined with a bicinchoninic acid (BCA) method (Thermo Scientific) according to the manufacturer's specifications. Prepared samples were heated to 100 °C for 5 min; for each sample the same amount of total protein (20–30 μg) was added to a well of 4–15% mini-protean TGX precast gels polyacrylamide gel (Bio-Rad Hercules, CA, USA) and resolved by SDS-PAGE. The separated proteins were transferred to a nitrocellulose membrane (Bio-Rad). The membranes were blocked for 1 h in Tris-buffered saline (10 mM Tris-HCl pH 7.5 and 0.15 M NaCl) containing 0.1% (v/v) Tween 20 and 5% (w/v) bovine serum albumin (BSA) (Sigma-Aldrich), and then probed at room temperature (RT) for 1 h with primary antibodies against human tenascin-C (diluted 1:500; Abcam, Cambridge, UK #ab3970), human E-cadherin (diluted 1:2000, Abcam #ab76055), human EDA-fibronectin (diluted 1:400, Abcam #ab6328), human collagen I (diluted 1:200 Abcam #ab88147), human collagen III (diluted 1:500 Abcam #ab6310) human α-SMA (diluted 1:1000, Sigma #A5228), human α-tubulin (diluted 1:5000, Sigma Aldrich # T6199), human vinculin (diluted 1:5000, Abcam #ab129002) and human β-actin (diluted 1:5000, Sigma #A1978). Immunoreactive bands were detected with IgG horseradish peroxidase-conjugated secondary antibodies (anti-mouse

diluted 1:1000; and anti-rabbit diluted 1:1000) (Dako, Glostrup, Denmark) and visualized by enhance chemiluminescence detection reagents ECL Western blotting kit (Bio-Rad) according to the manufacturer's instructions in a luminescent image analyzer (LAS 3000 Fujifilm) and were then scanned for densitometry analysis (Multi Gauge software, Fujifilm). Results were expressed as a ratio of band density to total β-actin, vinculin or α-tubulin.

RNA extraction and real-time polymerase chain reaction (RT-PCR)

Total RNA was isolated from cultured cells, after treatment with TGF–β, pirfenidone and rapamycin following the same protocol explained above, using the Qiagen RNeasy Mini Kit (Qiagen, Valencia, CA, USA) according to the manufacturer's recommendations. Samples were digested with DNase I (Qiagen) to remove contaminating genomic DNA. RNA concentration and purity of each sample were measured using UV spectrophotometry. A total of 1 μg of RNA was reverse-transcribed using the iScript cDNA synthesis kit (Bio Rad) with oligo deoxythymidine and random hexamer primers. The reverse transcriptase reaction proceeded in a total volume of 20 μl in a conventional thermal cycler (Bio-Rad) at 25 °C for 5 min, followed by 30 min at 42 °C and 5 min at 85 °C. Reaction volumes of 20 μl were placed in 384-well optical reaction plates with adhesive covers (ABI Prism™ Applied Biosystems, Foster City, CA, USA) using SYBR Green PCR Master Mix and specific sequence primers (Sigma). Glyceraldehyde-3-phosphate dehydrogenase (GADPH) mRNA amplified from the same samples served as the internal control. Samples were heated to 95 °C for 10 min and then PCR amplification was achieved by 40 cycles at 95 °C for 15 s and 60 °C for 1 min using the ABI Prism 7900 (Applied Biosystems). The relative expression of each targeted gene was normalized by subtracting the corresponding housekeeping genes (β-actin, GADPH, HPRT and RNA18s) threshold cycle (Ct) value using the comparative CT method ($\Delta\Delta C_t$ methods).

Cell migration assay

Cell migration was monitored from a confluent area to an area that was mechanically denuded of cells (scratch-wound assay). Cells were grown in 6-well plates (Nunc) to a confluent monolayer and then serum-deprived for 24 h. After the medium was discarded, a scratch was created in a straight line across the cells with a p20 pipette tip. The plates were then rinsed with phosphate buffered saline (PBS) to remove the suspended cells and incubated with the specific media supplemented with TGF–β (5 ng/ml), pirfenidone (1 mg/ml), rapamycin (1 μg/ml) or the combination of the three agents. Twenty-four and 72 h after the treatment, cells were monitored and photographed under a light microscope, and the distance cover by the cells in the wound closure was analyzed with Image J software (https://imagej.nih.gov/ij/ National Institute of Health NIH, Bethesda, MD, USA). Cells treated with drug-free medium were considered as controls.

Statistical analysis

All results are expressed as mean ± SEM of independent experiments. Statistical analysis was performed in Graph Pad Prism 5.01 (Graph Pad Software, San Diego, CA, USA). Significance is indicated as follows: $*p < 0.05$, $**p < 0.01$, $***p < 0.001$. * indicates the comparison between samples treated with TGF–β and all the other conditions: TGF–β versus untreated samples (control); TGF–β versus rapamycin and pirfenidone (rapa/pirfe); and samples treated with TGF–β in combination with rapamycin (TGF–β/rapa); pirfenidone (TGF–β/pirfe) or both (TGF–β/rapa/pirfe). $^{\#}p < 0.05$, $^{\#\#}p < 0.01$, $^{\#\#\#}p < 0.001$. # indicates significant differences between control versus samples treated with rapamycin and pirfenidone in absence of TGF–β.

Results

Pirfenidone and rapamycin are well tolerated by human lung fibroblasts and alveolar epithelial cells

Cell viability was assayed with the WST reagent in fibroblasts and A549 cells cultured in 96-well plates and treated with TGF–β (5 ng/ml), pirfenidone (1 mg/ml) and rapamycin (1 µg/ml) for 72 h. The cell toxicity assay demonstrated that pirfenidone and rapamycin, in addition to the combination of the 2 agents with TGF–β (5 ng/ml), did not cause cellular death when compared to untreated cells (control) and were well tolerated for the treatment period of 72 h (Fig. 1). We then selected the doses of 1 mg/ml for pirfenidone, in accordance with the results obtained by other Groups [7, 9, 23–27], 1 µg/ml rapamycin and 5 ng/ml of TGF–β to be used in the following studies for a treatment period of 72 h.

Pirfenidone and rapamycin treatment inhibits ECM protein expression in lung fibrotic fibroblasts

Fibroblasts were obtained from IPF patients submitted to lung biopsies for the diagnosis of interstitial disease. After the cultures were established, we stimulated the cells with TGF–β (5 ng/ml), pirfenidone (1 mg/ml) and rapamycin (1 µg/ml). Besides the treatment of rapamycin and pirfenidone without TGF–β, rapamycin alone with TGF–β, pirfenidone alone with TGF–β and the combination of rapamycin and pirfenidone with TGF–β for 72 h. Western blot and RT-PCR were performed to analyze the protein and gene expression of the different markers involved in the fibrotic process.

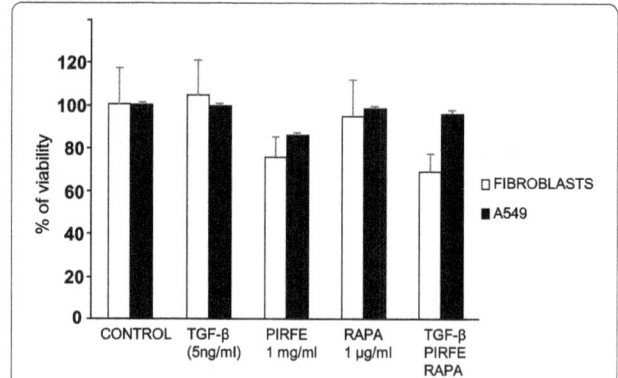

Fig. 1 Effect of TGF–β, pirfenidone and rapamycin on the viability of lung primary fibroblasts and A549 cells. Primary lung fibroblasts and bronchial epithelial human cells (A549) were incubated with pirfenidone (1 mg/ml) and rapamycin (1 µg/ml) in addition to the combination of the two agents with TGF–β (5 ng/ml) for 72 h, viability was measured with the WST reagent. No significant cytotoxic effect was observed for any combinatory treatments. The bars represent the mean values ± SEM of viability % related to control samples in three different experiments

We observed a significant decrease in tenascin-c, and collagen III when cells were incubated with pirfenidone or rapamycin.

Tenascin-c

Previous studies conducted by our Group [28] and others [29] have shown a clear induction of tenascin-c in the fibrotic fibroblasts from IPF patients compared to other interstitial diseases. We wanted to test the effect of pirfenidone and rapamycin on tenascin-c in lung fibroblasts from IPF patients treated with the pro-fibrotic factor TGF–β. As shown in Fig. 2a, b, we found clear inhibition of protein and gene expression levels when cells were treated with both drugs. The response of the treatment in the presence of TGF–β were clearer in both the gene expression analysis and the protein level. However, the effect was likely mediated by rapamycin. Furthermore, the incubation with pirfenidone and rapamycin in absence of TGF–β resulted in a significant decrease of tenascin-c, as compared control cells with rapamycin-pirfenidone treatment.

Fibronectin

Another component of the ECM that plays an important role in the maintenance of lung homeostasis and wound healing is fibronectin (FN). Due to its implication in the development of pulmonary fibrosis and its pro-fibrotic role in IPF, we analyzed the protein and gene expression of FN in lung fibroblasts. As shown in Fig. 2c, we observed a significant increase of protein level in TGF–β stimulated fibroblasts when compared to the control. However, we found a non-significant reduction in the FN protein expression when cells were incubated with pirfenidone and rapamycin. The gene expression of

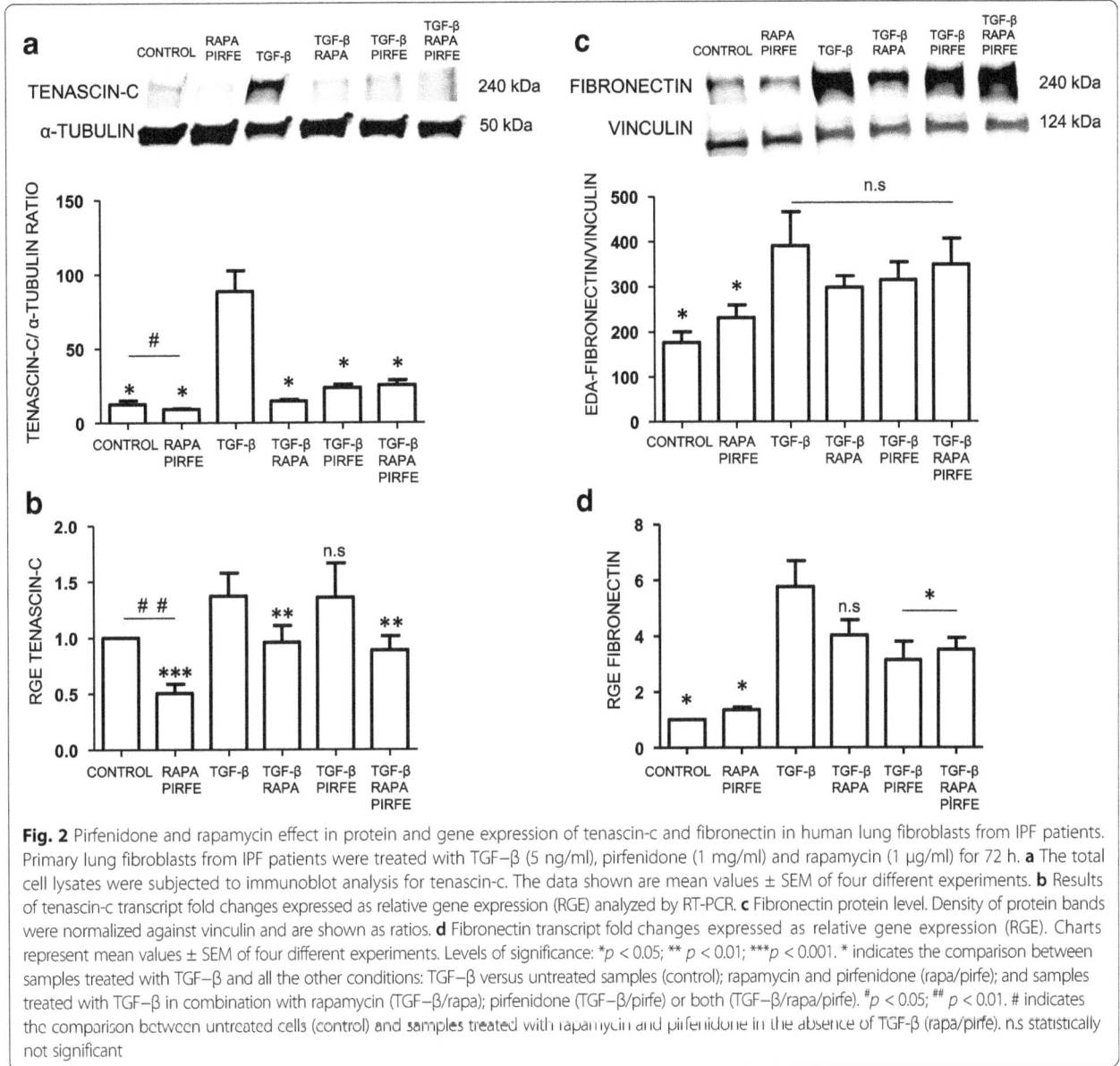

Fig. 2 Pirfenidone and rapamycin effect in protein and gene expression of tenascin-c and fibronectin in human lung fibroblasts from IPF patients. Primary lung fibroblasts from IPF patients were treated with TGF–β (5 ng/ml), pirfenidone (1 mg/ml) and rapamycin (1 μg/ml) for 72 h. **a** The total cell lysates were subjected to immunoblot analysis for tenascin-c. The data shown are mean values ± SEM of four different experiments. **b** Results of tenascin-c transcript fold changes expressed as relative gene expression (RGE) analyzed by RT-PCR. **c** Fibronectin protein level. Density of protein bands were normalized against vinculin and are shown as ratios. **d** Fibronectin transcript fold changes expressed as relative gene expression (RGE). Charts represent mean values ± SEM of four different experiments. Levels of significance: *$p < 0.05$; ** $p < 0.01$; ***$p < 0.001$. * indicates the comparison between samples treated with TGF–β and all the other conditions: TGF–β versus untreated samples (control); rapamycin and pirfenidone (rapa/pirfe); and samples treated with TGF–β in combination with rapamycin (TGF–β/rapa); pirfenidone (TGF–β/pirfe) or both (TGF–β/rapa/pirfe). #$p < 0.05$; ## $p < 0.01$. # indicates the comparison between untreated cells (control) and samples treated with rapamycin and pirfenidone in the absence of TGF–β (rapa/pirfe). n.s statistically not significant

fibronectin induced by TGF–β was clearly inhibited by the combination of pirfenidone and rapamycin, but the effect might likely be due to the action of pirfenidone (Fig. 2d). Moreover, when cells were stimulated with rapamycin and pirfenidone in absence of TGF–β we observed a slight increase of protein and gene expression of fibronectin but this was not statistically significant.

Collagen type I and III

The overexpression of collagen in fibrotic lungs has been shown to be a key factor in tissue dysfunction. Following the same protocol, we analyzed the levels of collagen type I (COL1A1) and collagen type III (COL3A1) in lung fibroblasts when they were stimulated with TGF–β,

pirfenidone and rapamycin for 72 h. The combination of pirfenidone and rapamycin with or without TGF–β did not alter the high basal levels of COL1A1 protein expression in fibroblasts from IPF patients. This high level of protein expression in control samples could due to the fibroblasts´ origin from fibrotic lung areas. On the other hand, levels of COL3A1 protein were inhibited by the treatment of rapamycin and pirfenidone in the presence of TGF–β. Furthermore, the gene expression of both collagen-I and III after treatment with TGF–β was abolished by pirfenidone or rapamycin, the most definitive response to the combined treatment of pirfenidone and rapamycin after TGF–β was found in collagen III (Fig. 3a, b, c, d).

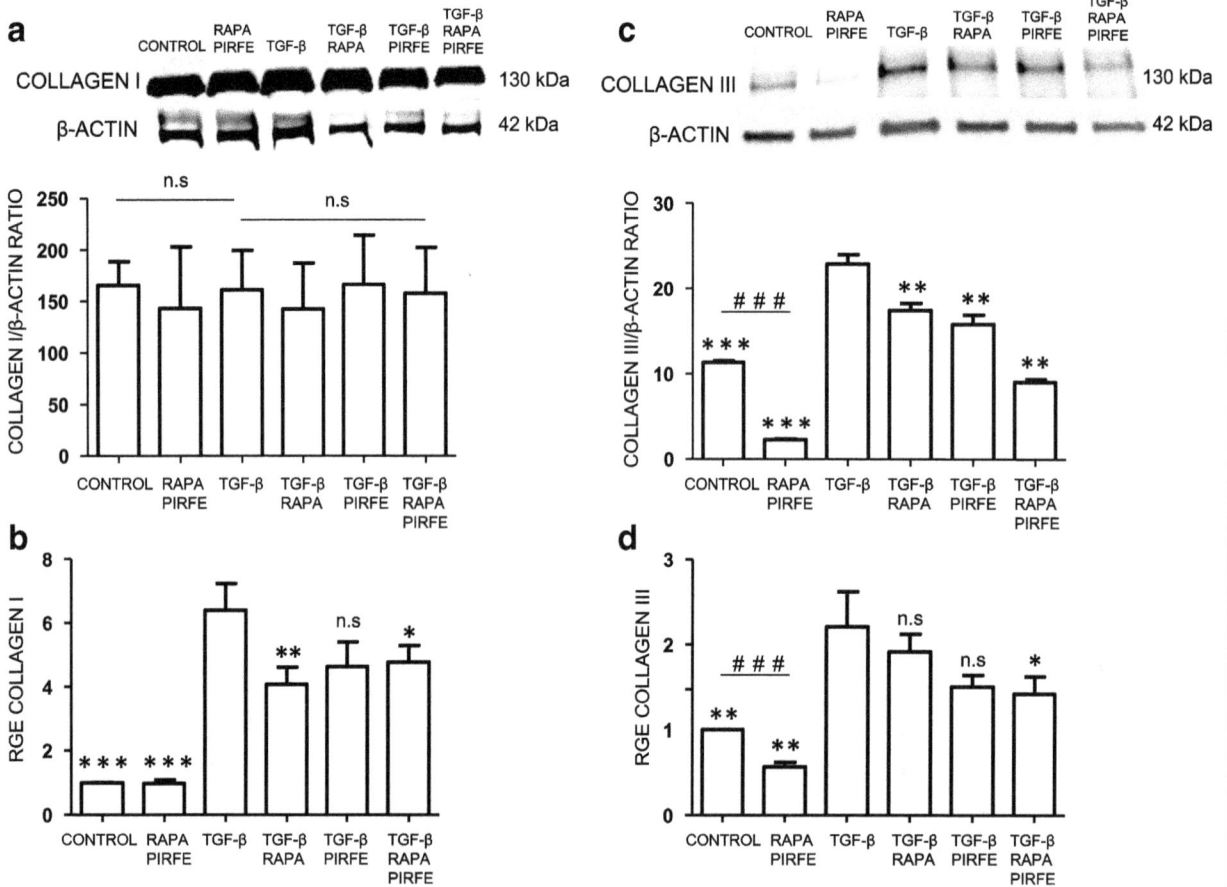

Fig. 3 Collagen I and III gene expression are decreased by pirfenidone and rapamycin, while only the protein expression level of collagen III is inhibited by pirfenidone and rapamycin. Primary lung fibroblasts from IPF patients were treated with TGF–β (5 ng/ml), pirfenidone (1 mg/ml) and rapamycin (1 μg/ml) for 72 h. **a** Densitometric analysis expressed as mean ± SEM and a representative blot showing the unchanged effect in COL1A1 levels by pirfenidone and rapamycin. **b** COL1A1 gene expression measured by RT-PCR was decreased by pirfenidone and rapamycin in IPF fibroblasts. Bars represent mean ± SEM values of the transcript fold changes expressed by relative gene expression (RGE) of four different experiments. **c** COL3A1 protein expression decreases with the combination treatment of rapamycin and pirfenidone. Bars expressed as mean ± SEM values. Treated samples with rapamycin and pirfenidone in the absence of TGF–β show a significant decrease of the protein compare to controls. **d** COL3A1 gene expression showing a significant decrease when cells were treated with rapamycin and pirfenidone combination treatment. Levels of significance: *$p < 0.05$; ** $p < 0.01$; ***$p < 0.001$. * indicates the comparison between samples treated with TGF–β and all the other conditions: TGF–β versus untreated samples (control); rapamycin and pirfenidone (rapa/pirfe); and samples treated with TGF–β in combination with rapamycin (TGF–β/rapa); pirfenidone (TGF–β/pirfe) or both (TGF–β/rapa/pirfe). ### $p < 0.001$. # indicates the comparison between untreated cells (control) and samples treated with rapamycin and pirfenidone (rapa/pirfe). n.s statistically not significant

The fibroblast to myofibroblast transition is inhibited by pirfenidone and rapamycin treatment combination

We studied the gene and protein expression of α-SMA as an indicator for fibroblast transformation into fibrotic active myofibroblasts. As expected, fibroblasts from fibrotic lungs showed a high protein expression of α-SMA, and the treatment with TGF–β increased α-SMA gene expression (Fig. 4a, b). This increase was significantly reduced with the treatment of pirfenidone and rapamycin, although pirfenidone alone had a clearer inhibitory effect. Interestingly, cells treated with both drugs in the absence of TGF–β also showed a significant decrease of α-SMA levels when compared to control samples. These results suggest that the transformation

of fibroblasts to myofibroblasts in IPF fibroblasts is inhibited by pirfenidone and rapamycin, but the effect was mainly due to the action of pirfenidone.

Pirfenidone and rapamycin treatment prevent fibroblast migration

We performed the scratch assay with primary lung fibroblasts from IPF patients. After the scar, cells were treated with TGF–β (5 ng/ml), pirfenidone (1 mg/ml), rapamycin (1 μg/ml) and the combination of all three agents for 24 and 72 h with the medium supplemented with 2% and 10% of FBS, as explained above. The cell migration assay, analyzed with Image J software, showed a decreased number of migrated cells after a scratch wound

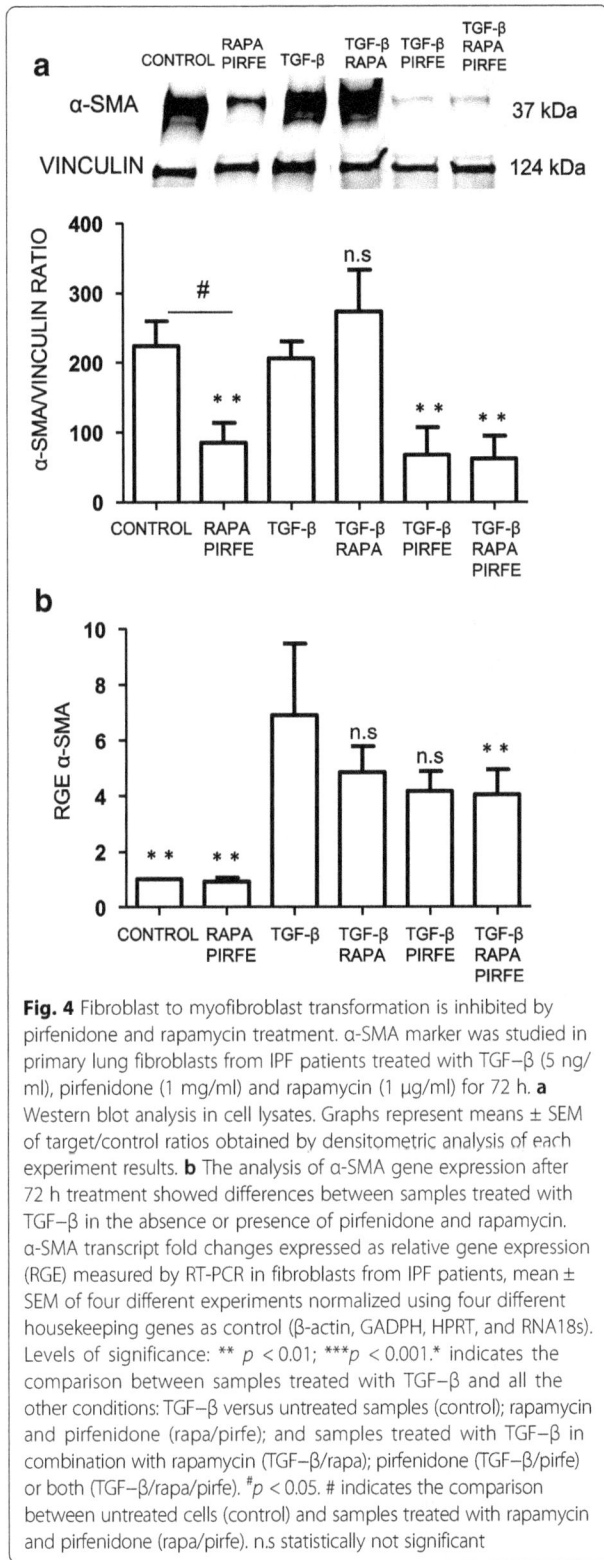

Fig. 4 Fibroblast to myofibroblast transformation is inhibited by pirfenidone and rapamycin treatment. α-SMA marker was studied in primary lung fibroblasts from IPF patients treated with TGF−β (5 ng/ml), pirfenidone (1 mg/ml) and rapamycin (1 μg/ml) for 72 h. **a** Western blot analysis in cell lysates. Graphs represent means ± SEM of target/control ratios obtained by densitometric analysis of each experiment results. **b** The analysis of α-SMA gene expression after 72 h treatment showed differences between samples treated with TGF−β in the absence or presence of pirfenidone and rapamycin. α-SMA transcript fold changes expressed as relative gene expression (RGE) measured by RT-PCR in fibroblasts from IPF patients, mean ± SEM of four different experiments normalized using four different housekeeping genes as control (β-actin, GADPH, HPRT, and RNA18s). Levels of significance: ** $p < 0.01$; ***$p < 0.001$.* indicates the comparison between samples treated with TGF−β and all the other conditions: TGF−β versus untreated samples (control); rapamycin and pirfenidone (rapa/pirfe); and samples treated with TGF−β in combination with rapamycin (TGF−β/rapa); pirfenidone (TGF−β/pirfe) or both (TGF−β/rapa/pirfe). #$p < 0.05$. # indicates the comparison between untreated cells (control) and samples treated with rapamycin and pirfenidone (rapa/pirfe). n.s statistically not significant

was made across the cells and treated with pirfenidone and rapamycin or the combination of both agents when compared with untreated cells or cells stimulated with only TGF−β. In control and TGF−β treated samples,

fibroblasts filled the scratch as early as 24 h after the start of incubation. In contrast, when cells were treated with pirfenidone and rapamycin, the migration took up to 72 h. The same protocol was repeated in a culture medium supplemented with 2% (Fig. 5a) and 10% (Fig. 5b) FBS to ensure that the FBS was not interfering with the migration process in control and treated cells. As shown in the graph, the same motility pattern was observed with the different concentrations of FBS assayed.

Pirfenidone and rapamycin inhibit the synthesis of pro-fibrotic markers induced by TGF-β in alveolar epithelial cells

In order to study the effect of pirfenidone and rapamycin in lung epithelium, we conducted the same protocol explained above for primary fibroblasts with A549 cells. Culture cells were incubated with TGF−β (5 ng/ml), pirfenidone (1 mg/ml) and rapamycin (1 μg/ml) for 72 h, and after the incubation period, cells were collected and total RNA and protein were extracted.

Tenascin-c

The tenascin-c levels from A549 cells incubated with TGF−β, pirfenidone and rapamycin for 72 h were analyzed western blot and RT-PCR. We found a significant decrease of tenascin-c in cells incubated with pirfenidone and rapamycin in absence of TGF−β. However, there was only a slight decrease of tenascin-c level in cells treated with rapamycin after TGF−β, indicating the role of this drug in inhibiting the protein expression of this ECM protein. (Fig. 6a, b).

Fibronectin

We analyzed the protein expression of FN in A549 cells. Western blot indicated that treatment with pirfenidone and rapamycin decreased the induced FN protein levels (Fig. 6c), and treatment with both drugs alone resulted in a partial inhibition of FN. Moreover, when FN transcript was analyzed by RT-PCR, we found that pirfenidone and rapamycin combined treatment reduced the increased levels induced by TGF−β, although the difference did not reach statistical significance (Fig. 6d), supporting the results obtained in the protein expression analysis.

Collagen type I and III

We also examined the effect of pirfenidone and rapamycin treatment in the synthesis of collagen when alveolar epithelial cells were stimulated with TGF−β. We observed an increase of COL1A1 and COL3A1 protein with TGF−β that was inhibited by the presence of pirfenidone and rapamycin, but the addition of both drugs did result in a lower decrease of only the collagen type III protein (Fig. 7a, c). We then studied the gene expression of COL1A1 and COL3A1 in

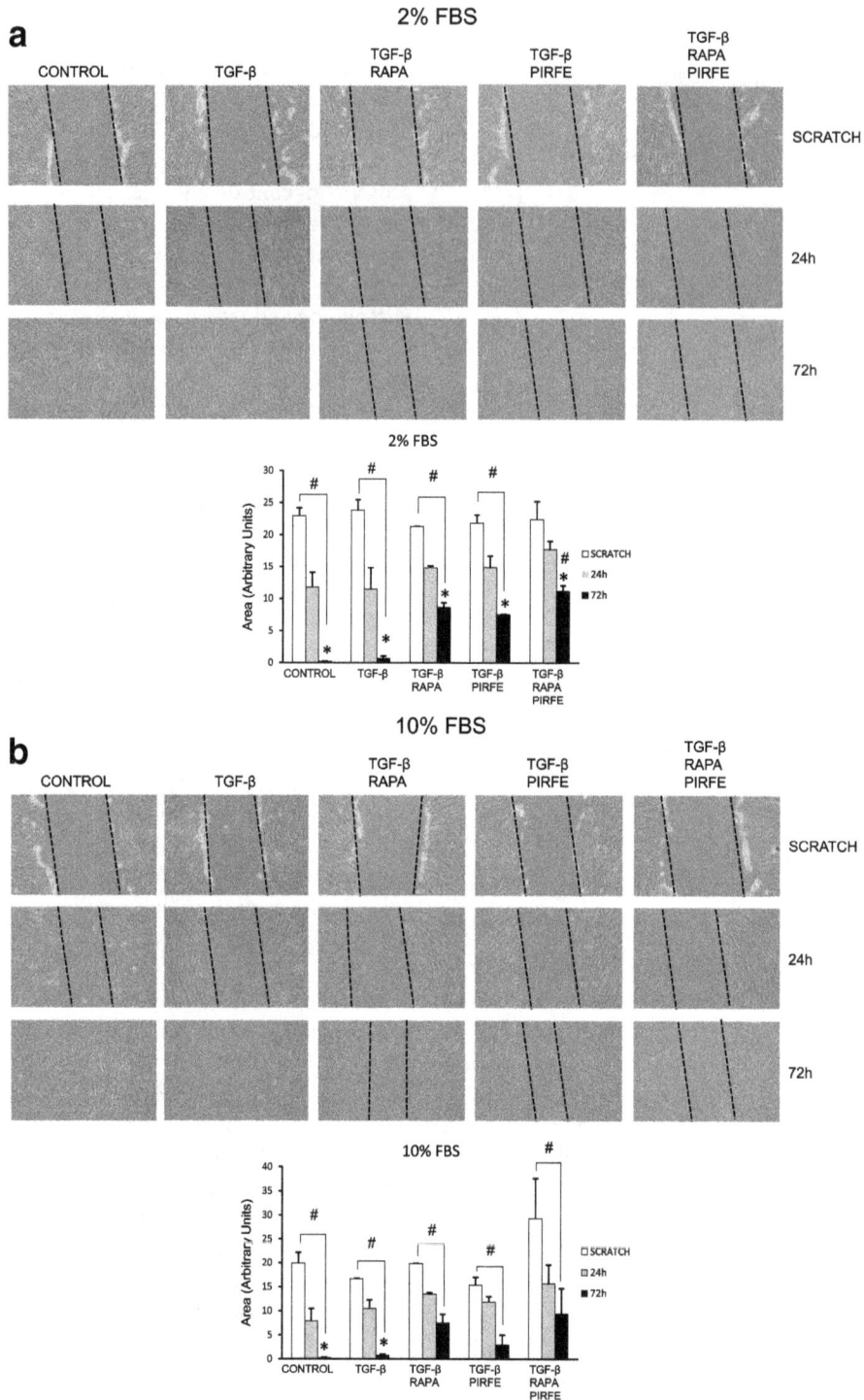

Fig. 5 Pirfenidone and rapamycin inhibited the TGF–β-induced migration of human IPF lung fibroblasts. Cell migration assay were performed in fibroblasts from IPF patients incubated with TGF–β (5 ng/ml), rapamycin (1 µg/ml) and pirfenidone (1 mg/ml). Images show that cell migration occurred within 72 h from culture scratch in medium containing 2% (**a**) and 10% (**b**) fetal bovine serum (FBS) in the presence of TGF–β, combination of TGF–β and rapamycin, TGF–β and pirfenidone, and the combination of TGF–β, rapamycin and pirfenidone. The uncovered area has been quantified by the ImageJ Software at each time point and represented in the graphs as mean values ± SEM of three different experiments. Magnification, 100X. Levels of significance; * indicates the statistical significance between all conditions assayed at 72 h time point. # indicates the significance between scratch and 24 and 72 h time points for each treatment conditions

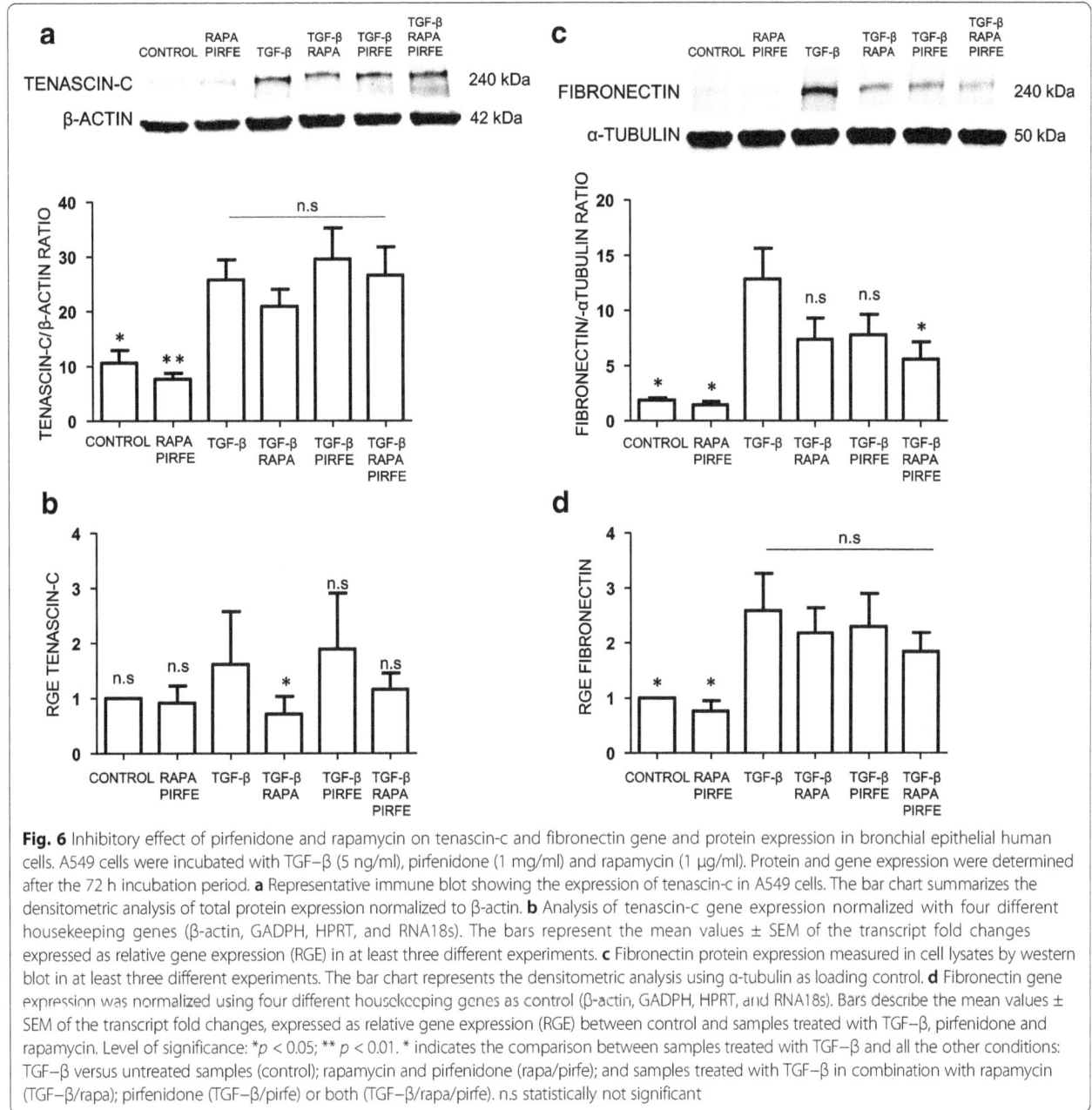

Fig. 6 Inhibitory effect of pirfenidone and rapamycin on tenascin-c and fibronectin gene and protein expression in bronchial epithelial human cells. A549 cells were incubated with TGF–β (5 ng/ml), pirfenidone (1 mg/ml) and rapamycin (1 μg/ml). Protein and gene expression were determined after the 72 h incubation period. **a** Representative immune blot showing the expression of tenascin-c in A549 cells. The bar chart summarizes the densitometric analysis of total protein expression normalized to β-actin. **b** Analysis of tenascin-c gene expression normalized with four different housekeeping genes (β-actin, GADPH, HPRT, and RNA18s). The bars represent the mean values ± SEM of the transcript fold changes expressed as relative gene expression (RGE) in at least three different experiments. **c** Fibronectin protein expression measured in cell lysates by western blot in at least three different experiments. The bar chart represents the densitometric analysis using α-tubulin as loading control. **d** Fibronectin gene expression was normalized using four different housekeeping genes as control (β-actin, GADPH, HPRT, and RNA18s). Bars describe the mean values ± SEM of the transcript fold changes, expressed as relative gene expression (RGE) between control and samples treated with TGF–β, pirfenidone and rapamycin. Level of significance: *$p < 0.05$; ** $p < 0.01$. * indicates the comparison between samples treated with TGF–β and all the other conditions: TGF–β versus untreated samples (control); rapamycin and pirfenidone (rapa/pirfe); and samples treated with TGF–β in combination with rapamycin (TGF–β/rapa); pirfenidone (TGF–β/pirfe) or both (TGF–β/rapa/pirfe). n.s statistically not significant

the same samples, and found that both genes increased their expression with TGF–β after 72 h of treatment. Pirfenidone and rapamycin combination significantly inhibited the collagen type III transcript induced by TGF–β (Fig. 7b, d).

Pirfenidone and rapamycin treatment does not revert the epithelial to mesenchymal transition (EMT) pathway activated by TGF–β in A549 cells

To gain deeper insight into the role of the combination pirfenidone and rapamycin treatment in the inhibition of the EMT pathway activated by TGF–β, E-cadherin marker was studied in A549 cells after 72 h of treatment with TGF–β and both drugs.

E-cadherin

When the epithelial cell marker E-cadherin was analyzed, we observed that TGF–β inhibited the synthesis of both protein and gene expression, indicating an activation of EMT in A549 cells. Treatment with pirfenidone and rapamycin alone did not significantly affect the E-cadherin expression. However, the effect of these drugs in combination with TGF–β failed to recover the synthesis level of E-cadherin (Fig. 8a, b).

Discussion

Pirfenidone is currently one of the primary choices for the treatment of IPF in clinical practice, however, it does

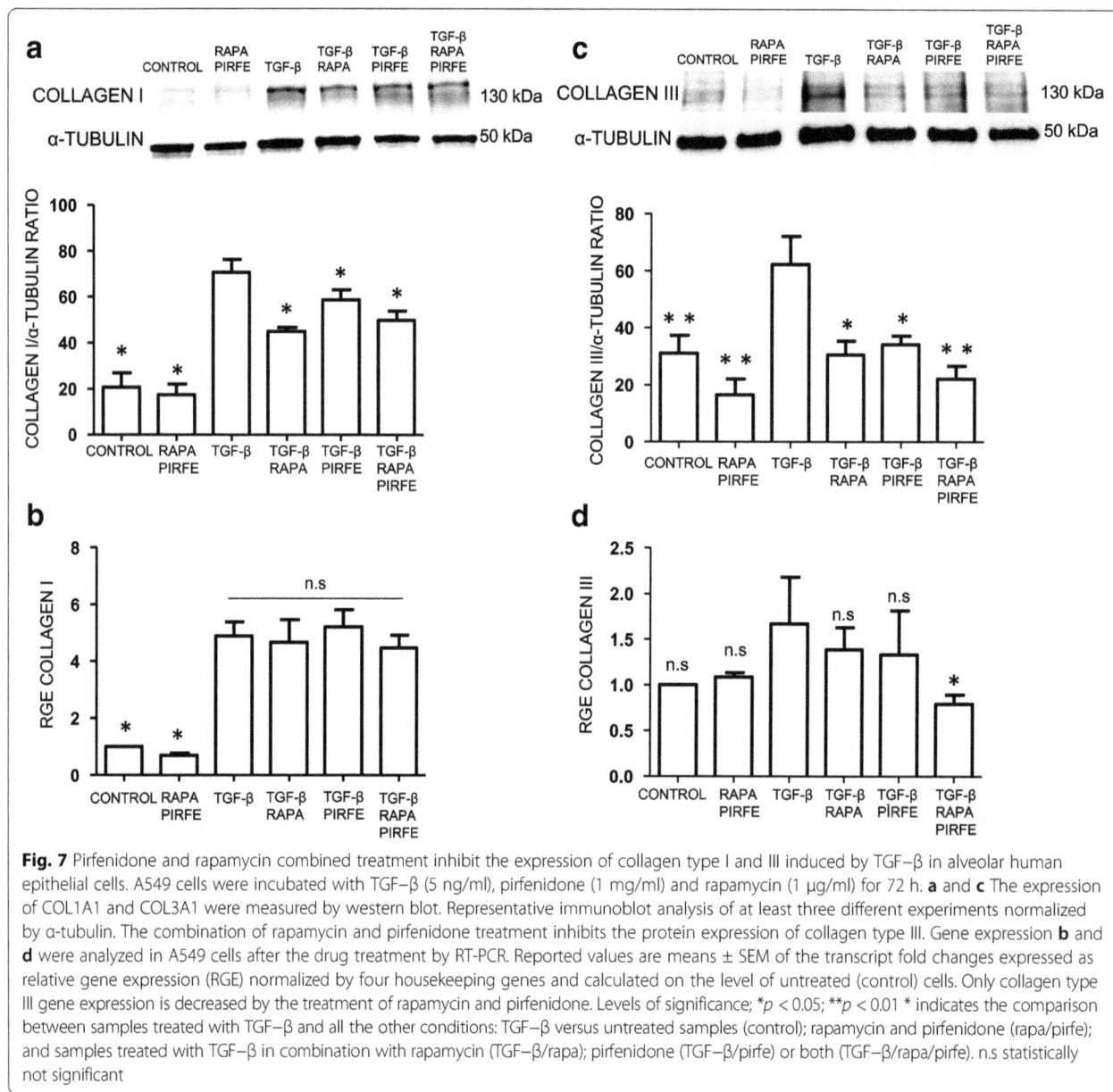

Fig. 7 Pirfenidone and rapamycin combined treatment inhibit the expression of collagen type I and III induced by TGF–β in alveolar human epithelial cells. A549 cells were incubated with TGF–β (5 ng/ml), pirfenidone (1 mg/ml) and rapamycin (1 μg/ml) for 72 h. **a** and **c** The expression of COL1A1 and COL3A1 were measured by western blot. Representative immunoblot analysis of at least three different experiments normalized by α-tubulin. The combination of rapamycin and pirfenidone treatment inhibits the protein expression of collagen type III. Gene expression **b** and **d** were analyzed in A549 cells after the drug treatment by RT-PCR. Reported values are means ± SEM of the transcript fold changes expressed as relative gene expression (RGE) normalized by four housekeeping genes and calculated on the level of untreated (control) cells. Only collagen type III gene expression is decreased by the treatment of rapamycin and pirfenidone. Levels of significance; *$p < 0.05$; **$p < 0.01$ * indicates the comparison between samples treated with TGF–β and all the other conditions: TGF–β versus untreated samples (control); rapamycin and pirfenidone (rapa/pirfe); and samples treated with TGF–β in combination with rapamycin (TGF–β/rapa); pirfenidone (TGF–β/pirfe) or both (TGF–β/rapa/pirfe). n.s statistically not significant

not stop or cure the disease completely, suggesting that a combination with other compounds involved in different pathways could be required in order to modify the fatal outcome [14].

In this context, this study was designed to test the potential role of the combination treatment of pirfenidone with rapamycin to improve the anti-fibrotic in vitro effect. Our cytotoxic assay showed no statistically significant changes in cell viability between control and treated cells, suggesting that the used concentration of pirfenidone and rapamycin had no cytotoxic effect. Both drugs have already been used separately, with different clinical indications and satisfactory tolerance [14–16]. It has been reported that pirfenidone exhibits an inhibitory

effect on a host of cell types in concentrations ranging from 0.2 to 2.0 mg/ml with no cytotoxic effect in vitro [24], and the drug is being administered orally at a daily dose of 2403 mg with tolerable degree of adverse effects in patients with pulmonary fibrosis [9]. Rapamycin, meanwhile, is already being used in cancer, transplant and LAM. An analog of rapamycin, everolimus, did not demonstrate benefit for IPF in a previous study [30]. However, everolimus and rapamycin present a different clinical profile in other diseases [31], and this indicates that choosing the correct mTOR inhibitor should be considered carefully. Rapamycin prevents and inhibits progression of ongoing pulmonary fibrosis caused by expression of TGF–α and increased epidermal growth

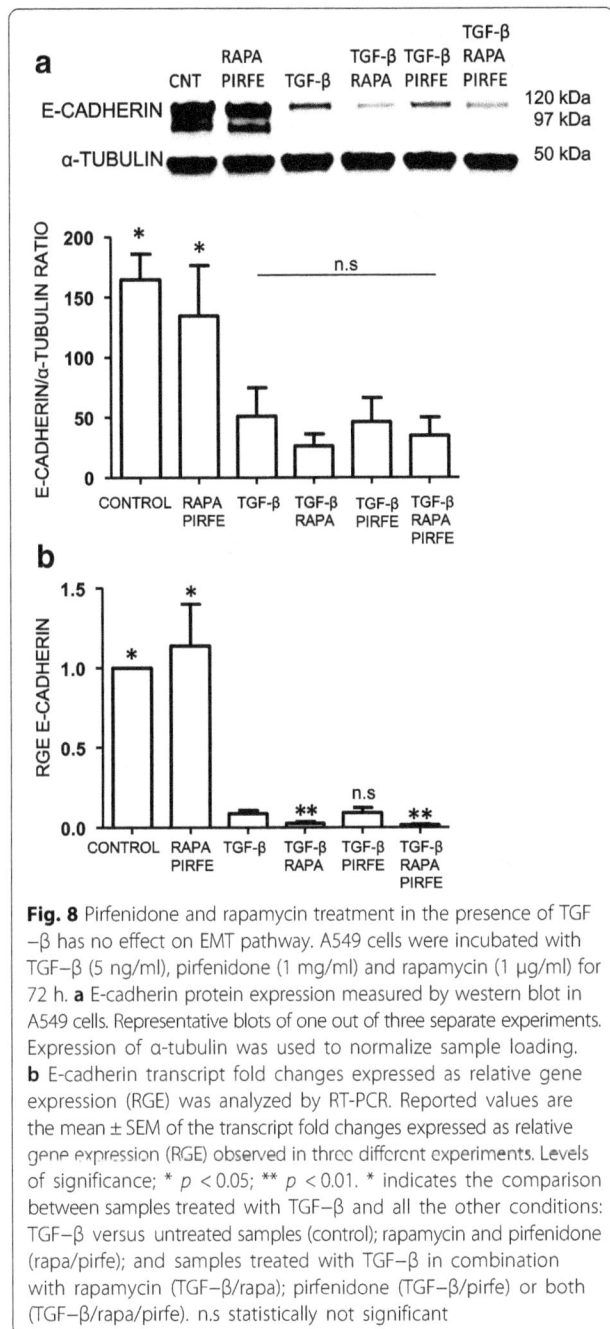

Fig. 8 Pirfenidone and rapamycin treatment in the presence of TGF–β has no effect on EMT pathway. A549 cells were incubated with TGF–β (5 ng/ml), pirfenidone (1 mg/ml) and rapamycin (1 μg/ml) for 72 h. **a** E-cadherin protein expression measured by western blot in A549 cells. Representative blots of one out of three separate experiments. Expression of α-tubulin was used to normalize sample loading. **b** E-cadherin transcript fold changes expressed as relative gene expression (RGE) was analyzed by RT-PCR. Reported values are the mean ± SEM of the transcript fold changes expressed as relative gene expression (RGE) observed in three different experiments. Levels of significance; * $p < 0.05$; ** $p < 0.01$. * indicates the comparison between samples treated with TGF–β and all the other conditions: TGF–β versus untreated samples (control); rapamycin and pirfenidone (rapa/pirfe); and samples treated with TGF–β in combination with rapamycin (TGF–β/rapa); pirfenidone (TGF–β/pirfe) or both (TGF–β/rapa/pirfe). n.s statistically not significant

proteins. We incubated the cell cultures with pirfenidone and rapamycin in absence or presence of the pro-fibrotic cytokine TGF–β. We observed different effects of pirfenidone and rapamycin when we analyzed the expression of the main proteins involved in the fibrotic process. We found that there is an inhibitory effect in the synthesis and gene expression of the ECM proteins, indicating that the treatment together is more efficient that the use of a single drug. The results indicated that rapamycin was able to inhibit the protein and gene expression of tenascin-c, and collagen I in fibroblasts and epithelial cells treated with TGF–β. On the other hand, pirfenidone succeeded in inhibiting the increase of fibronectin and α-sma in primary lung fibroblasts. These aggregated findings together demonstrated that each drug acts in different pathways and the use of both compounds would increase the anti-fibrotic range of action. Therefore, the drug combination increased the anti-fibrotic in vitro effect although a synergic effect was minimally present. Further studies are needed to better understand the role of each drug to inhibit the fibrotic process. These findings reveal the importance for a combined therapy that may result in a more efficient treatment to inhibit the ECM over-expression in the fibrotic process. The important role of both fibronectin and collagen in regulating the homeostasis of extracellular matrix and the inhibitory effect of pirfenidone in TGF–β stimulated fibroblasts has been reported [33]. Although pirfenidone has been shown to inhibit the synthesis of fibronectin and collagen in several studies, there is a discrepancy between the obtained results from protein and gene expression [34]. We demonstrate that the combination of pirfenidone with rapamycin produces more efficient results in the regulation of TGF–β-induced ECM over-expression, and highlights the importance of finding a new combinatory therapy for the treatment of pulmonary fibrosis.

Another important finding is the clear inhibition of TGF–β -induced myofibroblast transformation when fibroblasts are stimulated with pirfenidone and rapamycin, although the main effect is likely due to the action of pirfenidone. As shown in Fig. 4a, b, α-SMA was inhibited when cells were treated with both agents in the absence or presence of TGF–β, indicating a decrease in TGF–β -induced over-expression. Myofibroblasts are the last cells recruited to repair tissue damage; however, uncontrolled accumulation of this type of cell halts the healing process, resulting in the fibrotic and dysfunctional tissue. On the other hand, in agreement with other groups [35, 36], we found that pirfenidone and rapamycin failed to revert the EMT transition triggered by TGF–β in alveolar epithelial cells, as shown the studies of E-cadherin marker expression in A549 cells (Fig. 8). The discrepancy in the results we obtained in epithelial cells could be due

factor receptor (EGFR) signaling [21]. Currently, rapamycin is being evaluated in a clinical trial for IPF. Furthermore, the mTOR pathway is a hallmark of aging, and recent studies have shown it to be overexpressed in the fibrotic lungs of patients with a more detrimental progression [32].

Previous studies performed by our Group have shown the importance of ECM protein expression in the fibrotic process that occurs in IPF lungs [28]. In this study, we tested the combination of pirfenidone and rapamycin treatment to abolish the synthesis of ECM to the use of A549 cell line. It has been reported that even when these cells are standardized in in vitro models of EMT, some factors must still be taken into account when analyzing data obtained in this cell line [7]. We would need to confirm our results in primary human type II alveolar epithelial cells from IPF patients to better understand the potential effects of pirfenidone and rapamycin on these cells.

The inhibition of cell migration by pirfenidone has been reported by other groups [9, 33] whose results are consistent with our findings in lung fibroblasts stimulated with TGF–β and then treated with pirfenidone and rapamycin. Furthermore, when cells were stimulated with both drugs simultaneously, migration was inhibited up to the last time point assayed (72 h). These results support the role of both combined agents to avoid the uncontrolled migration of fibroblasts in the injured tissue. In vivo experimental studies would be required to support the beneficial anti-fibrotic effect of pirfenidone and rapamycin combination.

Conclusions

In summary, the present results open a new line of research into the potential of pirfenidone and rapamycin combination as a better anti-fibrotic approach and future treatment strategies.

Abbreviations
BCA: Bicinchonic acid; ECM: Extracellular matrix protein; EGFR: Epidermal growth factor receptor signaling; ELISA: Enzyme-linked immunosorbent assay; EMT: Epithelial to mesenchymal transition; FBS: Fetal bovine serum; FN: Fibronectin; FVC: Forced vital capacity; GADPH: Glyceraldehyde-3-phosphate dehydrogrenase; HPRT: Hypoxanthine-guanine phosphoribosyltransferase; IPF: Idiopathic Pulmonary Fibrosis; ITS: Insulin human transferrin and sodium selenite; LAM: lymphangioleiomiomatosis; mTOR: Mammalian target of rapamycin; PBS: Phosphate buffered saline; RIPA: Radio immunoprecipitation assay; RT-PCR: Real-time polymerase chain reaction; TGF: Transforming growth factor; α-SMA: α-Smooth muscle actin

Funding
This study was supported by Proyectos de Investigación en Salud del Instituto de Salud Carlos III (FIS PI 15/00710), Hoffmann-La Roche.

Author's contributions
Conceived and designed the experiments: AMW, MMM. Performed the experiments: AMW, CM. Analyzed the data: AMW, VVZ, MMM. Contributed reagents/materials/analysis tools: CM, RL, PL, IE. Wrote the paper: AMW, MMM. Revision of the manuscript: JD, ES, MMM. All the authors read and approved the final version of the manuscript.

Competing interests
Hoffmann-La Roche supported this work by providing pirfenidone and part of research founding. The authors declare that they have no competing interests.

Author details
[1]Department of Pneumology, Bellvitge University Hospital, Barcelona, Spain. [2]Pneumology Research Group, IDIBELL, University of Barcelona, Barcelona, Spain. [3]Research Network in Respiratory Diseases (CIBERES), ISCIII, Madrid, Spain. [4]Department of Pathology, Bellvitge University Hospital, Barcelona, Spain. [5]Department of Thoracic Surgery, Bellvitge University Hospital, Barcelona, Spain. [6]Servei de Diagnostic per la Imatge El Prat (SDPI El Prat) Department of Radiology, Bellvitge University Hospital, Barcelona, Spain. [7]Department of Penumology, Son Espases University Hospital, Palma de Mallorca, Spain. [8]Laboratori de Pneumologia Experimental (Lab. 4126). IDIBELL, Pavelló de Govern. Campus de Bellvitge, Universitat de Barcelona, Hospital de Bellvitge, Carrer de la Feixa Llarga, 08907 L'Hospitalet de Llobregat, Barcelona, Spain.

References
1. Fernandez IE, Eickelberg O. New cellular and molecular mechanisms of lung injury and fibrosis in idiopathic pulmonary fibrosis. Lancet. 2012;380(9842):680–8. https://doi.org/10.1016/s0140-6736(12)61144-1. Epub 2012/08/21. PubMed PMID: 22901889.
2. King TE Jr, Pardo A, Selman M. Idiopathic pulmonary fibrosis. Lancet. 2011;378(9807):1949–61. https://doi.org/10.1016/s0140-6736(11)60052-4. Epub 2011/07/02. PubMed PMID: 21719092.
3. Blaauboer ME, Boeijen FR, Emson CL, Turner SM, Zandieh-Doulabi B, Hanemaaijer R, et al. Extracellular matrix proteins: a positive feedback loop in lung fibrosis? Matrix Biol. 2014;34:170–8. https://doi.org/10.1016/j.matbio.2013.11.002. Epub 2013/12/03. PubMed PMID: 24291458.
4. Raghu G, Rochwerg B, Zhang Y, Garcia CA, Azuma A, Behr J, et al. An official ATS/ERS/JRS/ALAT clinical practice guideline: treatment of idiopathic pulmonary fibrosis. An update of the 2011 clinical practice guideline. Am J Respir Crit Care Med. 2015;192(2):e3–19. https://doi.org/10.1164/rccm.201506-1063ST. Epub 2015/07/16. PubMed PMID: 26177183.
5. Noble PW, Albera C, Bradford WZ, Costabel U, Glassberg MK, Kardatzke D, et al. Pirfenidone in patients with idiopathic pulmonary fibrosis (CAPACITY): two randomised trials. Lancet. 2011;377(9779):1760–9. https://doi.org/10.1016/s0140-6736(11)60405-4. Epub 2011/05/17. PubMed PMID: 21571362.
6. King TE Jr, Bradford WZ, Castro-Bernardini S, Fagan EA, Glaspole I, Glassberg MK, et al. A phase 3 trial of pirfenidone in patients with idiopathic pulmonary fibrosis. N Engl J Med. 2014;370(22):2083–92. https://doi.org/10.1056/NEJMoa1402582. Epub 2014/05/20. PubMed PMID: 24836312.
7. Hisatomi K, Mukae H, Sakamoto N, Ishimatsu Y, Kakugawa T, Hara S, et al. Pirfenidone inhibits TGF-beta1-induced over-expression of collagen type I and heat shock protein 47 in A549 cells. BMC Pulm Med. 2012;12:24. https://doi.org/10.1186/1471-2466-12-24. Epub 2012/06/15. PubMed PMID: 22694981; PubMed Central PMCID: PMCPMC3403980.
8. Adamali HI, Maher TM. Current and novel drug therapies for idiopathic pulmonary fibrosis. Drug Des Devel Ther. 2012;6:261–72. https://doi.org/10.2147/dddt.s29928. Epub 2012/10/12. PubMed PMID: 23055696; PubMed Central PMCID: PMCPMC3463380.
9. Lin X, Yu M, Wu K, Yuan H, Zhong H. Effects of pirfenidone on proliferation, migration, and collagen contraction of human Tenon's fibroblasts in vitro. Invest Ophthalmol Vis Sci. 2009;50(8):3763–70. https://doi.org/10.1167/iovs.08-2815. Epub 2009/03/07. PubMed PMID: 19264889.
10. Oku H, Shimizu T, Kawabata T, Nagira M, Hikita I, Ueyama A, et al. Antifibrotic action of pirfenidone and prednisolone: different effects on pulmonary cytokines and growth factors in bleomycin-induced murine pulmonary fibrosis. Eur J Pharmacol. 2008;590(1–3):400–8. https://doi.org/10.1016/j.ejphar.2008.06.046. Epub 2008/07/05. PubMed PMID: 18598692.
11. Macias-Barragan J, Sandoval-Rodriguez A, Navarro-Partida J, Armendariz-Borunda J. The multifaceted role of pirfenidone and its novel targets. Fibrogenesis Tissue Repair. 2010;3:1. https://doi.org/10.1186/1755-1536-3-16. Epub 2010/09/03. PubMed PMID: 20809935; PubMed Central PMCID: PMCPMC2944211.
12. Choi K, Lee K, Ryu SW, Im M, Kook KH, Choi C. Pirfenidone inhibits transforming growth factor-beta1-induced fibrogenesis by blocking nuclear translocation of Smads in human retinal pigment epithelial cell line ARPE-19. Mol Vis. 2012;18:1010–20. Epub 2012/05/03. PubMed PMID: 22550395; PubMed Central PMCID: PMCPMC3339036.
13. Costabel U, Bendstrup E, Cottin V, Dewint P, Egan JJ, Ferguson J, et al. Pirfenidone in idiopathic pulmonary fibrosis: expert panel discussion on the management of drug-related adverse events. Adv Ther. 2014;31(4):375–91. https://doi.org/10.1007/s12325-014-0112-1. Epub 2014/03/19. PubMed PMID: 24639005; PubMed Central PMCID: PMCPMC4003341.

14. Wells A. Combination therapy in idiopathic pulmonary fibrosis: the way ahead will be hard. Eur Respir J. 2015;45(5):1208–10. https://doi.org/10.1183/09031936.00043915. Epub 2015/05/02. PubMed PMID: 25931482.

15. Yates DH. mTOR treatment in lymphangioleiomyomatosis: the role of everolimus. Expert Rev Respir Med. 2016;10(3):249–60. https://doi.org/10.1586/17476348.2016.1148603. Epub 2016/02/06. PubMed PMID: 26847859.

16. AM T-DS, Moss J. Clinical features, epidemiology, and therapy of lymphangioleiomyomatosis. Clin Epidemiol. 2015;7:249–57. https://doi.org/10.2147/clep.s50780. Epub 2015/04/22. PubMed PMID: 25897262; PubMed Central PMCID: PMCPMC4396456.

17. Hartford CM, Ratain MJ. Rapamycin: something old, something new, sometimes borrowed and now renewed. Clin Pharmacol Ther. 2007;82(4):381–8. https://doi.org/10.1038/sj.clpt.6100317. Epub 2007/08/31. PubMed PMID: 17728765.

18. Bridle KR, Popa C, Morgan ML, Sobbe AL, Clouston AD, Fletcher LM, Crawford DH. Rapamycin inhibits hepatic fibrosis in rats by attenuating multiple profibrogenic pathways. Liver Transpl. 2009;15:1315–24. https://doi.org/10.1002/lt.21804.

19. Swaminathan S, Arbiser JL, Hiatt KM, High W, Abul-Ezz S, Horn TD, Shah SV. Rapid improvement of nephrogenic systemic fibrosis with rapamycin therapy: possible role of phospho-70-ribosomal-S6 kinase. J Am Acad Dermatol. 2010;62:343–5. https://doi.org/10.1016/j.jaad.2009.04.022.

20. Gao Y, Xu X, Ding K, Liang Y, Jiang D, Dai H. Rapamycin inhibits transforming growth factor beta1-induced fibrogenesis in primary human lung fibroblasts. Yonsei Med J. 2013;54(2):437–44. https://doi.org/10.3349/ymj.2013.54.2.437. Epub 2013/02/01. PubMed PMID: 23364979; PubMed Central PMCID: PMCPMC3576000.

21. Korfhagen TR, Le Cras TD, Davidson CR, Schmidt SM, Ikegami M, Whitsett JA, et al. Rapamycin prevents transforming growth factor-alpha-induced pulmonary fibrosis. Am J Respir Cell Mol Biol. 2009;41(5):562–72. https://doi.org/10.1165/rcmb.2008-0377OC. Epub 2009/02/27. PubMed PMID: 19244201; PubMed Central PMCID: PMCPMC2778163.

22. Chang W, Wei K, Ho L, Berry GJ, Jacobs SS, Chang CH, et al. A critical role for the mTORC2 pathway in lung fibrosis. PLoS One. 2014;9(8):e106155. https://doi.org/10.1371/journal.pone.0106155. Epub 2014/08/28. PubMed PMID: 25162417; PubMed Central PMCID: PMCPMC4146613.

23. Nakayama S, Mukae H, Sakamoto N, Kakugawa T, Yoshioka S, Soda H, Oku H, Urata Y, Kondo T, Kubota H, Nagata K, Kohno S. Pirfenidone inhibits the expression of HSP47 in TGF-beta1-stimulated human lung fibroblasts. Life Sci. 2008;82:210–7. https://doi.org/10.1016/j.lfs.2007.11.003.

24. Shin JM, Park JH, Park IH, Lee HM. Pirfenidone inhibits transforming growth factor β1-induced extracellular matrix production in nasal polyp-derived fibroblasts. Am J Rhinol Allergy. 2015;29:408–13. https://doi.org/10.2500/ajra.2015.29.4221.

25. Lee K, Young Lee S, Park SY, Yang H. Antifibrotic effect of pirfenidone on human pterygium fibroblasts. Curr Eye Res. 2014;39(7):680–5. https://doi.org/10.3109/02713683.2013.867063. Epub 2014 Jan 8.

26. Yang Y, Ye Y, Lin X, Wu K, Yu M. Inhibition of pirfenidone on TGF-beta2 induced proliferation, migration and epithlial-mesenchymal transition of human lens epithelial cells line SRA01/04. PLoS One. 2013;8(2):e56837. https://doi.org/10.1371/journal.pone.0056837. Epub 2013 Feb 21.

27. Shi Q, Liu X, Bai Y, Cui C, Li J, Li Y, Hu S, Wei Y. In vitro effects of pirfenidone on cardiac fibroblasts: proliferation, myofibroblast differentiation, migration and cytokine secretion. PLoS One. 2011;6(11):e28134. https://doi.org/10.1371/journal.pone.0028134. Epub 2011 Nov 23.

28. Vicens-Zygmunt V, Estany S, Colom A, Montes-Worboys A, Machahua C, Sanabria AJ, et al. Fibroblast viability and phenotypic changes within glycated stiffened three-dimensional collagen matrices. Respir Res. 2015;16:82. https://doi.org/10.1186/s12931-015-0237-z. Epub 2015/07/02. PubMed PMID: 26126411; PubMed Central PMCID: PMCPMC4494165.

29. Kaarteenaho-Wiik R, Tani T, Sormunen R, Soini Y, Virtanen I, Pääkkö P. Tenascin immunoreactivity as a prognostic marker in usual interstitial pneumonia. Am J Respir Crit Care Med. 1996;154(2 Pt 1):511–8.

30. Malouf MA, Hopkins P, Snell G, Glanville AR. An investigator-driven study of everolimus in surgical lung biopsy confirmed idiopathic pulmonary fibrosis. Respirology. 2011;16(5):776–83. https://doi.org/10.1111/j.1440-1843.2011.01955.x. Epub 2011/06/28. PubMed PMID: 21362103; PubMed Central PMCID: PMC21362103.

31. MacKeigan JP, Krueger DA. Differentiating the mTOR inhibitors everolimus and sirolimus in the treatment of tuberous sclerosis complex. Neuro-Oncology. 2015;17(12):1550–9. https://doi.org/10.1093/neuonc/nov152. Epub 2015/08/19. PubMed PMID: 26289591; PubMed Central PMCID: PMC4633932.

32. Park JS, Park HJ, Park YS, Lee SM, Yim JJ, Yoo CG, et al. Clinical significance of mTOR, ZEB1, ROCK1 expression in lung tissues of pulmonary fibrosis patients. BMC Pulm Med. 2014;14:168. https://doi.org/10.1186/1471-2466-14-168. Epub 2014/11/02. PubMed PMID: 25358403; PubMed Central PMCID: PMCPMC4233073.

33. Stahnke T, Kowtharapu BS, Stachs O, Schmitz KP, Wurm J, Wree A, Guthoff RF, Hovakimyan M. Suppression of TGF-β pathway by pirfenidone decreases extracellular matrix deposition in ocular fibroblasts in vitro. PLoS One. 2017;12:e0172592.

34. Knüppel L, Ishikawa Y, Aichler M, Heinzelmann K, Hatz R, Behr J, Walch A, Bächinger HP, Eickelberg O, Novel Antifibrotic A. Mechanism of Nintedanib and Pirfenidone. Inhibition of collagen fibril assembly. Staab-Weijnitz CA. Am J Respir Cell Mol Biol. 2017;57:77–90. https://doi.org/10.1165/rcmb.2016-0217OC.

35. Dawes LJ, Sleeman MA, Anderson IK, Reddan JR, Wormstone IM. TGFb/Smad4-dependent and -independent regulation of human lens epithelial cells. Invest Ophthalmol Vis Sci. 2009;50:5318–5327.

36. Kasai H, Allen JT, Mason RM, Kamimura T, Zhang Z. TGF-beta1 induces human alveolar epithelial to mesenchymal cell transition (EMT). Respir Res. 2005;6:56. https://doi.org/10.1186/1465-9921-6-56. Epub 2005/06/11. PubMed PMID: 15946381; PubMed Central PMCID: PMCPMC1177991.

Management of acute respiratory failure in interstitial lung diseases: overview and clinical insights

Paola Faverio[1]*[iD], Federica De Giacomi[1], Luca Sardella[1], Giuseppe Fiorentino[2], Mauro Carone[3], Francesco Salerno[3], Jousel Ora[4], Paola Rogliani[4], Giulia Pellegrino[5], Giuseppe Francesco Sferrazza Papa[5], Francesco Bini[6], Bruno Dino Bodini[7], Grazia Messinesi[1], Alberto Pesci[1] and Antonio Esquinas[8]

Abstract

Background: Interstitial lung diseases (ILDs) are a heterogeneous group of diseases characterized by widespread fibrotic and inflammatory abnormalities of the lung. Respiratory failure is a common complication in advanced stages or following acute worsening of the underlying disease. Aim of this review is to evaluate the current evidence in determining the best management of acute respiratory failure (ARF) in ILDs.

Methods: A literature search was performed in the Medline/PubMed and EMBASE databases to identify studies that investigated the management of ARF in ILDs (the last search was conducted on November 2017).

Results: In managing ARF, it is important to establish an adequate diagnostic and therapeutic management depending on whether the patient has an underlying known chronic ILD or ARF is presenting in an unknown or de novo ILD. In the first case both primary causes, such as acute exacerbations of the disease, and secondary causes, including concomitant pulmonary infections, fluid overload and pulmonary embolism need to be investigated. In the second case, a diagnostic work-up that includes investigations in regards to ILD etiology, such as autoimmune screening and bronchoalveolar lavage, should be performed, and possible concomitant causes of ARF have to be ruled out. Oxygen supplementation and ventilatory support need to be titrated according to the severity of ARF and patients' therapeutic options. High-Flow Nasal oxygen might potentially be an alternative to conventional oxygen therapy in patients requiring both high flows and high oxygen concentrations to correct hypoxemia and control dyspnea, however the evidence is still scarce. Neither Non-Invasive Ventilation (NIV) nor Invasive Mechanical Ventilation (IMV) seem to change the poor outcomes associated to advanced stages of ILDs. However, in selected patients, such as those with less severe ARF, a NIV trial might help in the early recognition of NIV-responder patients, who may present a better short-term prognosis. More invasive techniques, including IMV and Extracorporeal Membrane Oxygenation, should be limited to patients listed for lung transplant or with reversible causes of ARF.

Conclusions: Despite the overall poor prognosis of ARF in ILDs, a personalized approach may positively influence patients' management, possibly leading to improved outcomes. However, further studies are warranted.

Keywords: Interstitial lung diseases, Idiopathic pulmonary fibrosis, Acute respiratory failure, Invasive ventilation, Non-invasive ventilation, High-flow nasal cannula

* Correspondence: paola.faverio@unimib.it
[1]Dipartimento Cardio-Toraco-Vascolare, University of Milan Bicocca, Respiratory Unit, San Gerardo Hospital, ASST di Monza, Via Pergolesi 33, 20900 Monza, Italy
Full list of author information is available at the end of the article

Background

Interstitial lung diseases (ILDs) are a heterogeneous group of diseases that includes more than 200 entities characterized by widespread fibrotic and/or inflammatory abnormalities of the lung parenchyma, Fig. 1 [1, 2]. Respiratory failure is a common complication in advanced stages or following acute worsening of ILDs and can be classified on the basis of different parameters, including time of onset (acute or chronic), severity (mild to severe), and causes (reversible or irreversible).

Aim of this review is to evaluate the current evidence in determining the best management of acute respiratory failure (ARF) in ILDs.

Methods

A search of relevant medical literature in the English language was conducted in Medline/PubMed and EMBASE databases including observational and interventional studies from 1990 through November 2017. Keywords used to perform the research are reported in Table 1. Studies targeting children and editorials, narrative, and conference abstracts have been excluded. For the purpose of this review, any kind of ILD was included in the search.

Results and discussion

Epidemiology and risk factors

In recent times, ILDs definitions and classifications have been extensively revised [2], therefore it is difficult to provide precise epidemiological data for each class of ILD. In the present review we will mostly address idiopathic pulmonary fibrosis (IPF), which is the most widely studied ILD.

From a study conducted in New Mexico, USA, it was estimated that the prevalence of ILDs was approximately 81 / 100,000 in men and 64 / 100,000 in females [3]. The same study showed a higher incidence in males (31.5 per 100,000 / year) than females (26.1 per 100,000 / year) [3]. Both prevalence and incidence vary greatly depending on the specific type of ILD considered. In particular, although classified as rare diseases, the two most frequently diagnosed ILDs are IPF and sarcoidosis.

IPF has a prevalence of 0.5–27 / 100,000 and an incidence of 0.22–8.8 / 100,000 inhabitants worldwide [4]. When focusing on European data, the prevalence of IPF is 1.25–23.4 / 100,000, and the annual incidence 0.22–7.4 / 100,000 [5]. The incidence of acute exacerbation (AE) of IPF ranges between 0 and 21% according to

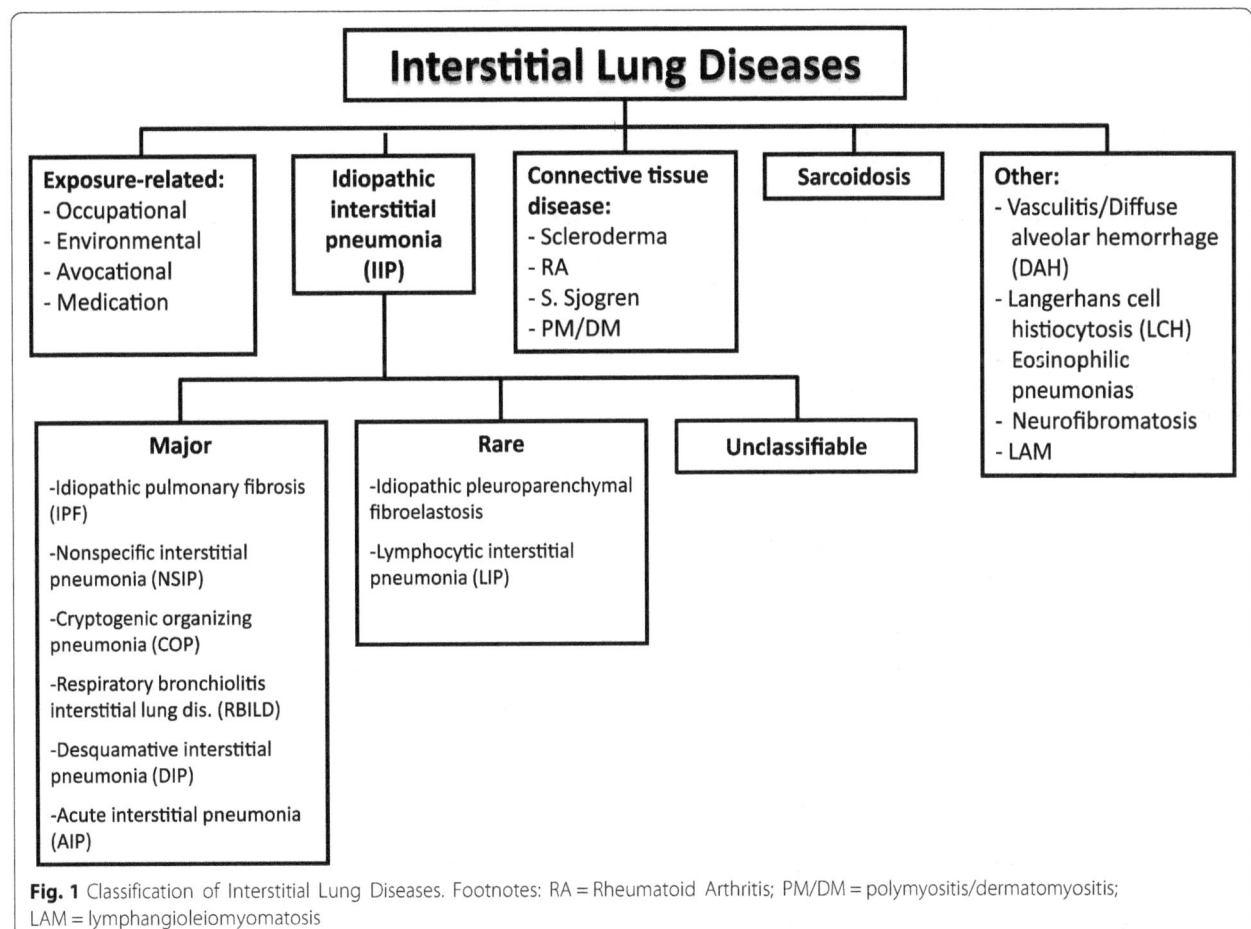

Fig. 1 Classification of Interstitial Lung Diseases. Footnotes: RA = Rheumatoid Arthritis; PM/DM = polymyositis/dermatomyositis; LAM = lymphangioleiomyomatosis

Table 1 Keywords used to perform the research

interstitial lung diseases outcomes, interstitial lung diseases prognosis, interstitial lung diseases (OR IPF OR NSIP OR CTD-ILD OR chronic HP OR acute idiopathic interstitial pneumonia) AND (ventilation OR invasive ventilation OR mechanical ventilation OR invasive mechanical ventilation), non-invasive ventilation AND interstitial lung diseases (OR IPF OR NSIP OR CTD-ILD OR chronic HP OR acute idiopathic interstitial pneumonia), (high flow oxygen OR high-flow nasal cannula OR oxygen therapy OR oxygen supplementation) AND interstitial lung diseases, ((non-invasive ventilation) AND respiratory failure) AND interstitial lung diseases, ((non-invasive ventilation) AND respiratory failure) AND idiopathic pulmonary fibrosis, acute respiratory failure AND interstitial lung disease (OR IPF OR NSIP OR CTD-ILD OR chronic HP OR acute idiopathic interstitial pneumonia), acute respiratory worsening AND interstitial lung disease (OR IPF OR NSIP OR CTD-ILD OR chronic HP OR acute idiopathic interstitial pneumonia), acute exacerbation AND interstitial lung disease (OR IPF OR NSIP OR CTD-ILD OR chronic HP OR acute idiopathic interstitial pneumonia).

different cohorts [6–26], and predominantly occurs in advanced stages of the disease [13, 27–29]. This highly variable incidence is probably due to differences in study design (prospective vs retrospective), definition of AE and statistical methodology [30]. Recognized risk factors for AE of IPF (AE-IPF) are lower forced vital capacity and diffusion capacity of carbon monoxide as well as reduced walked distance at 6-min walking test [13, 24, 27, 30–32], worsening respiratory gas exchange [31], higher dyspnea scores [30], greater disease extent on high-resolution computed tomography (HRCT) as well as presence and extent of honeycombing and traction bronchiectasis [33], presence of gastroesophageal reflux disease [34, 35], exposure to air pollution [36], presence of pulmonary hypertension [30], specific genetic variants [37], drug toxicity, bronchoalveolar lavage [38], surgical lung biopsy [39, 40], and surgery, radiotherapy or chemotherapy for concomitant lung cancer [28, 41–43]. Other non-validated risk factors are elevated baseline serum Krebs von der Lungen-6 (KL-6) [44, 45], increased body mass index [24], younger age [30], and concomitant coronary artery disease [27], whereas data on smoke exposure and emphysema as risk factors are discordant [13].

Outcome of different interstitial lung diseases

IPF is the ILD with the worst prognosis, having a median survival of 2 to 3 years from the time of diagnosis [46]. In 2003 in the USA, the mortality rate related to IPF was 61.2 deaths per 1,000,000 in men and 54.5 deaths per 1,000,000 in women [47]. AE-IPF is the most common cause of mortality in IPF cohorts [48, 49], accounting for over half of all hospitalizations [48] and up to 40% of all deaths [13]. Prognosis of AE-IPF is extremely poor with a in-hospital mortality rate around 50% in less severe patients and higher than 90% in those requiring Intensive Care Unit (ICU) admission [12, 13, 50–55].

Connective tissue disease related ILD (CTD-ILD) has a better prognosis compared to IPF, as emerged from a UK study by *Navaratnam* et al. [56], with a median

survival of 6.5 vs 3.1 years in patients with IPF. Among ILDs, sarcoidosis is the one with the best prognosis; *Thomeer* et al. compared the mortality of different forms of ILDs in a tertiary care hospital setting: the 5-year survival of patients with sarcoidosis was 91.6% compared to 69.7% for CTD-ILD and 35% for IPF [57].

Despite the high mortality associated to ARF in all ILDs, IPF showed higher one-year mortality after hospitalization for acute respiratory worsening compared to patients with other fibrotic ILDs, (87% vs 71%, respectively) [58]. Median survival after an AE-IPF ranges between 22 days and 4.2 months [13, 24].

Underlying pathophysiology of acute respiratory failure in interstitial lung diseases

ARF may occur as an acute/subacute presentation of ILD or may complicate the clinical course of a previously diagnosed ILD or unknown ILD as the result of the rapid decline of respiratory function caused by an accelerated worsening of the underlying interstitial process, the socalled AE, or because of superimposed complications, such as pulmonary thromboembolism, heart failure and infection [13].

AE-ILD might be the consequence of an intrinsic acceleration of the fibroproliferative process or a response to occult or known external events (e.g. infection, micro-aspiration or mechanical stretch such as lung biopsies) [30].

The histopathological hallmark of AE-ILDs, particularly AE-IPF, is diffuse alveolar damage (DAD), superimposed on the histological pattern of the underlying ILD [11, 59–61]. DAD presents histologically with two subsequent phases, an acute/exudative phase followed by an organizing/proliferative phase, that sometimes evolves in a final fibrotic stage.

The acute exudative phase is characterized by relatively sparse inflammatory cells and predominant hyaline membranes along alveolar septa with accentuation in alveolar ducts. In the organizing/proliferative phase, the hyaline membranes are incorporated into the alveolar septa through phagocytosis by macrophages or granulation tissue formation by proliferating myofibroblasts. Finally, the interstitium is thickened by loose myxoid fibroblastic tissue, causing altered pulmonary gas exchange mainly by diffusion impairment and ventilation-perfusion (V/Q) mismatch.

Acute respiratory failure etiologies and diagnostic work-up

In patients with ARF and ILD three possible scenarios have to be distinguished:

a)   ARF in known chronic ILDs

AE was firstly described in IPF patients with reported median survival time after the event of 3 to 4 months [13, 27], even shorter in patients requiring invasive mechanical ventilation (IMV) [62].

The definition of AE-IPF has recently been revised as an acute (less than 1 month in duration) and clinically significant respiratory deterioration in a previously diagnosed IPF patient, associated with the presence of new widespread alveolar infiltrates on HRCT and exclusion of alternative etiologies (including infection, heart failure, pulmonary embolism, and, less frequently, pneumothorax, drug toxicity and diffuse alveolar hemorrhage - DAH -), [30]. Questionably, this new definition removes the distinction between idiopathic and so-called triggered AE because considered irrelevant to patients' outcome. Nevertheless, identifying the trigger of AE may influence patients' management [58, 63].

AE may complicate the clinical course of other fibrosing ILDs, such as chronic hypersensitivity pneumonitis (CHP) [64–66], and non-specific interstitial pneumonia (NSIP) both idiopathic and secondary to CTD-ILD [61, 67–69].

The incidence of AE in CTD-ILDs depends on the underlying CTD (as an example, AE are more common in ILD secondary to Rheumatoid Arthritis) and AE may occur regardless of flares of the extrathoracic manifestations and in spite of the immunosuppressive treatment.

In clinical practice, a diagnostic work-up based on laboratory exams, CT scan (angioCT if pulmonary embolism is suspected), and bronchoscopy may be recommended in patients with ARF in a known ILD to evaluate all possible scenarios, Fig. 2.

b) Unknown chronic ILD presenting with ARF

Although less commonly than in a previously diagnosed ILD, ARF may also represent the clinical onset of an undiagnosed and unsuspected ILD. Possible ILDs presenting with this clinical manifestation are IPF, NSIP, CHP, CTD-ILDs, DAH and drug-toxicity [11, 13, 68, 70, 71].

In a previously apparently healthy patient presenting with ARF, the assessment of past medical history and symptoms, perhaps underestimated by the patient himself,

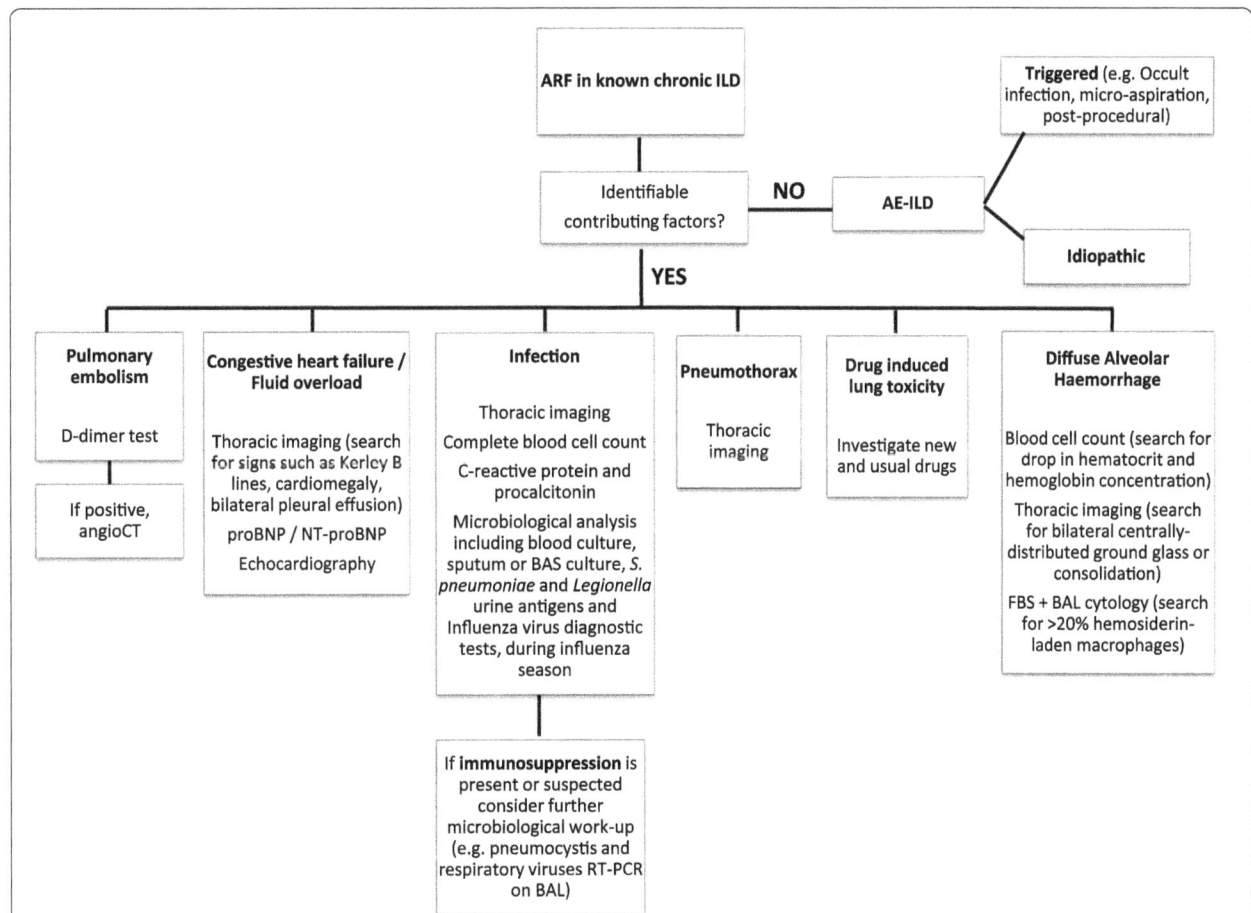

Fig. 2 Diagnostic work-up of acute respiratory failure in a known Interstitial Lung Disease. Footnotes: ARF = acute respiratory failure; ILD = interstitial lung disease; AE-ILD = acute exacerbation of ILD; CT = computed tomography; NT-proBNP = N-terminal pro b-type natriuretic peptide; FBS = fiberoptic bronchoscopy; BAS = bronchial aspirate; BAL = bronchoalveolar lavage; RT-PCR = real-time polymerase chain reaction

is mandatory. Physical examination and laboratories (e.g. digital clubbing and polyglobulia) may reveal a long-standing respiratory failure or extrapulmonary manifestations of an underlying CTD or systemic vasculitis. However, the absence of extrapulmonary signs does not exclude an underlying CTD, as pulmonary manifestations may precede by months or years the more typical systemic manifestations, especially in rheumatoid arthritis, systemic lupus erythematosus, and polymyositis-dermatomyositis (lung-dominant ILD) [72]. Therefore, complete autoimmune serology screening, inclusive of myositis-specific autoantibodies, might be helpful.

HRCT, performed as part of the initial assessment of ARF, should be carefully assessed to identify the presence of signs of architectural distortion such as traction bronchiectasis, lung volume loss and honeycombing, considered suggestive of a pre-existing ILD.

Bronchoscopy with bronchoalveolar lavage (BAL) and, in selected cases, lung biopsies may be useful in establishing the diagnosis of the underlying ILD. The indication for bronchoscopic assessment and the choice of the procedure to perform should be carefully discussed in each case, considering ARF severity, the potentially related complications and the risk to trigger an AE.

In unknown ILDs presenting with ARF and in de novo acute ILDs, as shown in the next section, the diagnostic work-up should always include both investigations on primary ILD (autoantibody panel and bronchoscopic procedures when respiratory gas exchange allows it) and investigations on concomitant conditions that may cause ARF, as summarised in Fig. 3.

c) De novo acute ILD presenting with ARF

ARF may also represent the clinical onset of a de novo rapidly progressive ILD. In the differential diagnosis the following should be considered: acute interstitial pneumonia (AIP), cryptogenic organizing pneumonia (COP), acute eosinophilic pneumonia (AEP), and drug-induced ILD [73], and, less frequently, acute hypersensitivity pneumonia, DAH in the setting of a de novo vasculitis, de novo CTD-ILD and lepidic adenocarcinoma with lymphangitic carcinomatosis.AIP, formerly known as Hamman-Rich syndrome, is a rare and fulminant form of diffuse lung injury with a clinical presentation similar to acute respiratory distress syndrome (ARDS), whose etiology remains uncertain [74]. The in-hospital mortality rate is greater than 50% and the majority of patients who survive dies within six months of presentation [75, 76].

In 10–15% of cases, COP may present with a rapidly progressive course, mimicking ARDS [77]. The diagnosis is made by ruling out infectious causes of pneumonia and documenting typical pathological changes in tissue obtained by lung biopsies demonstrating fibroblastic

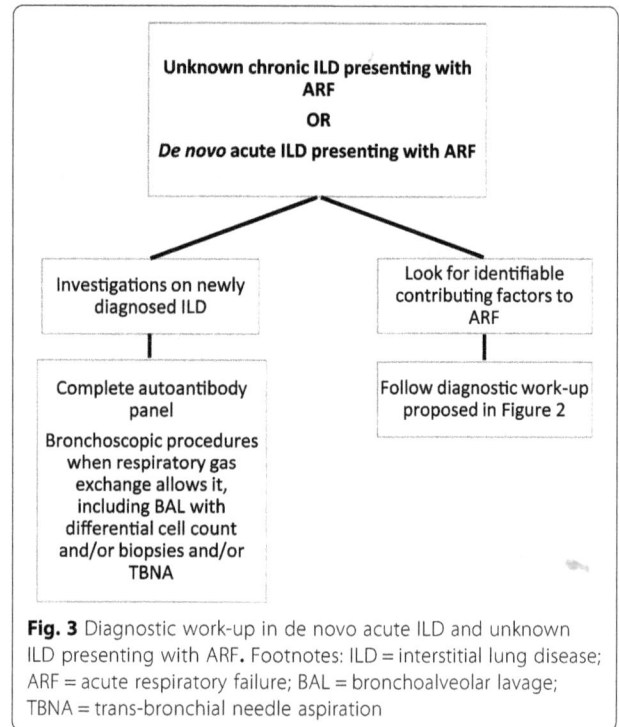

Fig. 3 Diagnostic work-up in de novo acute ILD and unknown ILD presenting with ARF. Footnotes: ILD = interstitial lung disease; ARF = acute respiratory failure; BAL = bronchoalveolar lavage; TBNA = trans-bronchial needle aspiration

polyps, sometimes associated with endoalveolar fibrin deposits, the so-called acute fibrinous organizing pneumonia (AFOP). The majority of patients recovers completely with corticosteroid therapy but relapses are common [78, 79].

AEP occurs in previously healthy individuals and is characterized by pulmonary eosinophilia (more than 25% eosinophils on BAL differential cell count) or eosinophilic pneumonia on lung biopsy with or without peripheral eosinophilia [80].

Many chemotherapeutic (e.g. bleomycin and busulfan) and non-chemotherapeutic agents (e.g. amiodarone, nitrofurantoin, and statins) may cause lung toxicity manifesting with ARF. The diagnosis of a drug-induced acute ILD is challenging, and it is supported by the temporal relationship between the first use of the medication and symptoms onset, spontaneous clinical improvement after the discontinuation of the drug and recurrence of symptoms on re-challenge [81].

Although acute hypersensitivity pneumonitis is most commonly self-limited, it can also present with ARF. It should be suspected when there is a temporal association with the exposure to an inhaled antigen known to trigger hypersensitivity reactions, and in the presence of an upper-lobe predominant process accompanied by lymphocytic alveolitis [82, 83].

Diffuse alveolar haemorrhage presents with three possible histopathologic patterns: pulmonary capillaritis, most frequently encountered in granulomatosis with polyangiitis, bland pulmonary haemorrhage and DAD due to drugs or inhalation of toxic chemicals [84].

Possible diagnostic work-up for this presentation of ILDs is summarised in Fig. 3.

Initial evaluation of the severity of respiratory failure and how to choose the site and intensity of care

ARF represents a true clinical and ethical challenge, given the lack of benefit of IMV in the majority of patients with ARF and ILDs [54], the high susceptibility of these patients to ventilator-induced lung injury (VILI) [54, 85], and, subsequently, the high mortality rate of ILD patients in the ICU [86–88]. Despite the majority of studies having been conducted on AE-IPF [86, 87], it appears that AEs of non-IPF forms of ILD do not differ in terms of prognosis [88]; furthermore, the duration of the underlying ILD from diagnosis to ICU admission has not shown to correlate with mortality. The unique definitive treatment option for pharmacologically refractory advanced stage ILDs is lung transplant [89], and the decision to proceed to intensive life support measures in these patients cannot withstand the patient's precedent enlisting. In rarer cases, a patient may be listed de novo upon ICU admission, in the form of a salvage transplant. To this aim, while waiting for lung transplant, IMV, and more recently ExtraCorporeal Membrane Oxygenation (ECMO) [90], have shown to be lifesaving options. Therefore, patients presenting with ARF on an underlying ILD should be addressed to centers specialized in ILD and disposing of a respiratory high dependency unit (HDU) and an ICU with ECMO experience; in case the patient is on the lung transplant list, he/she should be referred to the local transplant center [89, 91].

In respiratory HDUs, non-invasive ventilation (NIV) is effectively used to decrease work of breathing in patients such as those with exacerbation of chronic obstructive pulmonary disease (COPD). However, in most ILD cases with ARF the excessive work of breathing cannot be managed by NIV alone, and studies suggesting a definitive clinical benefit of NIV in ILDs are still lacking, as shown in the following sections of this review. Furthermore, a recent study on a large single-center cohort of NIV patients, showed that the presence of diffuse ILD was associated with increased mortality [92]. In this scenario, NIV could have a role in selected patients, such as survivors from an AE-ILD, as a bridge to transplant [89, 93], or to reduce patient discomfort after the onset of ARF in those who are not candidate to lung transplant, while establishing other supportive measures [94]. We will discuss specific indications and contraindications together with the available evidence in regards to various oxygenation and ventilation methods in the following sections.

Finally, given the poor prognosis, patients with end-stage ILD with no indication to transplant and aggressive life-support should not die in an acute care setting, but offered palliation and end-of-life supportive care [95]. Furthermore, all patients in advanced stages of ILD that are not candidates to invasive treatments should receive appropriate counseling about the prognosis of the disease and the possible supportive measures available.

In conclusion, site of care in ILD patients with ARF may include a wide range of choices from an ICU with ECMO to palliation centers. Clinicians, with the support of a multidisciplinary team (e.g. pulmonologist and intensivist), should be prepared to promptly recognize a possible candidate to lung transplant from one who may benefit from comfort and supportive measures alone.

Acute respiratory failure treatment

a) Oxygen therapy and high-flow nasal cannula

Oxygen supplementation is the mainstay of treatment of ARF in ILDs. In the acute setting, different kinds of oxygen therapy are available, from simple nasal cannulae to face masks, including high concentration oxygen with reservoir mask and Venturi mask.

Patients with ILDs in advanced stages or during AE have a high degree of diffusion impairment and V/Q mismatch and require high oxygen concentrations to achieve satisfactory respiratory gas exchange. The risk of hypercapnia in these patients is usually minimal, and at the very end stages [96].

In some conditions, patients' needs can be higher and the oxygen flows provided by conventional therapy may be lower than inspiratory peak flows. Humidified High-Flow Nasal Cannula (HFNC) oxygen therapy is a disposal, which may provide very high flows (up to 60 L/min) and utilizes an air oxygen blend allowing from 21 to 100% FIO_2 delivery [97].

This modality of oxygen delivery may offer several advantages in comparison to the usual oxygen therapy, since it provides both steady FIO_2, and, theoretically, an anatomical oxygen reservoir within the nasopharynx and oropharynx, by virtue of a carbon dioxide wash-out effect due to high oxygen flow [98–101]. This more efficient carbon dioxide elimination together with reduced dead space results in a reduced ventilatory drive that, ultimately, leads to a decreased respiratory rate and work of breathing [101, 102]. There is also a continuous positive airway pressure (CPAP) effect which provides an upper airway extending pressure that ranges between 3.2 and 7.4 cmH_2O with the mouth closed and leads to an increased end-expiratory lung volume [103, 104]. Finally, the heated humidification facilitates secretion clearance, increasing patients' comfort and maintaining mucosal integrity

[105, 106]. Although there is increasing evidence in neonatal and paediatric settings [107], the utility of HFNC in ILDs is unknown.

A recent systematic review analyzed the effect of HFNC vs conventional oxygen therapy or NIV in adults including 11 randomised control trials (RCTs) and concluded that HFNC use was associated with reduction in intubation rate, need for IMV and rate of escalation of respiratory support when compared to conventional oxygen therapy [108]. When HFNC was compared to NIV, no differences in the rate of intubation and escalation of respiratory support was observed. No difference was found in mortality between HFNC and conventional oxygen therapy or NIV utilization. However, inclusion criteria, as well as endpoints and etiology of ARF, were different among studies, leading to the impossibility to draw certain conclusions. In particular, none of the studies explicitly evaluated patients with ILDs.

No studies have yet assessed the effectiveness of HFNC in patients with ARF in ILD, with the exception of a case series. *Horio* et al. described three patients with AE of interstitial pneumonia and unsatisfactory respiratory gas exchange with no rebreathing face masks, who were successfully treated with HFNC [109].

In conclusion, HFNC in ILD patients might potentially be an alternative to conventional oxygen therapy in patients requiring both high concentration of oxygen and high-flow gas to correct hypoxemia and control dyspnea and tachypnea. However, the evidence is very scarce and RCTs are needed to establish the real efficacy of this oxygen delivery method.

b) Non-invasive ventilation

The outcome of patients with ARF and ILDs ventilated in the ICU is very poor and IMV proved to be mostly futile [54]. Current IPF guidelines recommend that the majority of patients with respiratory failure should not receive IMV [46]. The reason of this finding lies in the fact that both the underlying structural lung disease and the precipitating condition causing ARF have a high likelihood of being irreversible and progressive. The pathogenic mechanisms causing AE-ILD have not yet been fully understood, thus, there are no treatments that have proven to be effective in RCTs. In this scenario, NIV may be applied in the hope to treat or stabilize the cause of ARF, minimizing complications and the poor outcome connected with endotracheal intubation (ETI) and IMV [110].

A few studies and case series have evaluated the application of NIV in ARF in ILDs. Two case series by *Yokoyama and colleagues* and *Vianello* et al. reported similar results in IPF patients with ARF [111, 112]. On one hand, a minority of patients benefited from NIV application

(5/11–45% - and 8/18–44%, in the cohorts of *Yokoyama* and *Vianello*, respectively), and, in those who responded, the use of NIV was associated with better outcomes, including avoidance of ETI and better survival. On the other hand, patients who failed NIV died within 3 months, regardless of ETI.

Gungor and colleagues evaluated the use of NIV both in IPF and in other ILDs with better overall prognosis, including CTD and silicosis [113], however, they found similar outcomes to the previously cited cohorts of IPF patients [111, 112], with a higher mortality rate and NIV failure in those who needed continuous NIV compared to those that were able to tolerate NIV interruptions for feeding.

NIV responsiveness was associated with less severe ARF and patients' condition in most series [94, 111–114]. Furthermore, *Yokoyama* et al. in a study on 38 patients with ARF in ILDs, including IPF, CTD-ILD and drug-induced ILD, reported that early NIV initiation during the acute phase was associated with better 30-day survival [114], indicating that early optimization of supportive care, including oxygenation, may improve patients' management and short-term outcomes.

A further step was attempted by *Aliberti and colleagues* who evaluated NIV responsiveness in patients with ILD and ARF in a multicentre study, stratifying the results according to the cause of ARF and the underlying radiological pattern of ILD [115]. NIV showed to improve oxygenation in patients with pneumonia, but not in those with AE; however, this positive effect on oxygenation did not translate into improved outcomes in patients with pneumonia compared to those with AE. No differences were observed in terms of radiological pattern. These results seem to suggest that, in spite of a better oxygenation in specific subgroups of patients, NIV outcomes do not depend on the radiological pattern or underlying cause of ARF. In fact, even if the precipitating factors are promptly recognized and treated, most cases show an irreversible deterioration of baseline conditions.

In conclusion, despite the high rate of NIV failure in patients with ARF in ILDs, in selected patients, such as those with less severe respiratory failure, an early NIV trial might facilitate the recognition of NIV-responder patients, who may present better short-term clinical outcomes. However, NIV responsiveness does not seem to impact on the poor prognosis related to the underlying disease: one-year mortality rate in NIV-responder patients was ≥70% in all the studies evaluated [94, 111, 112].

The main difficulties encountered when applying NIV on patients with ILDs and some practical tips to overcome them are summarised in Table 2.

c) Invasive mechanical ventilation

Table 2 Clinical aspects of Non-Invasive Ventilation in Interstitial Lung Diseases

Problem	Tip for solution
High pressures required to obtain ideal tidal volume in fibrotic lung with risk of pneumothorax	- Tolerate low tidal volumes with higher respiratory rate to obtain acceptable minute ventilation - Low to moderate PEEP levels to avoid overdistension of "healthy" lung units
High respiratory rate that hampers patient-ventilator adaptation	- Titrate drugs to control respiratory rate, e.g. opiates (morphine or fentanyl)§
Intense breathlessness reported by patients especially in the acute phase	- Titrate drugs to control respiratory rate, e.g. opiates (morphine or fentanyl)§ - Rapid inspiratory curve - Increase FIO2

Footnotes: PEEP = positive end expiratory pressure; FIO2 = fraction of inspired oxygen
§ Matsumoto T, Tomii K, Tachikawa R, Otsuka K, Nagata K, Otsuka K, et al. Role of sedation for agitated patients undergoing noninvasive ventilation: clinical practice in a tertiary referral hospital. Bmc Pulm Med. 2015 Jul 13;15:71

During an episode of severe ARF, patients might need intensive care support, including ETI and IMV. Multiple retrospective studies have taken into account patients with IPF admitted to the ICU for ARF [11, 54, 55, 86, 87, 116, 117]. In all the reported studies, IMV was associated with negative clinical outcomes, in some cases with an in-hospital mortality higher than 90%. In some cohorts causes of ARF were divided into reversible, such as pneumonia, and irreversible, mainly AE-ILD. In the absence of reversible causes, patients did not seem to benefit from IMV, and, in these cases, some authors advised against the use of IMV, with the exception of patients listed for lung transplant [55].

A study by *Mollica* et al. in 2010 compared IMV to NIV or spontaneous breathing in patients with ARF and IPF [94]. Although both ventilatory strategies improved PaO2/FIO2 ratio, in comparison to spontaneous breathing, the authors reported a global in-hospital mortality of 85%, that rose up to 100% in patients treated with IMV.

Other authors evaluated the use of IMV in ARF in non-IPF fibrotic ILDs. *Molina-Molina* et al. assessed 20 patients with fibrotic ILDs (14 with IPF and 6 with CTD-ILD) who required IMV [118]: similarly to cohorts with only IPF patients, IMV was associated with 100% in-hospital mortality.

Vincent et al. and *Gaudry and colleagues*, described the same scenario from a different point of view [119, 120]. Both authors described IPF and fibrotic-NSIP patients with ARF treated with NIV or IMV. *Vincent* et al. observed that by dividing their cases into two successive time periods (the first period from 1999 to 2004 and the second from 2005 to 2009), the patient's prognosis improved in the second time period compared to the first [119].

Despite all the limitations of this study, the authors hypothesized that some of the improvements introduced in the years, including lung-protective ventilatory parameters with lower tidal volumes and plateau pressures and earlier admission to the ICU, might have changed the outcomes of these patients, suggesting that not all patients are doomed to poor short-term outcomes. *Gaudry* et al., while observing a poor prognosis in most cases (21 out of 27 patients, 85%, died during hospitalization), found that a small subgroup of patients survived (6 cases) and some of them were able to reach pulmonary transplant (2 patients, 7%), confirming that IMV might be indicated in very selected patients candidate to lung transplant [120].

One of the mechanisms involved in the poor prognosis of mechanically ventilated patients with advanced fibrotic ILDs is VILI [88, 120]. The forces applied through IMV can cause pathophysiological alterations culminating in the disruption of cell membranes and cell-cell contacts, particularly in those patients with inhomogeneously injured lungs, such as in ARDS [121]. The fibrotic lung might be subject to a similar VILI as a consequence of baro- and volutrauma. *Nava and colleagues* assessed the respiratory mechanics of end-stage fibrotic ILDs during IMV and reported an approximately fourfold increase in the elastance of the respiratory system compared to normal anaesthetised subjects [122]; the values reported were even higher than those in patients with ARDS [122]. This marked increase in lung elastance is mainly due to the "stiffness" of the fibrotic lung. At the same time, the authors also observed that the resistance of the respiratory system was markedly increased compared with the values reported for normal subjects (although to a lesser extent than COPD patients) [122]. This finding reflects similar observations by *West and colleagues* that reported in patients with fibrotic lung diseases an increased resistive work in association with a higher work of breathing in comparison to normal subjects [123].

In conclusion, despite the low quality of the evidence available, IMV in patients with IPF and advanced fibrotic ILDs that develop ARF seems to be contraindicated, because of the high short-term mortality. However, it is necessary to differentiate some subgroups of patients, such as those with a potentially reversible cause of ARF or those listed for lung transplant, on whom prognostic data are less accurate and indications to IMV should be assessed on a case-by-case basis.

d) Extracorporeal membrane oxygenation

ECMO, referring to an extracorporeal circuit that directly oxygenates and removes carbon dioxide from the blood, may be considered in refractory severe ARF when positive-pressure ventilation, in combination with other ventilatory strategies such as prone positioning and neuromuscular block, results in unacceptable levels of hypoxemia, hypercapnia and acidemia [124].

ECMO in ILDs might be considered in patients with severe respiratory failure secondary to a potentially reversible cause of deterioration (e.g., infection or pulmonary embolism) and if the patient is a candidate for lung transplant [125].

The recent improvements in ECMO technology have allowed some centres to use less invasive ECMO or other extracorporeal devices to liberate patients from IMV and successfully bridge them to lung transplantation [125].

Trudzinski et al. reported their experience with ILD patients treated with ECMO for ARF [90]. ECMO was only used when patients were considered potential candidates for lung transplant or when two intensivists agreed on a potentially reversible pulmonary cause of ARF (e.g., acute infection on previous chronic ILD). Indications for veno-venous ECMO in the 21 patients included in the study were: refractory hypoxemia or uncompensated hypercapnia in ARDS despite optimization of IMV, or refractory hypoxemia despite maximal non-invasive therapies in patients considered "at risk of intubation". In the latter case, ECMO was used to prevent intubation, and referred to as "awake-ECMO", meaning the use of ECMO in awake, non-intubated, spontaneously breathing patients. The authors reported that out of the 21 patients treated with ECMO, six (29%) underwent lung transplant and two (10%) died on the waiting list after 9 and 63 days on ECMO. Of the 15 patients who did not undergo lung transplantation, 14 died after a mean time on ECMO of 40 days. These results confirm that in the absence of effective therapeutic perspectives (e.g. transplantation), ECMO is unable to prevent the irreversible progression of the underlying disease and does not improve mortality in patients with severe ARF and ILDs.

Fuehner et al. were the first to compare the outcomes of awake-ECMO patients with terminal respiratory or cardiopulmonary failure candidate to lung transplant to a historical cohort of patients treated with conventional IMV as bridge to transplant [126]. The duration of awake-ECMO and IMV were similar between the 2 groups (median 9 and 15 days, respectively), as well as the mortality rate on ECMO and IMV before a donor organ was available (23 and 29%, respectively). Results were encouraging, with a 6-month survival rate after transplantation of 80% in the "awake-ECMO" group vs 50% in the mechanically ventilated group.

A strategy based on ECMO to avoid IMV might potentially offer numerous benefits, including prevention of VILI and ventilator-associated pneumonia, preservation of oral feeding, spontaneous coughing, and social interaction, and allowance of early rehabilitation [127]. However, extracorporeal support devices are frequently linked to complications, including vessel perforation, bleeding, and

infections. The main complications reported in *Trudzinski*'s cohort were bleeding (3 cases, 14%) and cannulation placement (2 cases, 13%), while in *Fuehner*'s cohort were bleeding requiring transfusions (8 cases, 31%), sepsis-like syndrome (5 cases, 19%), intractable coughing requiring ETI (2 cases, 8%).

Of all the available forms of extracorporeal gas exchange, partial lung support, also known as extracorporeal CO_2 removal (ECCO2R) or respiratory dialysis, has shown some interesting results [128]. Recently, $ECCO_2R$ has been proposed as an intervention to eliminate CO2 from the blood of patients undergoing NIV who are unable to achieve adequate gas exchange despite optimization of ventilatory settings [129]. *Vianello* et al. described the successful management of an IPF patient with ARF using a pump-assisted veno-venous system for $ECCO_2R$ as an alternative to ETI following NIV failure [130]. The authors were able to minimize the complications most commonly related to ECMO by using a small single veno-venous dual lumen catheter. However, both clinicians' experience and the technology behind $ECCO_2R$ still need to be improved before its use can be widely implemented in clinical practice.

In conclusion, extracorporeal lung support might allow to prevent or reduce the invasiveness of IMV, and, therefore, minimize the risk of "triggering" fatal deterioration of the underlying chronic process, such as VILI. However, ECMO alone does not change the poor outcome associated with severe ARF in ILDs, and, given the high costs and risk of complications, should be limited to patients with a potential good short-term prognosis, e.g. those listed for lung transplant.

Conclusions

ARF is a feared complication in ILDs, both for its difficult management and diagnostic work-up and the poor prognosis.

Oxygen supplementation and ventilatory support have proven to be ineffective in modifying the prognosis of the disease in the absence of effective therapeutic options. Less invasive techniques, including HFNC oxygen and NIV, might be used in less severe cases to correct hypoxemia and control dyspnea, while, invasive techniques, such as IMV and ECMO, should be limited to patients listed for lung transplant or with reversible causes of ARF.

Abbreviations

AE: Acute exacerbation; AE-IPF: AE of IPF; AEP: Acute eosinophilic pneumonia; AFOP: Acute fibrinous organizing pneumonia; AIP: Acute interstitial pneumonia; ARDS: Acute respiratory distress syndrome; ARF: Acute respiratory failure; BAL: Bronchoalveolar lavage; CHP: Chronic hypersensitivity pneumonitis; COP: Cryptogenic organizing pneumonia; COPD: Chronic obstructive pulmonary disease; CPAP: Continuous positive airway pressure; CTD-ILD: Connective tissue disease related ILD; DAD: Diffuse alveolar damage; DAH: Diffuse alveolar hemorrhage; ECCO2R: Extracorporeal CO_2 removal; ECMO: ExtraCorporeal Membrane Oxygenation; ETI: Endotracheal intubation; HDU: High dependency unit; HFNC: High-Flow Nasal Cannula; HRCT: High-resolution computed tomography; ICU: Intensive care unit; ILD: Interstitial lung disease; IMV: Invasive mechanical ventilation; IPF: Idiopathic pulmonary fibrosis; NIV: Non-invasive ventilation; NSIP: Non-specific interstitial pneumonia; RCT: Randomised control trial; V/Q: Ventilation-perfusion; VILI: Ventilator-induced lung injury

Authors' contributions
Study concept and design: PF, GM, and AP; acquisition of data: all authors; drafting of the manuscript: all authors; critical revision of the manuscript for important intellectual content: all authors; and read and approved the final manuscript: all authors.

Competing interests
The authors declare that they have no competing interests.

Author details
[1]Dipartimento Cardio-Toraco-Vascolare, University of Milan Bicocca, Respiratory Unit, San Gerardo Hospital, ASST di Monza, Via Pergolesi 33, 20900 Monza, Italy. [2]UOC di Fisiopatologia e Riabilitazione Respiratoria, AO Ospedali dei Colli Monaldi, Naples, Italy. [3]UOC Pulmonology and Pulmonary Rehabilitation, Istituti Clinici Scientifici Maugeri, IRCCS di Cassano Murge (BA), Cassano delle Murge, Italy. [4]Division of Respiratory Medicine, University Hospital Tor Vergata, Rome, Italy. [5]Dipartimento di Scienze Neuroriabilitative, Casa di Cura del Policlinico, Milan, Italy. [6]Department of Internal Medicine, UOC Pulmonology, Ospedale ASST-Rhodense, Garbagnate Milanese, Italy. [7]Pulmonology Unit, Ospedale Maggiore della Carità, University of Piemonte Orientale, Novara, Italy. [8]Internsive Care Unit, Hospital Morales Meseguer, Múrcia, Spain.

References
1. Ryerson CJ, Collard HR. Update on the diagnosis and classification of ILD. Curr Opin Pulm Med. 2013;19:453–9.
2. Travis WD, Costabel U, Hansell DM, King TE, Lynch DA, Nicholson AG, et al. An official American Thoracic Society/European Respiratory Society statement: update of the international multidisciplinary classification of the idiopathic interstitial pneumonias. Am J Respir Crit Care Med. 2013;188:733–48.
3. Coultas DB, Zumwalt RE, Black WC, Sobonya RE. The epidemiology of interstitial lung diseases. Am J Respir Crit Care Med. 1994;150:967–72.
4. Kaunisto J, Salomaa E-R, Hodgson U, Kaarteenaho R, Myllärniemi M. Idiopathic pulmonary fibrosis–a systematic review on methodology for the collection of epidemiological data. Bmc Pulm Med. 2013;13:53.
5. Nalysnyk L, Cid-Ruzafa J, Rotella P, Esser D. Incidence and prevalence of idiopathic pulmonary fibrosis: review of the literature. Eur Respir Rev Off J Eur Respir Soc. 2012;21:355–61.
6. Azuma A, Nukiwa T, Tsuboi E, Suga M, Abe S, Nakata K, et al. Double-blind, placebo-controlled trial of pirfenidone in patients with idiopathic pulmonary fibrosis. Am J Respir Crit Care Med. 2005;171:1040–7.
7. Noble PW, Albera C, Bradford WZ, Costabel U, Glassberg MK, Kardatzke D, et al. Pirfenidone in patients with idiopathic pulmonary fibrosis (CAPACITY): two randomised trials. Lancet Lond. Engl. 2011;377:1760–9.
8. Daniels CE, Lasky JA, Limper AH, Mieras K, Gabor E, Schroeder DR, et al. Imatinib treatment for idiopathic pulmonary fibrosis: randomized placebo-controlled trial results. Am J Respir Crit Care Med. 2010;181:604–10.
9. Kubo H, Nakayama K, Yanai M, Suzuki T, Yamaya M, Watanabe M, et al. Anticoagulant therapy for idiopathic pulmonary fibrosis. Chest. 2005;128:1475–82.
10. Demedts M, Behr J, Buhl R, Costabel U, Dekhuijzen R, Jansen HM, et al. High-dose acetylcysteine in idiopathic pulmonary fibrosis. N Engl J Med. 2005;353:2229–42.
11. Kim DS, Park JH, Park BK, Lee JS, Nicholson AG, Colby T. Acute exacerbation of idiopathic pulmonary fibrosis: frequency and clinical features. Eur Respir J. 2006;27:143–50.
12. Kishaba T, Tamaki H, Shimaoka Y, Fukuyama H, Yamashiro S. Staging of acute exacerbation in patients with idiopathic pulmonary fibrosis. Lung. 2014;192:141–9.
13. Song JW, Hong S-B, Lim C-M, Koh Y, Kim DS. Acute exacerbation of idiopathic pulmonary fibrosis: incidence, risk factors and outcome. Eur Respir J. 2011;37:356–63.
14. Taniguchi H, Ebina M, Kondoh Y, Ogura T, Azuma A, Suga M, et al. Pirfenidone in idiopathic pulmonary fibrosis. Eur Respir J. 2010;35:821–9.
15. Idiopathic Pulmonary Fibrosis Clinical Research Network, Martinez FJ, de Andrade JA, Anstrom KJ, King TE, Raghu G. Randomized trial of acetylcysteine in idiopathic pulmonary fibrosis. N Engl J Med. 2014;370:2093–101.
16. Richeldi L, Costabel U, Selman M, Kim DS, Hansell DM, Nicholson AG, et al. Efficacy of a tyrosine kinase inhibitor in idiopathic pulmonary fibrosis. N Engl J Med. 2011;365:1079–87.
17. Richeldi L, du Bois RM, Raghu G, Azuma A, Brown KK, Costabel U, et al. Efficacy and safety of nintedanib in idiopathic pulmonary fibrosis. N Engl J Med. 2014;370:2071–82.
18. King TE, Albera C, Bradford WZ, Costabel U, Hormel P, Lancaster L, et al. Effect of interferon gamma-1b on survival in patients with idiopathic pulmonary fibrosis (INSPIRE): a multicentre, randomised, placebo-controlled trial. Lancet Lond Engl. 2009;374:222–8.
19. King TE, Bradford WZ, Castro-Bernardini S, Fagan EA, Glaspole I, Glassberg MK, et al. A phase 3 trial of pirfenidone in patients with idiopathic pulmonary fibrosis. N Engl J Med. 2014;370:2083–92.
20. King TE, Brown KK, Raghu G, du Bois RM, Lynch DA, Martinez F, et al. BUILD-3: a randomized, controlled trial of bosentan in idiopathic pulmonary fibrosis. Am J Respir Crit Care Med. 2011;184:92–9.
21. King TE, Behr J, Brown KK, du Bois RM, Lancaster L, de Andrade JA, et al. BUILD-1: a randomized placebo-controlled trial of bosentan in idiopathic pulmonary fibrosis. Am J Respir Crit Care Med. 2008;177:75–81.
22. Raghu G, Behr J, Brown KK, Egan JJ, Kawut SM, Flaherty KR, et al. Treatment of idiopathic pulmonary fibrosis with ambrisentan: a parallel, randomized trial. Ann Intern Med. 2013;158(9):641.
23. Noth I, Anstrom KJ, Calvert SB, de Andrade J, Flaherty KR, Glazer C, et al. A placebo-controlled randomized trial of warfarin in idiopathic pulmonary fibrosis. Am J Respir Crit Care Med. 2012;186:88–95.
24. Kondoh Y, Taniguchi H, Katsuta T, Kataoka K, Kimura T, Nishiyama O, et al. Risk factors of acute exacerbation of idiopathic pulmonary fibrosis. Sarcoidosis Vasc Diffuse Lung Dis Off J Wasog. 2010;27:103–10.
25. Idiopathic Pulmonary Fibrosis Clinical Research Network, Zisman DA, Schwarz M, Anstrom KJ, Collard HR, Flaherty KR, et al. A controlled trial of sildenafil in advanced idiopathic pulmonary fibrosis. N Engl J Med. 2010;363:620–8.
26. Idiopathic Pulmonary Fibrosis Clinical Research Network, Raghu G, Anstrom KJ, King TE, Lasky JA, Martinez FJ. Prednisone, azathioprine, and N-acetylcysteine for pulmonary fibrosis. N Engl J Med. 2012;366:1968–77.
27. Collard HR, Yow E, Richeldi L, Anstrom KJ, Glazer C, investigators IPF. Suspected acute exacerbation of idiopathic pulmonary fibrosis as an outcome measure in clinical trials. Respir Res. 2013;14:73.
28. Suzuki H, Sekine Y, Yoshida S, Suzuki M, Shibuya K, Yonemori Y, et al. Risk of acute exacerbation of interstitial pneumonia after pulmonary resection for lung cancer in patients with idiopathic pulmonary fibrosis based on preoperative high-resolution computed tomography. Surg Today. 2011;41:914–21.
29. Shintani Y, Ohta M, Iwasaki T, Ikeda N, Tomita E, Kawahara K, et al. Predictive factors for postoperative acute exacerbation of interstitial pneumonia combined with lung cancer. Gen Thorac Cardiovasc Surg. 2010;58:182–5.
30. Collard HR, Ryerson CJ, Corte TJ, Jenkins G, Kondoh Y, Lederer DJ, et al. Acute exacerbation of idiopathic pulmonary fibrosis. An international working group report. Am J Respir Crit Care Med. 2016;194:265–75.
31. Kondoh Y, Taniguchi H, Ebina M, Azuma A, Ogura T, Taguchi Y, et al. Risk factors for acute exacerbation of idiopathic pulmonary fibrosis–extended analysis of pirfenidone trial in Japan. Respir. Investig. 2015;53:271–8.
32. Costabel U, Inoue Y, Richeldi L, Collard HR, Tschoepe I, Stowasser S, et al. Efficacy of Nintedanib in idiopathic pulmonary fibrosis across Prespecified subgroups in INPULSIS. Am J Respir Crit Care Med. 2016;193:178–85.

33. Akira M, Kozuka T, Yamamoto S, Sakatani M. Computed tomography findings in acute exacerbation of idiopathic pulmonary fibrosis. Am J Respir Crit Care Med. 2008;178:372–8.

34. Lee JS, Collard HR, Anstrom KJ, Martinez FJ, Noth I, Roberts RS, et al. Anti-acid treatment and disease progression in idiopathic pulmonary fibrosis: an analysis of data from three randomised controlled trials. Lancet Respir Med. 2013;1:369–76.

35. Lee JS, Song JW, Wolters PJ, Elicker BM, King TE, Kim DS, et al. Bronchoalveolar lavage pepsin in acute exacerbation of idiopathic pulmonary fibrosis. Eur Respir J. 2012;39:352–8.

36. Johannson KA, Vittinghoff E, Lee K, Balmes JR, Ji W, Kaplan GG, et al. Acute exacerbation of idiopathic pulmonary fibrosis associated with air pollution exposure. Eur Respir J. 2014;43:1124–31.

37. Spagnolo P, Cottin V. Genetics of idiopathic pulmonary fibrosis: from mechanistic pathways to personalised medicine. J Med Genet. 2017;54:93–9.

38. Sakamoto K, Taniguchi H, Kondoh Y, Wakai K, Kimura T, Kataoka K, et al. Acute exacerbation of IPF following diagnostic bronchoalveolar lavage procedures. Respir Med. 2012;106:436–42.

39. Bando M, Ohno S, Hosono T, Yanase K, Sato Y, Sohara Y, et al. Risk of acute exacerbation after video-assisted Thoracoscopic lung biopsy for interstitial lung disease. J Bronchology Interv Pulmonol. 2009;16:229–35.

40. Sakamoto S, Homma S, Mun M, Fujii T, Kurosaki A, Yoshimura K. Acute exacerbation of idiopathic interstitial pneumonia following lung surgery in 3 of 68 consecutive patients: a retrospective study. Intern. Med. Tokyo Jpn. 2011;50:77–85.

41. Mizuno Y, Iwata H, Shirahashi K, Takamochi K, Oh S, Suzuki K, et al. The importance of intraoperative fluid balance for the prevention of postoperative acute exacerbation of idiopathic pulmonary fibrosis after pulmonary resection for primary lung cancer. Eur J Cardio-Thorac Surg Off J Eur Assoc Cardio-Thorac Surg. 2012;41:e161–5.

42. Kenmotsu H, Naito T, Kimura M, Ono A, Shukuya T, Nakamura Y, et al. The risk of cytotoxic chemotherapy-related exacerbation of interstitial lung disease with lung cancer. J Thorac Oncol Off Publ Int Assoc Study Lung Cancer. 2011;6:1242–6.

43. Takeda A, Enomoto T, Sanuki N, Nakajima T, Takeda T, Sayama K, et al. Acute exacerbation of subclinical idiopathic pulmonary fibrosis triggered by hypofractionated stereotactic body radiotherapy in a patient with primary lung cancer and slightly focal honeycombing. Radiat Med. 2008;26:504–7.

44. Ohshimo S, Ishikawa N, Horimasu Y, Hattori N, Hirohashi N, Tanigawa K, et al. Baseline KL-6 predicts increased risk for acute exacerbation of idiopathic pulmonary fibrosis. Respir Med. 2014;108:1031–9.

45. Kishaba T, Shimaoka Y, Fukuyama H, Yoshida K, Tanaka M, Yamashiro S, et al. A cohort study of mortality predictors and characteristics of patients with combined pulmonary fibrosis and emphysema. BMJ Open. 2012;2

46. Raghu G, Rochwerg B, Zhang Y, Garcia CAC, Azuma A, Behr J, et al. An official ATS/ERS/JRS/ALAT clinical practice guideline: treatment of idiopathic pulmonary fibrosis. An update of the 2011 clinical practice guideline. Am J Respir Crit Care Med. 2015;192:e3–19.

47. Olson AL, Swigris JJ, Lezotte DC, Norris JM, Wilson CG, Brown KK. Mortality from pulmonary fibrosis increased in the United States from 1992 to 2003. Am J Respir Crit Care Med. 2007;176:277–84.

48. Natsuizaka M, Chiba H, Kuronuma K, Ōtsuka M, Kudo K, Mori M, et al. Epidemiologic survey of Japanese patients with idiopathic pulmonary fibrosis and investigation of ethnic differences. Am J Respir Crit Care Med. 2014;190:773–9.

49. Daniels CE, Yi ES, Ryu JH. Autopsy findings in 42 consecutive patients with idiopathic pulmonary fibrosis. Eur Respir J. 2008;32:170–4.

50. Agarwal R, Jindal SK. Acute exacerbation of idiopathic pulmonary fibrosis: a systematic review. Eur J Intern Med. 2008;19:227–35.

51. Huie TJ, Olson AL, Cosgrove GP, Janssen WJ, Lara AR, Lynch DA, et al. A detailed evaluation of acute respiratory decline in patients with fibrotic lung disease: aetiology and outcomes. Respirol Carlton Vic. 2010;15:909–17.

52. Tachibana K, Inoue Y, Nishiyama A, Sugimoto C, Matsumuro A, Hirose M, et al. Polymyxin-B hemoperfusion for acute exacerbation of idiopathic pulmonary fibrosis: serum IL-7 as a prognostic marker. Sarcoidosis Vasc. Diffuse lung dis. Off. J Wasog. 2011;28:113–22.

53. Simon-Blancal V, Freynet O, Nunes H, Bouvry D, Naggara N, Brillet P-Y, et al. Acute exacerbation of idiopathic pulmonary fibrosis: outcome and prognostic factors. Respir. Int. Rev. Thorac. Dis. 2012;83:28–35.

54. Rangappa P, Moran JL. Outcomes of patients admitted to the intensive care unit with idiopathic pulmonary fibrosis. Crit. Care Resusc. J. Australas. Acad. Crit Care Med. 2009;11:102–9.

55. Al-Hameed FM, Sharma S. Outcome of patients admitted to the intensive care unit for acute exacerbation of idiopathic pulmonary fibrosis. Can Respir J. 2004;11:117–22.

56. Navaratnam V, Ali N, Smith CJP, McKeever T, Fogarty A, Hubbard RB. Does the presence of connective tissue disease modify survival in patients with pulmonary fibrosis? Respir Med. 2011;105:1925–30.

57. Thomeer MJ, Vansteenkiste J, Verbeken EK, Demedts M. Interstitial lung diseases: characteristics at diagnosis and mortality risk assessment. Respir Med. 2004;98:567–73.

58. Moua T, Westerly BD, Dulohery MM, Daniels CE, Ryu JH, Lim KG. Patients with fibrotic interstitial lung disease hospitalized for acute respiratory worsening: a large cohort analysis. Chest. 2016;149:1205–14.

59. Ambrosini V, Cancellieri A, Chilosi M, Zompatori M, Trisolini R, Saragoni L, et al. Acute exacerbation of idiopathic pulmonary fibrosis: report of a series. Eur Respir J. 2003;22:821–6.

60. Collard HR, Moore BB, Flaherty KR, Brown KK, Kaner RJ, King TE, et al. Acute exacerbations of idiopathic pulmonary fibrosis. Am J Respir Crit Care Med. 2007;176:636–43.

61. Rice AJ, Wells AU, Bouros D, du Bois RM, Hansell DM, Polychronopoulos V, et al. Terminal diffuse alveolar damage in relation to interstitial pneumonias. An autopsy study Am J Clin Pathol. 2003;119:709–14.

62. Rush B, Wiskar K, Berger L, Griesdale D. The use of mechanical ventilation in patients with idiopathic pulmonary fibrosis in the United States: a nationwide retrospective cohort analysis. Respir Med. 2016;111:72–6.

63. Huie TJ, Olson AL, Cosgrove GP, Janssen WJ, Lara AR, Lynch DA, et al. A detailed evaluation of acute respiratory decline in patients with fibrotic lung disease: aetiology and outcomes. Respirol. Carlton Vic. 2010;15:909–17.

64. Churg A, Müller NL, Silva CIS, Wright JL. Acute exacerbation (acute lung injury of unknown cause) in UIP and other forms of fibrotic interstitial pneumonias. Am J Surg Pathol. 2007;31:277–84.

65. Olson AL, Huie TJ, Groshong SD, Cosgrove GP, Janssen WJ, Schwarz MI, et al. Acute exacerbations of fibrotic hypersensitivity pneumonitis: a case series. Chest. 2008;134:844–50.

66. Miyazaki Y, Tateishi T, Akashi T, Ohtani Y, Inase N, Yoshizawa Y. Clinical predictors and histologic appearance of acute exacerbations in chronic hypersensitivity pneumonitis. Chest. 2008;134:1265–70.

67. Suda T, Kaida Y, Nakamura Y, Enomoto N, Fujisawa T, Imokawa S, et al. Acute exacerbation of interstitial pneumonia associated with collagen vascular diseases. Respir Med. 2009;103:846–53.

68. Spagnolo P, Wuyts W. Acute exacerbations of interstitial lung disease: lessons from idiopathic pulmonary fibrosis. Curr Opin Pulm Med. 2017;23:411–7.

69. Park I-N, Kim DS, Shim TS, Lim C-M, Lee SD, Koh Y, et al. Acute exacerbation of interstitial pneumonia other than idiopathic pulmonary fibrosis. Chest. 2007;132:214–20.

70. Parambil JG, Myers JL, Ryu JH. Histopathologic features and outcome of patients with acute exacerbation of idiopathic pulmonary fibrosis undergoing surgical lung biopsy. Chest. 2005;128(5):3310.

71. Douglas WW, Tazelaar HD, Hartman TE, Hartman RP, Decker PA, Schroeder DR, et al. Polymyositis-dermatomyositis-associated interstitial lung disease. Am J Respir Crit Care Med. 2001;164:1182–5.

72. Tzelepis GE, Toya SP, Moutsopoulos HM. Occult connective tissue diseases mimicking idiopathic interstitial pneumonias. Eur Respir J. 2008;31:11–20.

73. Taniguchi H, Kondoh Y. Acute and subacute idiopathic interstitial pneumonias. Respirol. Carlton Vic. 2016;21:810–20.

74. Olson J, Colby TV, Elliott CG. Hamman-rich syndrome revisited. Mayo Clin Proc. 1990;65:1538–48.

75. Bouros D, Nicholson AC, Polychronopoulos V, du Bois RM. Acute interstitial pneumonia. Eur Respir J. 2000;15:412–8.

76. Vourlekis JS, Brown KK, Cool CD, Young DA, Cherniack RM, King TE, et al. Acute interstitial pneumonitis. Case series and review of the literature. Medicine (Baltimore). 2000;79:369–78.

77. Cohen AJ, King TE, Downey GP. Rapidly progressive bronchiolitis obliterans with organizing pneumonia. Am J Respir Crit Care Med. 1994;149:1670–5.

78. King TE, Mortenson RL. Cryptogenic organizing pneumonitis. The north American experience. Chest 1992;102:8S–13S.

79. Oymak FS, Demirbaş HM, Mavili E, Akgun H, Gulmez I, Demir R, et al. Bronchiolitis obliterans organizing pneumonia. Clinical and roentgenological features in 26 cases. Respir. Int. Rev. Thorac. Dis. 2005;72:254–62.

80. Philit F, Etienne-Mastroïanni B, Parrot A, Guérin C, Robert D, Cordier J-F. Idiopathic acute eosinophilic pneumonia: a study of 22 patients. Am J Respir Crit Care Med. 2002;166(9):1235.

81. Camus P, Bonniaud P, Fanton A, Camus C, Baudaun N, Foucher P. Drug-induced and iatrogenic infiltrative lung disease. Clin Chest Med. 2004;25:479–519. vi

82. Patel AM, Ryu JH, Reed CE. Hypersensitivity pneumonitis: current concepts and future questions. J Allergy Clin Immunol. 2001;108:661–70.

83. D'Ippolito R, Chetta A, Foresi A, Marangio E, Castagnaro A, Merliniaft S, et al. Induced sputum and bronchoalveolar lavage from patients with hypersensitivity pneumonitis. Respir Med. 2004;98:977–83.

84. Imoto EM, Lombard CM, Sachs DP. Pulmonary capillaritis and hemorrhage. A clue to the diagnosis of systemic necrotizing vasculitis. Chest. 1989;96:927–8.

85. Mallick S. Outcome of patients with idiopathic pulmonary fibrosis (IPF) ventilated in intensive care unit. Respir Med. 2008;102:1355–9.

86. Blivet S, Philit F, Sab JM, Langevin B, Paret M, Guérin C, et al. Outcome of patients with idiopathic pulmonary fibrosis admitted to the ICU for respiratory failure. Chest. 2001;120:209–12.

87. Saydain G, Islam A, Afessa B, Ryu JH, Scott JP, Peters SG. Outcome of patients with idiopathic pulmonary fibrosis admitted to the intensive care unit. Am J Respir Crit Care Med. 2002;166:839–42.

88. Fernández-Pérez ER, Yilmaz M, Jenad H, Daniels CE, Ryu JH, Hubmayr RD, et al. Ventilator settings and outcome of respiratory failure in chronic interstitial lung disease. Chest. 2008;133:1113–9.

89. Papiris SA, Manali ED, Kolilekas L, Kagouridis K, Triantafillidou C, Tsangaris I, et al. Clinical review: idiopathic pulmonary fibrosis acute exacerbations–unravelling Ariadne's thread. Crit. Care Lond. Engl. 2010;14:246.

90. Trudzinski FC, Kaestner F, Schäfers H-J, Fähndrich S, Seiler F, Böhmer P, et al. Outcome of patients with interstitial lung disease treated with extracorporeal membrane oxygenation for acute respiratory failure. Am J Respir Crit Care Med. 2016;193:527–33.

91. Bradley B, Branley HM, Egan JJ, Greaves MS, Hansell DM, Harrison NK, et al. Interstitial lung disease guideline: the British Thoracic Society in collaboration with the Thoracic Society of Australia and new Zealand and the Irish thoracic society. Thorax. 2008;63(Suppl 5):v1–58.

92. Gacouin A, Jouneau S, Letheulle J, Kerjouan M, Bouju P, Fillatre P, et al. Trends in prevalence and prognosis in subjects with acute chronic respiratory failure treated with noninvasive and/or invasive ventilation. Respir Care. 2015;60:210–8.

93. Trulock EP, Edwards LB, Taylor DO, Boucek MM, Mohacsi PJ, Keck BM, et al. The registry of the International Society for Heart and Lung Transplantation: twentieth official adult lung and heart-lung transplant report–2003. J. Heart lung transplant. Off. Publ. Int. Soc. Heart Transplant. 2003;22:625–35.

94. Mollica C, Paone G, Conti V, Ceccarelli D, Schmid G, Mattia P, et al. Mechanical ventilation in patients with end-stage idiopathic pulmonary fibrosis. Respiration. 2010;79:209–15.

95. Rajala K, Lehto JT, Saarinen M, Sutinen E, Saarto T, Myllärniemi M. End-of-life care of patients with idiopathic pulmonary fibrosis. Bmc Palliat Care. 2016;15:85.

96. O'Driscoll BR, Howard LS, Davison AG. British Thoracic Society. BTS guideline for emergency oxygen use in adult patients. Thorax. 2008;63(Suppl 6):vi1–68.

97. Spoletini G, Alotaibi M, Blasi F, Hill NS. Heated humidified high-flow nasal oxygen in adults: mechanisms of action and clinical implications. Chest. 2015;148:253–61.

98. Parke R, McGuinness S, Eccleston M. Nasal high-flow therapy delivers low level positive airway pressure. Br J Anaesth. 2009;103:886–90.

99. Ritchie JE, Williams AB, Gerard C, Hockey H. Evaluation of a humidified nasal high-flow oxygen system, using oxygraphy, capnography and measurement of upper airway pressures. Anaesth Intensive Care. 2011;39:1103–10.

100. Schreiber A, DI Marco F, Braido F, Solidoro P. High flow nasal cannula oxygen therapy, work in progress in respiratory critical care. Minerva Med. 2016;107:14–20.

101. Bräunlich J, Beyer D, Mai D, Hammerschmidt S, Seyfarth H-J, Wirtz H. Effects of nasal high flow on ventilation in volunteers, COPD and idiopathic pulmonary fibrosis patients. Respir Int Rev Thorac Dis. 2013;85:319–25.

102. Schwabbauer N, Berg B, Blumenstock G, Haap M, Hetzel J, Riessen R. Nasal high-flow oxygen therapy in patients with hypoxic respiratory failure: effect on functional and subjective respiratory parameters compared to conventional oxygen therapy and non-invasive ventilation (NIV). Bmc Anesth. 2014;14:66.

103. Chanques G, Riboulet F, Molinari N, Carr J, Jung B, Prades A, et al. Comparison of three high flow oxygen therapy delivery devices: a clinical physiological cross-over study. Minerva Anestesiol. 2013;79:1344–55.

104. Ward JJ. High-flow oxygen administration by nasal cannula for adult and perinatal patients. Respir Care. 2013;58:98–122.

105. Williams R, Rankin N, Smith T, Galler D, Seakins P. Relationship between the humidity and temperature of inspired gas and the function of the airway mucosa. Crit Care Med. 1996;24:1920–9.

106. Sztrymf B, Messika J, Bertrand F, Hurel D, Leon R, Dreyfuss D, et al. Beneficial effects of humidified high flow nasal oxygen in critical care patients: a prospective pilot study. Intensive Care Med. 2011;37:1780–6.

107. Wilkinson D, Andersen C, O'Donnell CPF, De Paoli AG, Manley BJ. High flow nasal cannula for respiratory support in preterm infants. Cochrane Database Syst Rev. 2016;2:CD006405.

108. Zhao H, Wang H, Sun F, Lyu S, An Y. High-flow nasal cannula oxygen therapy is superior to conventional oxygen therapy but not to noninvasive mechanical ventilation on intubation rate: a systematic review and meta-analysis. Crit Care Lond Engl. 2017;21:184.

109. Horio Y, Takihara T, Niimi K, Komatsu M, Sato M, Tanaka J, et al. High-flow nasal cannula oxygen therapy for acute exacerbation of interstitial pneumonia: a case series. Respir Investig. 2016;54:125–9.

110. Tomii K, Tachikawa R, Chin K, Murase K, Handa T, Mishima M, et al. Role of non-invasive ventilation in managing life-threatening acute exacerbation of interstitial pneumonia. Intern. Med. Tokyo Jpn. 2010;49:1341–7.

111. Yokoyama T, Kondoh Y, Taniguchi H, Kataoka K, Kato K, Nishiyama O, et al. Noninvasive ventilation in acute exacerbation of idiopathic pulmonary fibrosis. Intern Med. 2010;49:1509–14.

112. Vianello A, Arcaro G, Battistella L, Pipitone E, Vio S, Concas A, et al. Noninvasive ventilation in the event of acute respiratory failure in patients with idiopathic pulmonary fibrosis. J Crit Care. 2014;29:562–7.

113. Gungor G, Tatar D, Salturk C, Cimen P, Karakurt Z, Kirakli C, et al. Why do patients with interstitial lung diseases fail in the ICU? A 2-center cohort study. Respir Care. 2013;58:525–31.

114. Yokoyama T, Tsushima K, Yamamoto H, Koizumi T, Kubo K. Potential benefits of early continuous positive pressure ventilation in patients with rapidly progressive interstitial pneumonia. Respirol. Carlton Vic. 2012;17:315–21.

115. Aliberti S, Messinesi G, Gamberini S, Maggiolini S, Visca D, Galavotti V, et al. Non-invasive mechanical ventilation in patients with diffuse interstitial lung diseases. Bmc Pulm. Med. [Internet]. 2014; [cited 2017 Nov 26];14. Available from: https://doi.org/10.1186/1471-2466-14-194.

116. Fumeaux T, Rothmeier C, Jolliet P. Outcome of mechanical ventilation for acute respiratory failure in patients with pulmonary fibrosis. Intensive Care Med. 2001;27:1868–74.

117. Stern JB, Mal H, Groussard O, Brugière O, Marceau A, Jebrak G, et al. Prognosis of patients with advanced idiopathic pulmonary fibrosis requiring mechanical ventilation for acute respiratory failure. Chest. 2001;120:213–9.

118. Molina-Molina M, Badia JR, Marín-Arguedas A, Xaubet A, Santos MJ, Nicolás JM, et al. Outcomes and clinical characteristics of patients with pulmonary fibrosis and respiratory failure admitted to an intensive care unit. A study of 20 cases. Med Clin (Barc). 2003;121:63–7.

119. Vincent F, Gonzalez F, Do C-H, Clec'h C, Cohen Y. Invasive mechanical ventilation in patients with idiopathic pulmonary fibrosis or idiopathic non-specific interstitial pneumonia. Intern Med Tokyo Jpn. 2011;50:173–4. author reply 175

120. Gaudry S, Vincent F, Rabbat A, Nunes H, Crestani B, Naccache JM, et al. Invasive mechanical ventilation in patients with fibrosing interstitial pneumonia. J Thorac Cardiovasc Surg. 2014;147:47–53.

121. Uhlig U, Uhlig S. Ventilation-Induced Lung Injury. In: Terjung R, editor. Compr. Physiol. [Internet]. Hoboken: Wiley; 2011 [cited 2017 Nov 29]. Available from: https://doi.org/10.1002/cphy.c100004.

122. Nava S, Rubini F. Lung and chest wall mechanics in ventilated patients with end stage idiopathic pulmonary fibrosis. Thorax. 1999;54(5):390.

123. West JR, Alexander JK. Studies on respiratory mechanics and the work of breathing in pulmonary fibrosis. Am J Med. 1959;27:529–44.

124. Brodie D, Bacchetta M. Extracorporeal membrane oxygenation for ARDS in adults. N Engl J Med. 2011;365:1905–14.

125. Marasco SF, Lukas G, McDonald M, McMillan J, Ihle B. Review of ECMO (extra corporeal membrane oxygenation) support in critically ill adult patients. Heart Lung Circ. 2008;17(Suppl 4):S41–7.

126. Fuehner T, Kuehn C, Hadem J, Wiesner O, Gottlieb J, Tudorache I, et al. Extracorporeal membrane oxygenation in awake patients as bridge to lung transplantation. Am J Respir Crit Care Med. 2012;185:763–8.

127. Abrams D, Javidfar J, Farrand E, Mongero LB, Agerstrand CL, Ryan P, et al. Early mobilization of patients receiving extracorporeal membrane oxygenation: a retrospective cohort study. Crit. Care Lond. Engl. 2014;18:R38.

128. Barrett NA, Camporota L. The evolving role and practical application of extracorporeal carbon dioxide removal in critical care. Crit. Care Resusc. J. Australas. Acad Crit Care Med. 2017;19:62–7.

129. Braune S, Sieweke A, Brettner F, Staudinger T, Joannidis M, Verbrugge S, et al. The feasibility and safety of extracorporeal carbon dioxide removal to avoid intubation in patients with COPD unresponsive to noninvasive ventilation for acute hypercapnic respiratory failure (ECLAIR study): multicentre case-control study. Intensive Care Med. 2016;42:1437–44.

130. Vianello A, Arcaro G, Paladini L, Iovino S. Successful management of acute respiratory failure in an idiopathic pulmonary fibrosis patient using an extracorporeal carbon dioxide removal system. Sarcoidosis Vasc. Diffuse lung dis. Off. J Wasog. 2016;33:186–90.

Balloon pulmonary angioplasty – efficient therapy of chronic thromboembolic pulmonary hypertension in the patient with advanced sarcoidosis

Andrzej Labyk[1]*⬤, Dominik Wretowski[1], Sabina Zybińska-Oksiutowicz[1], Aleksandra Furdyna[1], Katarzyna Ciesielska[1], Dorota Piotrowska-Kownacka[2], Olga Dzikowska –Diduch[1], Barbara Lichodziejewska[1], Andrzej Biederman[3], Piotr Pruszczyk[1] and Marek Roik[1]

Abstract

Background: Approximately a quarter of patients with advanced sarcoidosis develop pulmonary hypertension (PH), which affects their prognosis. We report unusual case of confirmed chronic thromboembolic pulmonary hypertension (CTEPH) in a patient with stage IV sarcoidosis successfully treated with balloon pulmonary angioplasty (BPA).

Case presentation: A 65 years old male with a history of colitis ulcerosa, and pulmonary sarcoidosis diagnosed in 10 years before, on long term oral steroids, with a history of deep vein thrombosis and acute pulmonary embolism chronically anticoagulated was referred to our center due to severe dyspnea. On admission he presented WHO functional class IV, mean pulmonary artery pressure (mPAP) in right heart catheterization (RHC) was elevated to 54 mmHg. Diagnosis of CTEPH was definitely confirmed with typical V/Q scan, and with selective pulmonary angiography (PAG) completes by intravascular imagining (intravascular ultrasound, optical coherent tomography). The patient was deemed inoperable by CTEPH team and two sessions of BPA with multimodal approach resulted in significant clinical and haemodynamical improvement to WHO class II and mPAP decrease to 27 mmHg.

Conclusions: Balloon pulmonary angioplasty, rapidly developing method of treatment of inoperable CTEPH patients, is also extremely useful therapeutic tool in complex PH patients.

Keywords: Sarcoidosis, Chronic thromboembolic pulmonary hypertension, Balloon pulmonary angioplasty

Background

Approximately 26% of patients with advanced pulmonary sarcoidosis may develop pulmonary hypertension (PH), which is related with poor prognosis [1, 2]. According to current guidelines, patients with suspected PH should undergo detailed diagnostic workup and differential diagnosis among others should include chronic lung diseases leading to hypoxia and chronic thromboembolic pulmonary hypertension (CTEPH) [3]. We report an unusual challenging case of CTEPH in a patient with stage IV sarcoidosis.

Case presentation

A 65 years old male with history of colitis ulcerosa, and advanced sarcoidosis diagnosed 10 years before, on oral steroids was admitted to our department due to exertional dyspnea and right ventricular (RV) heart failure progressing since last 12 months to functional class IV. Two years earlier, he experienced the first severe decompensation of right heart function. At that time PH was diagnosed on echocardiography. RV to left ventricle (LV) ratio exceeded one (RV:LV - 39/32 mm); peak systolic tricuspid regurgitation gradient (TRPG) was 75 mmHg, and decreased tricuspid annular plane systolic excursion

* Correspondence: endrjulab@tlen.pl
[1]Center for Diagnostics and Treatment of Venous Thromboembolism, Department of Internal Medicine and Cardiology, Warsaw Medical University, Infant Jesus Hospital, Lindleya Street 4, 02-005 Warsaw, Poland
Full list of author information is available at the end of the article

(TAPSE) 15 mm indicated significant pressure overload and RV systolic dysfunction. Chest computed tomography (CT) revealed sarcoidosis progression, however no pulmonary thromboemboli were detected. After typical heart failure treatment with diuretics, ACE inhibitors, and steroid dose increase the patient improved and he was discharged home in a good clinical condition in WHO functional class II, with the diagnosis of PH due to sarcoidosis stage IV. One year later, due to acute dyspnea, worsening of RV function and unilateral leg swelling he underwent another chest CT, which this time showed fresh thrombi in the left segmental upper lobe pulmonary artery. Moreover, acute deep vein thrombosis was detected with lower limb compression ultrasound. Long term oral anticoagulation with rivaroxaban was started. Two years later the patient was referred to our center due to progressive functional deterioration. On admission he was in WHO functional class IV, saturation on room air was 85%, blood pressure 120/80 mmHg, heart rate 90 beats per minute. Mild peripheral edema was present. Distance covered in 6 min walk test (6MWT) was 100 m with desaturation to 77%. Plasma natriuretic peptide (NT-pro-BNP) concentration was elevated to 6239 pg/ml (normal range < 125 pg/ml). Echocardiography showed severe RV pressure overload with TRPG 95 mmHg, dilatation of both right atrium and ventricle. Preserved morphology and function of LV

was observed. Chest CT scan showed signs of advanced interstitial lung fibrosis (Fig. 1a) and calcified mediastinal lymph nodes (Fig. 1b). However, organized thrombi in both pulmonary were also detected (Fig. 1c and d). At that time multifactorial etiology of PH was considered: sarcoidosis with secondary PH and local in situ thrombosis, or CTEPH in a patient with stage IV sarcoidosis, and with deep vein thrombosis in the past. Lung perfusion scan with SPECT/CT showed bilateral perfusion defects which strongly suggested thromboembolic component of PH. Right heart catheterization (RHC) followed by selective pulmonary angiography (PAG) showed mean pulmonary artery pressure (mPAP) of 54 mmHg. Pulmonary artery wedge pressure (PAWP) was 6 mmHg and pulmonary vascular resistance (PVR) was 13,5 Wood Units. Selective PAG confirmed chronic thromboembolic lesions suggestive of CTEPH – left upper lobe artery occlusion, intravascular webs in right pulmonary artery (Fig. 2a). After experienced cardiac surgeon consultation, the patient was deemed inoperable due to advanced, sarcoidosis - related lung changes and propable complications regarding the use of extracorporeal circulation. He was finaly qualified for balloon pulmonary angioplasty (BPA).

BPA procedures were performed according the previously published protocol [4]. Importantly, in order to confirm intraluminal localization of thromboembolic

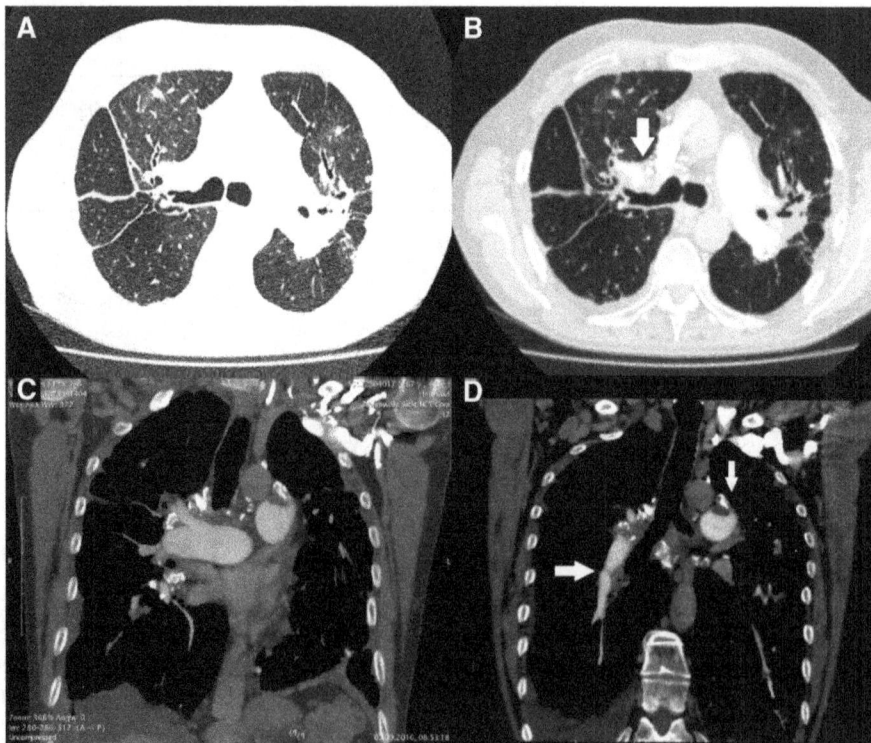

Fig. 1 a, b – interstitial lung fibrosis and calcified lymph nodes. **c, d** – organized thrombi in left and right pulmonary arteries

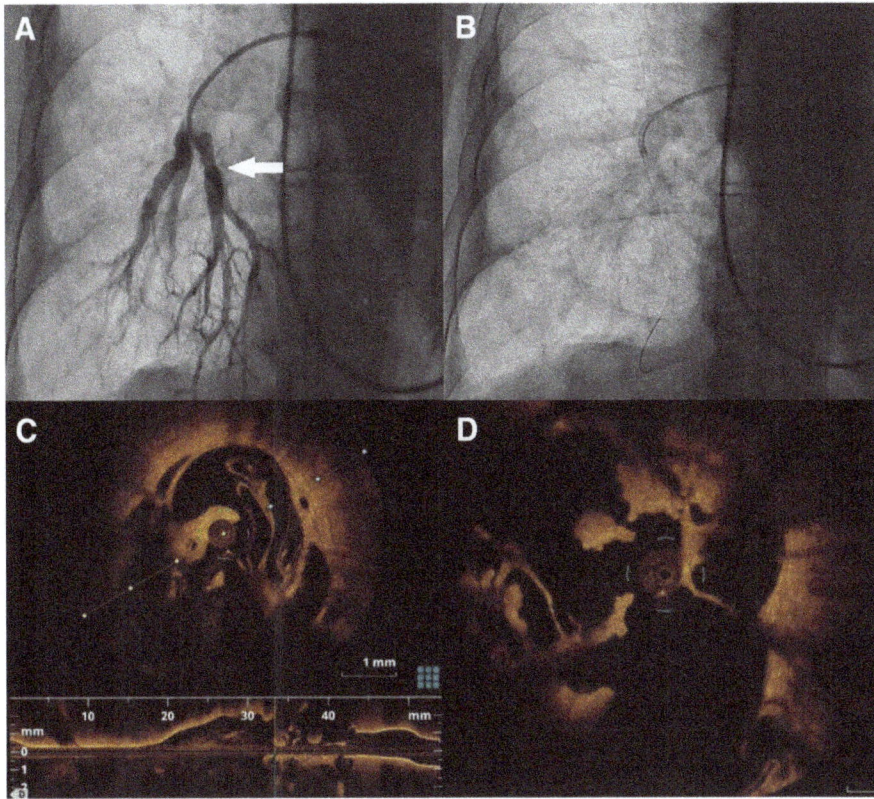

Fig. 2 a – initial selective right pulmonary artery angiography with intravascular web marked with arrow. **b, c** – intravascular web/organized thrombus in optical coherent tomography (OCT). **d** – guide wire with pressure catheter to assess pulmonary pressure ratio (PPR)

lesions intravascular imaging with optical coherence tomography (OCT) and intravascular ultrasound (IVUS) were performed. It allowed to definitely confirm organized thrombi (Fig. 2a – white arrow, 2C, 2D). With the use of pressure catheter we assessed hemodynamic significance of intrapulmonary lesions (Fig. 2b). Pulmonary pressure ratio (PPR, the ratio of the pressure distal to the lesion (Pd) divided by the pressure proximal to the lesion (Pp)) was assessed to optimize the BPA procedure and to minimize potential complications such as reperfusion pulmonary injury (RPI). PPR in arteries A9 and A10 was 0.19 and 0.22 – which suggested functional occlusion of both arteries. After simultaneous inflation of balloon catheters - "kissing balloon" technique (4.0x20mm and 4.0x27mm respectively), followed by proximal optimization with 7.0x30mm balloon catheter resulted in PPR 0.63 in A9 and 0.65 in A10 (Fig. 3, part A and D – green curve marking distal pressure). There were no periprocedural complications. Mean PAP after the first BPA procedure decreased from 52 mmHG to 40 mmHg. The second BPA session was performed 3 weeks later (left pulmonary artery), also without complications. Both procedures (3 segmental lesions in total) resulted in further hemodynamic and functional improvement, with mPAP drop to 27 mmHg at 12 months follow – up. Patient was still in functional class II WHO, echocardiography and 6MWT showed further improvement in clinical condition and RV function (Table 1).

Discussion and conclusions

Sarcoidosis related PH as is predominantly caused severe lung fibrosis or by compression of pulmonary arteries by mediastinal fibrosis and lymphadenopathy [1, 2, 5]. Pulmonary artery stenting was reported to be efficient in the treatment of pulmonary arteries compression in advanced sarcoidosis [5], while pharmacology with sildenafil or other PH specific dugs are of very limited short term efficacy [6, 7].

Presented case is probably one of the first available reports with initially suspected sarcoidosis related PH, which eventually was verified by pulmonary angiography and multimodal intravascular assessment as CTEPH. There are no data on optimal treatment in such challenging patients. After being deemed inoperable due to advanced sarcoidosis resulting in severe lung alterations, the patient was qualified to BPA procedure. Percutaneous catheter based method, is a rapidly developing therapeutic method for CTEPH patients. There is a growing evidence that in expert centers it is safe and effective, allowing normalization or near normalization of

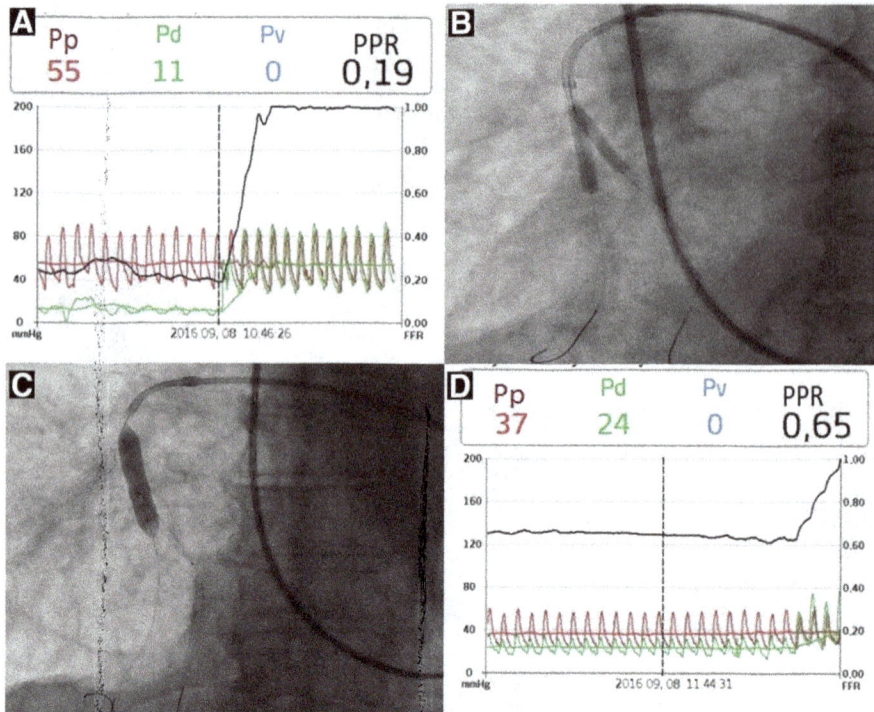

Fig. 3 a – PPR assessment before balloon pulmonary angioplasty, green curve nearly flat at first with rise after thrombus crossing. **b** – "kissing balloons" technique. **c** – proximal optimization with large balloon catheter. **d** – final PPR assessment, green curve showes restored pressure on safe level, preventing reperfusion pulmonary injury

mPAP in majority of treated cases [4, 8–13]. In our institution we have started BPA program in inoperable CTEPH in 2014. BPA procedures are performed according to the previously described protocol [4] with the use of pressure catheter, and in selected cases with OCT/IVUS intravascular imaging. Our data indicate that this

Table 1 Clinical and hemodynamical assessment before and after 2 BPA sessions

	Before treatment	At 12 months follow-up
WHO functional class	IV	II
NT-pro-BNP level (pg/ml)	6239	281
6MWT distance (m)	100	405
TRPG (mmHg)	95	31
RVSP (mmHg)	102	53
TAPSE (mm)	14	20
AcT (ms)	63	100
mPAP (mmHg)	54	27
CI (l/min/m²)	2.08	3.34
RAP (mmHg) systolic/diastolic/mean	14/10/9	5/3/1
PVR (Wood Units)	13.5	3.7

NT-pro-BNP natriuretic peptide concentration, *6MWT* 6 min walk test, *TRPG* tricuspid regurgitation peak gradient, *RVSP* right ventricle systolic pressure, *TAPSE* tricuspid annular plane excursion, *AcT* acceleration time, *mPAP* mean pulmonary artery pressure, *CI* cardiac index, *RAP* right atrial pressure, *PVR* pulmonary vascular resistance, *BPA* balloon pulmonary angioplasty

technique is safe and effective also in CTEPH high risk patients with severe comorbidities [14]. We are convinced that multimodal approach not only allowed to confirm CTEPH definitely in the patient with advanced sarcoidosis, but it also allowed to treat him and successfully and safely. We performed angioplasties of selected thromboembolic lesions, which were proved to be hemodynamically significant in multimodal assessment. Such fast improvement was also observed in other CTEPH patients treated with BPA. Based on our experience, it is related with initial treatment of the lesions in segmental artreries of lower lobes. In presented case, specific drug therapy (riociguat) was not avaliable at that time. Patient was on sildenafi (25 mg t.i.d.) and initial mPAP decreased only by 2 mmHg (54 mmHg in initial RHC versus 52 mmHg before first BPA session). Thus, only two BPA sessions resulted in mPAP reduction and significant clinical improvement. We think that BPA became a real therapeutic option in CTEPH patients, who are not candidates for surgery.

Abbreviations
6MWT: 6 min walk test; AcT: Acceleration time; BPA: Balloon pulmonary angioplasty; CI: Cardiac index; CT: Computed tomography; CTEPH: Chronic thromboembolic pulmonary hypertension; IVUS: Intravascular ultrasound; LV: Left ventricle; mPAP: Mean pulmonary artery pressure; NT-pro-BNP: Natriuretic peptide concentration; OCT: Optical coherent tomography; PAG: Pulmonary angiography; PAWP: Pulmonary artery wedge pressure; PH: Pulmonary hypertension; PPR: Pulmonary pressure ratio; PVR: Pulmonary

vascular resistance; RAP: Right atral pressure; RHC: Right heart catheterization; RPI: Reperfusion pulmonary injury; RV: Right ventricle; RVSP: Right ventricle systolic pressure; SPECT: Single-photon emission computed tomography; TAPSE: Tricuspid annular plane excursion; TRPG: Tricuspid regurgitation peak gradient

Funding

The authors declare that there was no funding regarding this manuscript.

Authors' contributions

AL – analysis and interpretation of patient's data, second operator in BPA procedures, leading contribution in writing the manuscript. DW, MR – first operators in BPA procedures, data analysis and interpretation, supervision, contribution in writing the manuscript. SZO, AF, KC – diagnostic work-up, follow-up, data collection. DPK – radiology studies assessment. ODD, BL – echocardiography assessment. AB – cardiac surgeon, consulted the patient. PP - contribution in writing the manuscript, supervision. All authors read and approved the final manuscript.

Competing interests

The authors declare that they have no competing interests.

Author details

[1]Center for Diagnostics and Treatment of Venous Thromboembolism, Department of Internal Medicine and Cardiology, Warsaw Medical University, Infant Jesus Hospital, Lindleya Street 4, 02-005 Warsaw, Poland. [2]Department of Radiology, Infant Jesus Hospital, Lindleya Street 4, 02-005 Warsaw, Poland. [3]Cardiac Surgery Department Medicover Hospital, Rzeczypospolitej 5 Avenue, 02-972 Warsaw, Poland.

References

1. Boucly A, Cottin V, Nunes H, et al. Management and long-term outcomes of sarcoidosis-associated pulmonary hypertension. Eur Respir J. 2017. https://doi.org/10.1183/13993003.00465-2017.

2. Baughman RP, Shlobin OA. Treatment of sarcoidosis-associated pulmonary hypertension: so close, and yet so far. Eur Respir J. 2017; https://doi.org/10.1183/13993003.01725-2017.

3. Galiè N, Humbert M, Vachiery JL, et al. 2015 ESC/ERS Guidelines for the diagnosis and treatment of pulmonary hypertension: The Joint Task Force for the Diagnosis and Treatment of Pulmonary Hypertension of the European Society of Cardiology (ESC) and the European Respiratory Society (ERS): Endorsed by: Association for European Paediatric and Congenital Cardiology (AEPC), International Society for Heart and Lung Transplantation (ISHLT). Eur Heart J. 2016;37(1):67–119.

4. Roik M, Wretowski D, Łabyk A, et al. Refined balloon pulmonary angioplasty driven by combined assessment of intra-arterial anatomy and physiology--Multimodal approach to treated lesions in patients with non-operable distal chronic thromboembolic pulmonary hypertension--Technique, safety and efficacy of 50 consecutive angioplasties. Int J Cardiol. 2016;203:228–35.

5. Hamilton-Craig CR, Slaughter R, McNeil K, et al. Improvement after angioplasty and stenting of pulmonary arteries due to sarcoid mediastinal fibrosis. Heart Lung Circ. 2009;18(3):222–5.

6. Toonkel RL, Borczuk AC, Pearson GD, et al. Sarcoidosis-associated fibrosing mediastinitis with resultant pulmonary hypertension: a case report and review of the literature. Respiration. 2010;79(4):341–5.

7. Kacprzak A, Szturmowicz M, Burakowska B, et al. Sarcoidosis-associated pulmonary hypertension treated with sildenafil - a case report. Adv Respir Med. 2017;85(5):258–63.

8. Mizoguchi H, Ogawa A, Munemasa M, et al. Refined balloon pulmonary angioplasty for inoperable patients with chronic thromboembolic pulmonary hypertension. Circ Cardiovasc Interv. 2012;5(6):748–55.

9. Kataoka M, Inami T, Hayashida K, et al. Percutaneous transluminal pulmonary angioplasty for the treatment of chronic thromboembolic pulmonary hypertension. Circ Cardiovasc Interv. 2012;5:756–62.

10. Sugimura K, Fukumoto Y, Satoh K, et al. Percutaneous transluminal pulmonary angioplasty markedly improves pulmonary hemodynamics and long-term prognosis in patients with chronic thromboembolic pulmonary hypertension. Circ J. 2012;76(2):485–8.

11. Inami T, Kataoka M, Shimura N, et al. Pressure-wire-guided percutaneous transluminal pulmonary angioplasty: a breakthrough in catheter-interventional therapy for chronic thromboembolic pulmonary hypertension. JACC Cardiovasc Interv. 2014;7(11):1297–306.

12. Roik M, Wretowski D, Łabyk A, et al. Optical coherence tomography of inoperable chronic thromboembolic pulmonary hypertension treated with refined balloon pulmonary angioplasty. Pol Arch Med Wewn. 2014;124(12): 742–3.

13. Roik M, Wretowski D, Rowiński O, et al. Refined balloon pulmonary angioplasty in inoperable chronic thromboembolic pulmonary hypertension--a multi-modality approach to the treated lesion. Int J Cardiol. 2014;177(3):e139–41.

14. Roik M, Wretowski D, Łabyk A, et al. Refined balloon pulmonary angioplasty-a therapeutic option in very elderly patients with chronic thromboembolic pulmonary hypertension. J Interv Cardiol. 2017;30(3):249–55.

Lower mortality after early supervised pulmonary rehabilitation following COPD exacerbations

Camilla Koch Ryrsø[1,2]* (iD), Nina Skavlan Godtfredsen[3,4], Linette Marie Kofod[5], Marie Lavesen[6], Line Mogensen[7], Randi Tobberup[8], Ingeborg Farver-Vestergaard[9], Henriette Edemann Callesen[2], Britta Tendal[2], Peter Lange[1,10,11] and Ulrik Winning Iepsen[1]

Abstract

Background: Pulmonary rehabilitation (PR), delivered as a supervised multidisciplinary program including exercise training, is one of the cornerstones in the chronic obstructive pulmonary disease (COPD) management. We performed a systematic review and meta-analysis to assess the effect on mortality of a supervised early PR program, initiated during or within 4 weeks after hospitalization with an acute exacerbation of COPD compared with usual post-exacerbation care or no PR program. Secondary outcomes were days in hospital, COPD related readmissions, health-related quality of life (HRQoL), exercise capacity (walking distance), activities of daily living (ADL), fall risk and drop-out rate.

Methods: We identified randomized trials through a systematic search using MEDLINE, EMBASE and Cocharne Library and other sources through October 2017. Risk of bias was assessed regarding randomization, allocation sequence concealment, blinding, incomplete outcome data, selective outcome reporting, and other biases using the Cochrane Risk of Bias tool.

Results: We included 13 randomized trials (801 participants). Our meta-analyses showed a clinically relevant reduction in mortality after early PR (4 trials, 319 patients; RR = 0.58 (95% CI: [0.35 to 0.98])) and at the longest follow-up (3 trials, 127 patients; RR = 0.55 (95% CI: [0.12 to 2.57])). Early PR reduced number of days in hospital by 4.27 days (1 trial, 180 patients; 95% CI: [− 6.85 to − 1.69]) and hospital readmissions (6 trials, 319 patients; RR = 0.47 (95% CI: [0.29 to 0.75])). Moreover, early PR improved HRQoL and walking distance, and did not affect drop-out rate. Several of the trials had unclear risk of bias in regard to the randomization and blinding, for some outcome there was also a lack of power.

Conclusion: Moderate quality of evidence showed reductions in mortality, number of days in hospital and number of readmissions after early PR in patients hospitalized with a COPD exacerbation. Long-term effects on mortality were not statistically significant, but improvements in HRQoL and exercise capacity appeared to be maintained for at least 12 months. Therefore, we recommend early supervised PR to patients with COPD-related exacerbations. PR should be initiated during hospital admission or within 4 weeks after hospital discharge.

Keywords: Chronic obstructive pulmonary disease, Supervised early pulmonary rehabilitation, Exacerbation of COPD, Hospital readmissions, Mortality, Systematic review

* Correspondence: camilla.koch.ryrsoe@regionh.dk; http://www.inflammation-metabolism.dk; http://aktivsundhed.dk
[1]The Centre of Inflammation and Metabolism and the Centre for Physical Activity Research, Rigshospitalet, University of Copenhagen, Blegdamsvej 9, DK-2100 Copenhagen, Denmark
[2]Danish Health Authority, Copenhagen, Denmark
Full list of author information is available at the end of the article

Background

Acute exacerbation in chronic obstructive pulmonary disease (AECOPD) is the most common reason for hospital admission among patients with chronic obstructive pulmonary disease (COPD) [1]. These events result in higher mortality and lower quality of life [2]. The estimated mortality rate within 90 days after hospitalization for AECOPD is approximately 3.6% (1.8–20.4%) while mortality rate during the first 2 years after admission for AECOPD is approximately 31.0% (18.8–45.4%) [3]. The estimated 30-day and 12-month readmission-rate after AECOPD hospitalization is approximately 19.2% [4] and 42.3% [5], respectively. Readmission following an AECOPD has a negative effect on physical performance by lowering exercise capacity, muscle strength and physical activity level, which patients may never fully recover from [6, 7]. Patients with frequent exacerbations may be prone to a more rapid decline in activities of daily living (ADL) and functional capacity, which is associated with reductions health-related quality of life (HRQoL) [6]. Repeated exacerbations may cause a *vicious circle* as physical inactivity and low exercise capacity are related to a higher risk of hospital readmission, regardless of the COPD severity [8].

Pulmonary rehabilitation (PR) has been suggested in AECOPD because of its known beneficial effects on exercise capacity, HRQoL and symptom burden in stable patients [9, 10]. It should be noted that the evidence in favor of PR in stable COPD is based on studies investigating supervised PR programs including exercise training for 6–12 weeks [11, 12], although at long-term follow-up, adherence to exercise training is low and effects are not maintained [13]. Likewise, studies have shown that early PR, initiated at the beginning of exacerbation treatment or within 3 weeks of initiation of exacerbation treatment, improves exercise capacity and HRQoL along with reductions in hospital readmissions [14] and mortality [15] compared with no PR. Based on evidence from randomized controlled trials (RCT), NICE guidelines from 2011 recommended the use of early PR in patients hospitalized with COPD exacerbations [16]. Yet, recent concerns have been raised about PR not being safe in AECOPD when initiated during the hospital admission [17]. Based on this new evidence, the 2017 guideline from the European Respiratory Society (ERS) and American Thoracic Society (ATS) recommend that PR is not initiated during hospitalization in patients with COPD related exacerbations, but is delayed until after hospital discharge (within 3 weeks) [18]. However, the ERS/ATS recommendation was based on both supervised and unsupervised PR programs, and interestingly, the potentially negative effects of early PR were mainly driven by studies providing unsupervised PR.

Therefore, our aim was to investigate the effect of a supervised early PR program, initiated during or within 4 weeks, in patients hospitalized with a COPD exacerbation compared with usual care. Our primary outcome was mortality at the end of PR and at the longest follow-up. Secondary outcomes were hospital readmission, days in hospital, HRQoL and exercise capacity. We followed the guidelines of the Grading of Recommendations Assessment, Development and Evaluation (GRADE) Working Group [19] in order to support clinical decision making in a national Danish setting where only supervised PR programs take place.

Methods

Protocol and registration

This review was among a series of reviews performed for a guideline developed by the Danish Health Authority. The population, intervention, control intervention (comparison) as well as critical and important outcomes (PICO) [20] were determined by the working-group members prior to our literature search. The methods and review process are a standardized part of the guideline development process within the Danish Health Authority. The methods handbook (in Danish) as well as the full guideline and more detail regarding the PICO can be accessed at www.sst.dk, the full guideline can also be found on https://app.magicapp.org/app#/guideline/2551.

Eligibility criteria

We considered studies eligible if they compared the effect of early supervised PR initiated during admission or within 4 weeks of hospital discharge (intervention) with no early pulmonary rehabilitation/usual care (comparison) in patients admitted and/or having been admitted to hospital with exacerbations of COPD (population). The PR was defined by a main component of supervised exercise training but could contain education, smoking cessation, nutritional support, management in activities of daily living (ADL) and physio-social support.

Studies providing inpatient pulmonary rehabilitation with exercise training was included if rehabilitation were continued after hospital discharge and/or a comprehensive rehabilitation program could be documented. Studies were excluded if they were not randomized or did not cover the predefined PICO. Our pre-specified outcomes were evaluated immediately after the end of intervention and at the longest follow up. Our primary outcome was mortality while secondary outcomes included number of days in hospital, number of COPD related hospital readmissions, health related quality of life (HRQoL), exercise capacity (walking tests), activities of daily living (ADL), falls and dropout.

Information sources and search strategy

A research librarian and search specialist performed the systematic literature search including the following databases:

Medline, Embase, Physiotherapy Evidence Database (PE-DRO), CINAHL, G-I-N international, NICE, National Guideline Clearinghouse, Surgical Implant Generation Network, Cochrane Library and OTseeker. The full search strategy is presented in Additional file 1.

This review is an update of a previous review. First, a comprehensive search for COPD rehabilitation guidelines and systematic reviews was conducted in July 2013, yielding a total of 2412 records. In November 2013, a second and more specific search (Medline, Embase and PEDRO) for RCTs was performed, in which 876 additional records were identified. An updated search for guidelines and systematic reviews was conducted in July 2017, covering the period from July 2013 to July 2017, where we identified 460 additional records. The search for primary studies was updated in October 2017, covering the period from December 2013 to October 2017. The search resulted in 1187 additional records (Fig. 1). All records were screened for relevant titles or abstracts, while reference lists of included studies were assessed for further eligible literature.

Study selection

Clinical guidelines identified in the first search were evaluated with the Appraisal of Guidelines for Research and Evaluation instrument version II (AGREE II) by two independent authors and disagreement was resolved through consensus (see Additional file 2). Likewise, systematic reviews were assessed with A Measurement Tool to Asses Systematic Reviews (AMSTAR) by three authors and disagreement was resolved through consensus (see Additional file 3). Based on these assessments we decided to include one clinical guideline [21] and two systematic reviews [14, 15]. From the second search, two authors independently evaluated the full text of all potentially eligible studies and decided whether to include or exclude each study based on the prespecified criteria.

Data analysis and risk of bias

Data on participants, study design, interventions and outcomes were extracted from the full-text reports of the included studies by two independent authors, using Covidence (Covidence systematic review software, Veritas

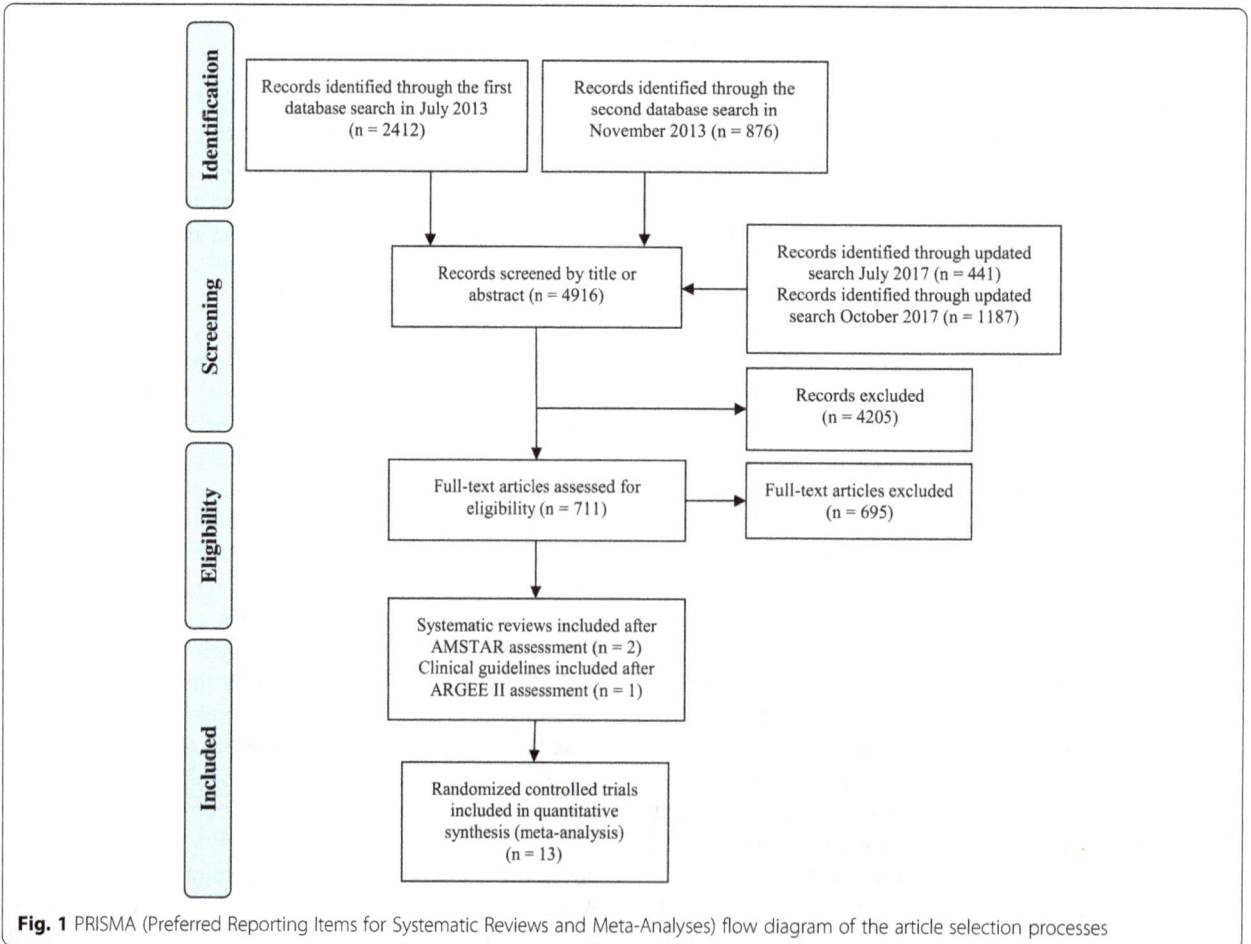

Fig. 1 PRISMA (Preferred Reporting Items for Systematic Reviews and Meta-Analyses) flow diagram of the article selection processes

Health Innovation, Melbourne, Australia. Available at www.covidence.org). Disagreement was resolved through consensus. Each included study was assessed using the Cochrane risk of bias tool [22]. Two independent authors performed the risk of bias assessment, and disagreement was resolved through discussion and consensus (see Additional file 4).

We used mean difference (MD) to calculate effect estimates for continuous outcomes if the same scale was used for a particular outcome. When pooling continuous outcome data from different scales a standardized mean difference (SMD) was calculated. Rate ratio and relative risk (RR) was used to calculate effects for dichotomous outcomes. Random-effects meta-analyses were performed as we expected variation in population, duration of intervention, and types of training between the included studies. Review Manager 5.3 software [23] was used for the statistical analyses and to produce forest plots. Heterogeneity in the effect estimate was determined using the I-square (I^2) statistic and values below 40% indicated low heterogeneity [24].

The quality of evidence for each outcome was assessed across the included studies as proposed by the GRADE Working Group [25]. A draft of the grading for each outcome using the GRADE criteria (i.e., risk of bias, inconsistency, indirectness, imprecision, and publication bias) was presented to the working group and the final grading was reached through discussion and consensus. The full guideline was then submitted to peer review and public hearing. For details on the hearing see www.sst.dk (in Danish).

Assessment of PR extensiveness
We assessed the extensiveness of the PR program in the included trials by following the statements and guidelines from BTS [26], ERS/ATS [10]), and as described in Puhan et al. [14] (see Additional file 5).

Results
Study selection
We identified 13 eligible primary RCTs for our analysis. These included a total of 801 participants who were in the recovery phase of a recent COPD exacerbation. Excluding dropouts (167 participants), 634 participants were included in our analysis. Nine of the 13 studies were included in a systematic Cochrane review [14]. Figure 1 summarizes the flow diagram of the two selection processes.

Included studies
Table 1 shows the characteristics of the included studies. In three studies [27–29] patients initiated an inpatient PR program within 4 to 8 days of hospital admission. In one study [30] patients began PR as either in- or outpatients and all continued as outpatients, in eight studies [31–38] the outpatient program was initiated within

one to four weeks after the inpatient exacerbation treatment and in one study [39] the outpatient rehabilitation was initiated after the "hospital at home" treatment of the exacerbation. In four studies [27, 29, 38, 39] the PR consisted of only supervised exercise training, whereas in the remaining nine studies [28, 30–37] PR consisted of supervised exercise training and education, smoking cessation, nutritional support, management in activities of daily living (ADL) and physio-social support. Duration of the different PR programs was ten days to six months, with training frequencies ranging from two to seven times a week, and exercise durations of 30–90 min per session. Table S1 in the Additional file 5 shows the extensiveness of the PR programs in the included trials. The participants followed an extensive PR program in ten of the included trials [27–31, 33–36, 38]. In the remaining three studies, the extensiveness of the PR was deemed as moderate [39], slightly extensive [37], and undescribed [32]. The control group received usual care consisting of optimal medical treatment. There were no reported differences in baseline characteristics of patients between groups in all of the included studies.

Risk of bias within studies
Figures 2, 3, 4, 5, 6, 7, 8, 9, 10, 11 and 12 and Additional file 4 shows risk of bias of the included studies. In nine studies [28, 29, 31, 32, 34–38] the allocation concealment was not described, while seven studies [27, 29, 31, 36–39] did not report the randomization process. Three studies [27, 34, 39] blinded the personnel, with only two of the studies [34, 39] blinding the outcome assessor. One study [27] was assessed as having a high risk of incomplete outcome data reporting due to a large dropout. Selective outcome reporting of outcome measures was detected in one study [34]. No other sources of bias were detected. Thus, the quality of evidence from all studies included was downgraded due to risk of bias (Table 2, Additional file 4).

Effect of the intervention
We preformed meta-analyses in ten of our predefined outcomes. Subgroup analyses were undertaken in order to reveal differences between PR initiated during admission or within one week after discharge and PR initiated between one and four weeks after discharge from hospital. For an overview of all the outcomes, our confidence in the estimates and our interpretations see Table 2 GRADE Evidence profile.

Mortality
Total mortality after end of treatment was reported in four of the included studies, including 319 randomized participants (early PR: $N = 163$; usual care: $N = 156$) [29, 32, 33, 37]. A total of 18 events were reported in the

Table 1 Characteristics of the included studies

Reference	Country	Study design	Setting, duration and frequency	Participants	Intervention	Intervention after discharge	Usual care	Notes	Outcomes	Dropouts
Behnke 2000 [27]	Germany	RCT	Setting: in- and outpatient Duration: hospital-based 10 days, home-based 6 months Frequency: 7/week	46 admitted patients with AECOPD (mean age: 64–68 years, FEV₁: 36% predicted). Comorbidities: not specified.	PR consisted of conventional therapy including 30 min of daily breath exercises with respirologists and hospital-based training. Exercise training consisted of daily 6MWT and 5 self-controlled walking sessions at 75% of the treadmill walking distance of the respective day.	Supervised home-based training for 6 mo.: walking training 3/day at 125% of the best 6MWD, health check every 2 weeks (mo. 0–3) followed by phone calls from mo. 3–6.	Usual care: standard inpatient care and community care with respirologists (30 min of daily breathing exercises) but without exercise training	Both groups (intervention and usual care) were supervised by the physician.	Mortality[b] Walking test[b] COPD related hospital readmissions[b] Dropout[a]	16 dropouts (8 in PR group and 8 in control group)
Daabis 2017 [31]	Egypt	RCT	Setting: outpatient Duration: 8 weeks Frequency: 3/week	30 admitted patients with AECOPD (mean age: 58–61 years, FEV₁: 53–56% of predicted). Comorbidities: not specified.	PR consisted of patient assessment, exercise training (ET), patient education including self-management of the disease, nutrition and lifestyle issues. Exercise training consisted of ET with 30-min of walking at the intensity of 75% 6MWT including 30-min of low-intensity RT.	Outpatient PR	Medical treatment.	All patients received standard treatment with optimal medical treatment.	HRQoL[a] Walking distance[a]	No dropouts reported
Deepak 2014 [32]	India	RCT	Setting outpatient Duration: 12 weeks	60 admitted patients with AECOPD (mean age: 59 years, FEV₁: 47–53% of predicted, 93% men). Comorbidities: not specified.	PR consisted of patient assessment, exercise testing, exercise training (mixture of limb strengthening and aerobic activities, tailored to individual baseline function), education, nutrition and psycho-social rehabilitation.	Outpatient PR	Conventional treatment without PR.	All patients received conventional management consisting of medical treatment.	HRQoL[a] Walking distance[a]	4 dropouts
Eaton 2009 [28]	New Zealand	RCT	Setting: in- and outpatient Duration: 8 weeks Frequency: 2/week	97 admitted patients with AECOPD (mean age: 70 years, FEV₁: 35–36% of predicted, 42–45% men). Comorbidities: Measured with Charlson index (PR group: 3.1; control: 3.2).	PR consisted of a daily 30-min structured, supervised exercise regimen that included walking and upper and lower limb strengthening exercises.	Hospital-based outpatient program consisting of 1-h sessions of supervised exercise training and educational sessions (e.g. coping with dyspnea, management of ADL, nutritional advises, airway clearance).	Usual care standardized in according with the ATS/ERS COPD guidelines and standardized advises on the benefits of exercise and maintaining daily activities.	All patients received usual care standardized in according with the ATS/ERS COPD guidelines.	Walking distance[a] COPD related hospital readmissions[b] Dropout[a]	13 dropouts (8 in PR group and 5 in control group)
Kirsten 1998 [29]	Germany	RCT	Setting: inpatient Duration: 10 days	31 admitted patients with AECOPD (mean	PR consisted of 6MWT each day and additional 5	Inpatient supervised walking	Usual care with optimal medical	All patients received standard	Walking test[a]	2 dropouts (not reported in which

Table 1 Characteristics of the included studies (Continued)

Reference	Country	Study design	Setting, duration and frequency	Participants	Intervention	Intervention after discharge	Usual care	Notes	Outcomes	Dropouts
			Frequency: 7/week		walking sessions per day at ≥75% of the respective walking distance.	sessions 5/day.	treatment.	medical treatment.		group)
Ko 2011 [34]	China	RCT	Setting: outpatient Duration: 8 weeks Frequency: 3/week	60 admitted patients with AECOPD (mean age: 73–74 years, FEV1: 41–46% of predicted, 98% men). Comorbidities: coronary artery disease, cardiac arrhythmic, heart failure, hypertension, diabetes.	PR consisted of supervised exercise training including treadmill, arm cycling, arm and leg strength training at 60–70% of VO_{2max} or HR_{max} and were advised to perform at least 20 min home exercises a day. Education on proper breathing techniques and how to cope with daily activities.	Supervised outpatient exercise training.	Usual care with instructions to perform regular exercise at home (walking and muscle stretching exercise).	Both groups were seen by the nurse specialist at the baseline assessment.	HRQoL[b] Mortality[a,b] Walking test[b] Dropout[a,b]	9 dropouts (5 in PR group and 4 in control group) at the end of treatment. 6 dropouts (2 in PR group and 4 in control group) at the longest follow-up.
Ko 2017 [33]	China	RCT	Setting: outpatient Duration: 8 weeks (1 year follow up) Frequency: 3/week	180 admitted patients with AECOPD (mean age: 75 years, FEV1: 42–47% of predicted, 94–97% men). Comorbidities: hypertension, type 2 diabetes, hyperlipidemia, ischemic heart disease, heart failure, old pulmonary tuberculosis.	PR consisted of education (smoking cessation, nutrition, technique of using medications, dyspnea management, self-management, psychological distress, exercise benefits and strategies, breathing and sputum-removal techniques) and individual physical training program to perform at home or a short course of outpatient PR.	Patients are offered supervised exercise training 3/week, if declining they are offered instructions for self-training, education, and telephone calls.	Usual care with medical treatment.	All patients received standard treatment with optimal medical therapy.	HRQoL[b] Mortality[a] Walking test[b] Days in hospital[a]	38 dropouts (17 in PR group and 21 in control group)
Man 2004 [35]	England	RCT	Setting: outpatient Duration: 8 weeks Frequency: 2/week	42 admitted patients with AECOPD (mean age: 70 years, FEV1: 37–42% of predicted, 40% men). Comorbidities: not specified.	Supervised multidisciplinary PR, 1-h of exercise (aerobic walking and cycling, strength training for the upper and lower limb) and 1-h of education (with an emphasis on self-management of the disease, nutrition and lifestyle issues).	Supervised multidisciplinary PR.	Usual care with optimal medical treatment.	All admitted patients received standard treatment and home diaries which included a disease specific information pack.	HRQoF[b] Mortality[b] Walking test[b] COPD related hospital readmissions[b] Dropout[a]	8 dropouts (3 in PR group and 5 in control group)
Murphy 2005 [39]	Ireland	RCT	Setting: outpatient home-based Duration: 6 weeks Frequency: 2/week	31 admitted patients with AECOPD (mean age: 65–67 years, FEV1: 38–42% of predicted, 65% men). Comorbidities: not specified.	PR consisted of 30–40-min supervised home-based exercise program including stepping up and down a stair, sitting to stand from a chair, upper limb strength exercises with low-impact elastic band at 3–5 on the	Supervised home-based exercise program.	Standard medical treatment without any form of PR exercises or lifestyle changes advice.	All patients received standard medical treatment.	Walking test[a] COPD related hospital readmissions[b] Dropout[a]	5 dropouts (3 in PR group and 2 in control group)

Table 1 Characteristics of the included studies (Continued)

Reference	Country	Study design	Setting, duration and frequency	Participants	Intervention	Intervention after discharge	Usual care	Notes	Outcomes	Dropouts
Puhan 2012 [30]	Switzerland	RCT	Setting: in- and outpatient Duration: 12 weeks Frequency: 24 sessions (range 18–36)	36 admitted patients with AECOPD (mean age: 67 years, FEV₁: 43–46% of predicted, 58% men). Comorbidities: cardiovascular, endocrine, musculoskeletal, other.	Borg breathlessness score. Early inpatient PR within 2 weeks after exacerbation, exercise training included endurance, strength and calisthenics training in addition with education (e.g. individual action plan, mediational use, exercise at home, coping with daily activities, smoking cessation).	Outpatient PR, exercise training included endurance, strength and calisthenics training in addition with education (as described under intervention).	Late PR starting 6 mo. after exacerbation, exercise training included endurance, strength and calisthenics training in addition with education.	Recommended number of exercise session 24 (ranged between 18 and 36).	Mortality[a] Dropout[a]	8 dropouts (4 in PR group and 4 in control group)
Revitt 2018 [37]	United Kingdom	RCT	Setting: inpatient Duration: 6 weeks Frequency: 2/week	28 admitted patients with AECOPD (mean age: 66 years; FEV₁: 1.18 l). Comorbidities: not specified.	Early PR within 4 weeks of discharge. PR consisted of individualized aerobic and resistance exercises and education on chest clearance and energy conservation.	Hospital-based PR.	Late PR initiated 7 weeks after discharge including exercise and education.	All patients received the same PR program.	Dropout[a]	11 dropouts (3 in control group prior to the program and 8 in PR group during the program)
Seymour 2010 [36]	United Kingdom	RCT	Setting: outpatient (hospital-led) Duration: 8 weeks Frequency: 2/week	60 admitted patients with AECOPD (mean age: 65-67 years, FEV₁: 52% of predicted, 45% men). Comorbidities: hypertension, type 2 diabetes, ischemic heart disease.	PR consisted of supervised exercise training including a mixture of limb strengthening and aerobic activities tailored to individual baseline function and education session (lasting 2 h).	Hospital-led supervised exercise training.	Usual care with optimal medical treatment.	All patients were provided with general information about COPD and offered outpatient appointments with their general practitioner or respiratory team.	HRQoF[b] Walking test[a] COPD related hospital readmissions[b] Dropout[b]	11 dropouts (7 in PR group and 4 in control group)
Troosters 2000 [38]	Belgium	RCT	Setting: outpatient Duration: 6 mo (18 mo follow up) Frequency: 2-3/week	100 patients with AECOPD referred to outpatient clinic (mean age: 60–63 years, FEV₁: 41–43% of predicted, 87% men). Comorbidities: not specified.	PR consisted of 90-min supervised ET and RT. ET consisting of cycling, treadmill walking, and stair climbing at 60–80% of initial W$_{max}$ during cycle ergometer/maximal walking speed. RT consisting of strength exercises for 5 muscle groups, 10 reps at 60% 1RM.	Supervised outpatient exercise training.	Usual medical care consisting of standard community care with respirologist.	During exercise training supplemental oxygen was given to maintain oxygen saturation above 90%.	Mortality[a] walking test[a] dropout[a,b]	30 dropouts (13 in PR group and 17 in control group) at the end of treatment 21 dropouts (11 in PR group and 10 in control group) at the longest follow-up.

AECOPD acute exacerbations of chronic obstructive pulmonary disease, COPD chronic obstructive pulmonary disease, CT combined training, ET endurance training, FEV₁ forced expiratory volume in 1 s, HR$_{max}$ maximum heart rate, HRQoL health related quality of life, RCT randomized controlled trial, 1RM one repetition maximum, RT resistance training, Reps repetitions, VO$_{2max}$ maximal oxygen uptake, W$_{max}$ maximal work load in Watts, 6MWD 6 min walking distance, 6MWT 6 min walking test

[a] After end of treatment
[b] After longest follow up

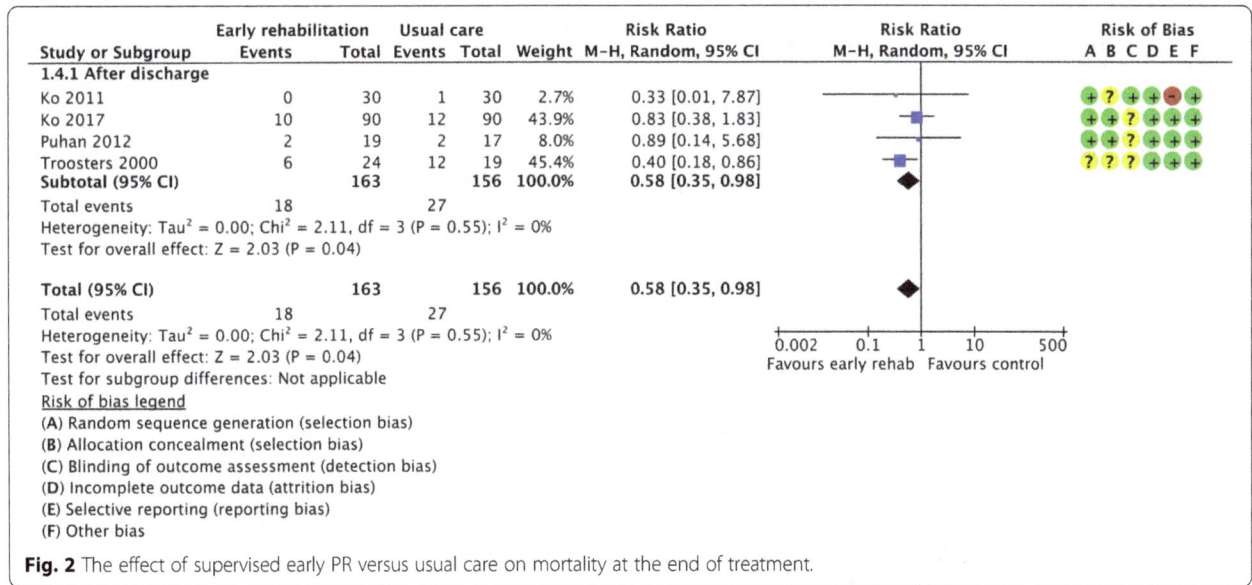

Study or Subgroup	Early rehabilitation Events	Total	Usual care Events	Total	Weight	Risk Ratio M–H, Random, 95% CI	Risk Ratio M–H, Random, 95% CI	Risk of Bias A B C D E F
1.4.1 After discharge								
Ko 2011	0	30	1	30	2.7%	0.33 [0.01, 7.87]		+ ? + + ● +
Ko 2017	10	90	12	90	43.9%	0.83 [0.38, 1.83]		+ + ? + + +
Puhan 2012	2	19	2	17	8.0%	0.89 [0.14, 5.68]		+ + ? + + +
Troosters 2000	6	24	12	19	45.4%	0.40 [0.18, 0.86]		? ? ? + + +
Subtotal (95% CI)		163		156	100.0%	0.58 [0.35, 0.98]		
Total events	18		27					

Heterogeneity: Tau^2 = 0.00; Chi^2 = 2.11, df = 3 (P = 0.55); I^2 = 0%
Test for overall effect: Z = 2.03 (P = 0.04)

| Total (95% CI) | | 163 | | 156 | 100.0% | 0.58 [0.35, 0.98] | | |
| Total events | 18 | | 27 | | | | | |

Heterogeneity: Tau^2 = 0.00; Chi^2 = 2.11, df = 3 (P = 0.55); I^2 = 0%
Test for overall effect: Z = 2.03 (P = 0.04)
Test for subgroup differences: Not applicable

Risk of bias legend
(A) Random sequence generation (selection bias)
(B) Allocation concealment (selection bias)
(C) Blinding of outcome assessment (detection bias)
(D) Incomplete outcome data (attrition bias)
(E) Selective reporting (reporting bias)
(F) Other bias

Fig. 2 The effect of supervised early PR versus usual care on mortality at the end of treatment.

early PR group, whereas 27 events were reported in the usual care group. We found a statistically significant reduction in mortality favoring PR (RR = 0.58 (95% CI: [0.35 to 0.98])), with low heterogeneity (Fig. 2). The quality of evidence was downgraded due to unclear sequence generation, allocation concealment and blinding together with selective outcome reporting (Table 2).

Total mortality at longest follow up was reported in three of the included studies, including 127 participants (early PR: $N = 64$; usual care: $N = 63$) [26, 33,

34]. Two events were reported in the early PR groups while four events were reported in the usual care group. We found no statistical significant difference between groups (RR = 0.55 (95% CI: [0.12 to 2.57])). Subgroup analysis showed no difference in effect between trials with PR initiated during admission and after discharge ($P = 0.70$) (Fig. 3). Our confidence in the effect estimate was downgraded due to unclear sequence generation and allocation concealment together with lack of precision, incomplete outcome data and selective reporting (Table 2).

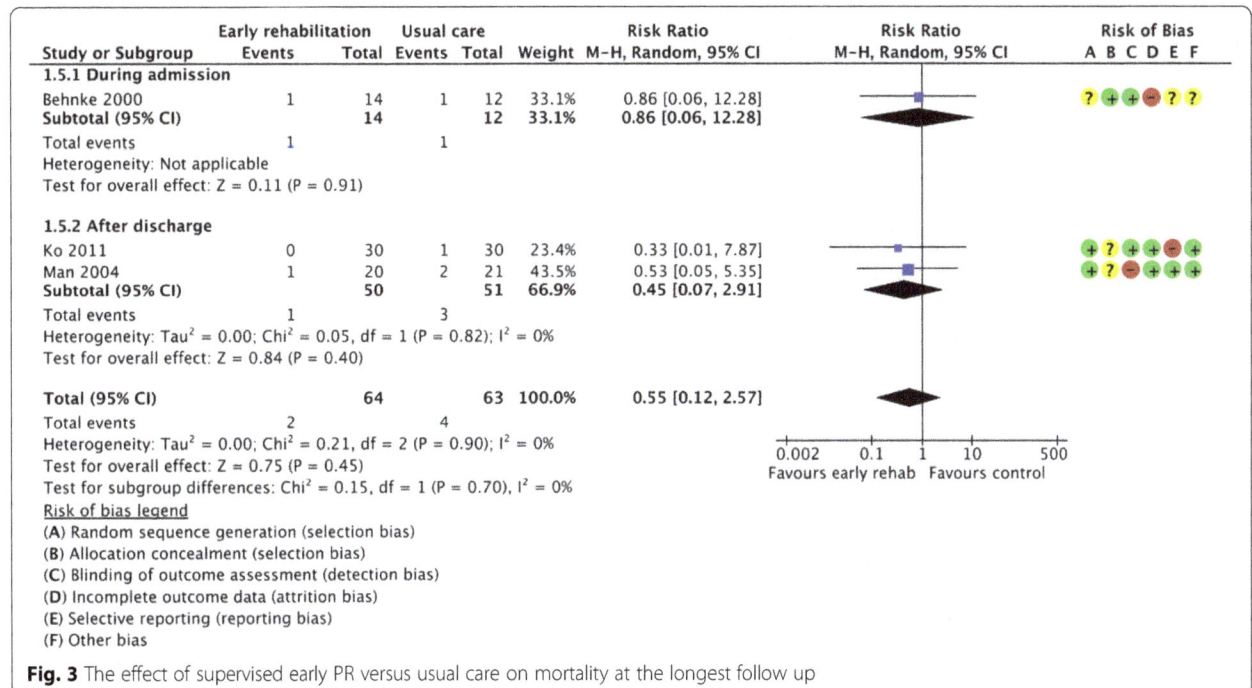

Study or Subgroup	Early rehabilitation Events	Total	Usual care Events	Total	Weight	Risk Ratio M–H, Random, 95% CI	Risk Ratio M–H, Random, 95% CI	Risk of Bias A B C D E F
1.5.1 During admission								
Behnke 2000	1	14	1	12	33.1%	0.86 [0.06, 12.28]		? + + ● ? ?
Subtotal (95% CI)		14		12	33.1%	0.86 [0.06, 12.28]		
Total events	1		1					

Heterogeneity: Not applicable
Test for overall effect: Z = 0.11 (P = 0.91)

1.5.2 After discharge								
Ko 2011	0	30	1	30	23.4%	0.33 [0.01, 7.87]		+ ? + + ● +
Man 2004	1	20	2	21	43.5%	0.53 [0.05, 5.35]		+ ? ● + + +
Subtotal (95% CI)		50		51	66.9%	0.45 [0.07, 2.91]		
Total events	1		3					

Heterogeneity: Tau^2 = 0.00; Chi^2 = 0.05, df = 1 (P = 0.82); I^2 = 0%
Test for overall effect: Z = 0.84 (P = 0.40)

| Total (95% CI) | | 64 | | 63 | 100.0% | 0.55 [0.12, 2.57] | | |
| Total events | 2 | | 4 | | | | | |

Heterogeneity: Tau^2 = 0.00; Chi^2 = 0.21, df = 2 (P = 0.90); I^2 = 0%
Test for overall effect: Z = 0.75 (P = 0.45)
Test for subgroup differences: Chi^2 = 0.15, df = 1 (P = 0.70), I^2 = 0%

Risk of bias legend
(A) Random sequence generation (selection bias)
(B) Allocation concealment (selection bias)
(C) Blinding of outcome assessment (detection bias)
(D) Incomplete outcome data (attrition bias)
(E) Selective reporting (reporting bias)
(F) Other bias

Fig. 3 The effect of supervised early PR versus usual care on mortality at the longest follow up

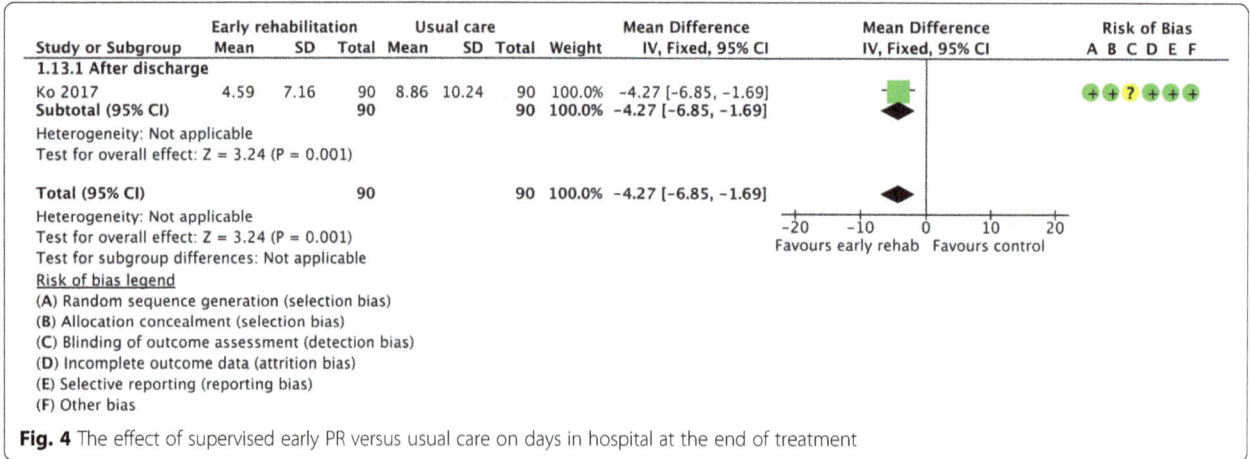

Fig. 4 The effect of supervised early PR versus usual care on days in hospital at the end of treatment

Days in hospital

One study investigated the effect of early PR on the number of days in hospital after the end of treatment and stated that early PR led to a statistically reduction of 4.27 days (95% CI: [−6.85 to −1.69]) in the number of days in hospitals (Fig. 4). Accordingly, our confidence in the effect estimate was downgraded due to inclusion of only one study (Table 2).

COPD related hospital readmissions

Six studies provided data from 365 participants on the number of COPD related hospital readmissions 3–12 months from baseline [27, 28, 33, 35, 36, 38]. The pooled effect estimate showed a decrease in the number of COPD related hospital readmissions favoring the early PR (RR = 0.47 (95% CI: [0.29 to 0.75])). Low heterogeneity (I^2 = 38%) was observed, and the subgroup analysis showed no difference in effect between trials with PR initiated during admission and after discharge (P = 0.93) (Fig. 5). The quality of evidence was downgraded due to unclear sequence generation and allocation concealment together with lack of blinding and incomplete outcome date (Table 2).

Health-related quality of life

The St. George's Respiratory Questionnaire (SGRQ) (scale from 0 to 100, lower is better) were used across

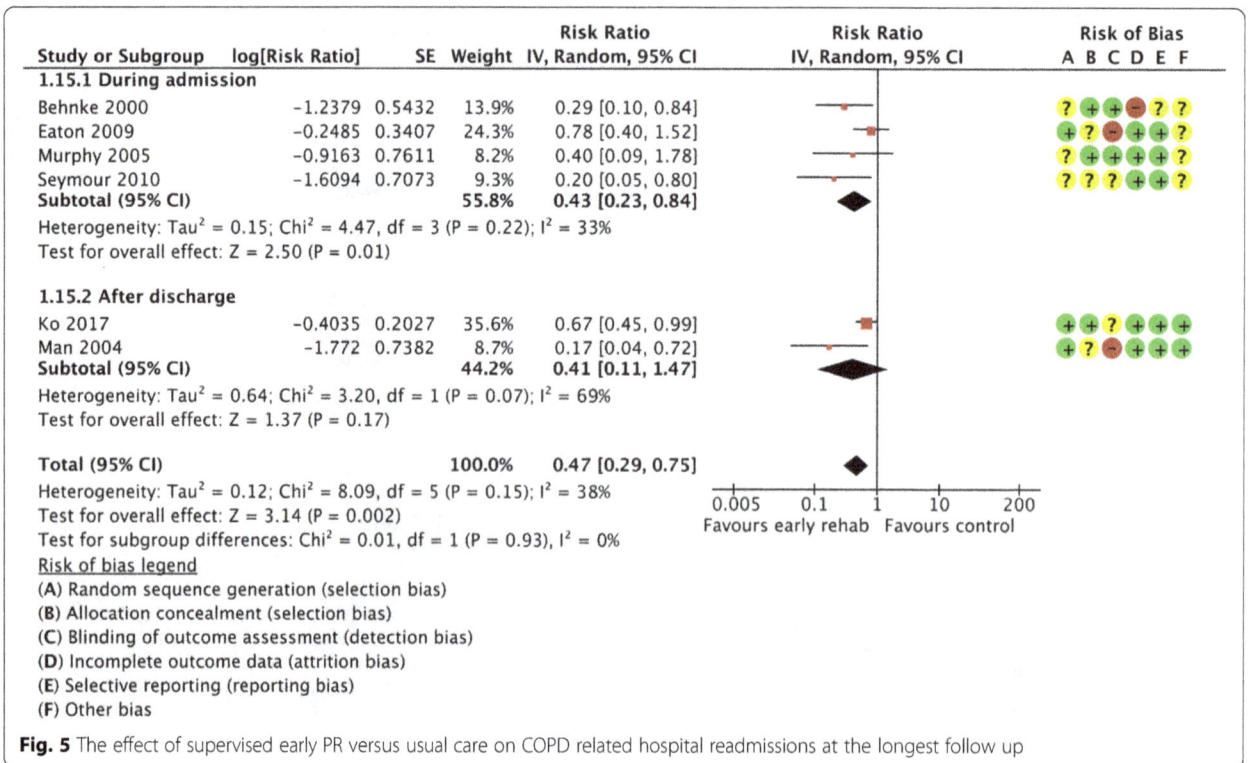

Fig. 5 The effect of supervised early PR versus usual care on COPD related hospital readmissions at the longest follow up

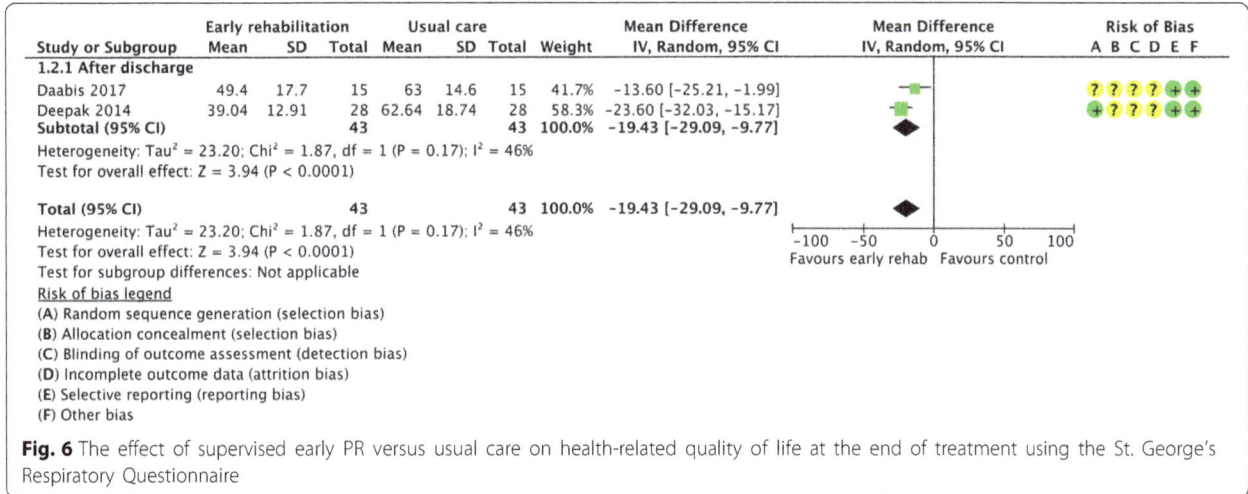

Study or Subgroup	Early rehabilitation			Usual care			Weight	Mean Difference IV, Random, 95% CI	Mean Difference IV, Random, 95% CI	Risk of Bias A B C D E F
	Mean	SD	Total	Mean	SD	Total				
1.2.1 After discharge										
Daabis 2017	49.4	17.7	15	63	14.6	15	41.7%	-13.60 [-25.21, -1.99]		? ? ? ? + +
Deepak 2014	39.04	12.91	28	62.64	18.74	28	58.3%	-23.60 [-32.03, -15.17]		+ ? ? ? + +
Subtotal (95% CI)			43			43	100.0%	-19.43 [-29.09, -9.77]		

Heterogeneity: Tau² = 23.20; Chi² = 1.87, df = 1 (P = 0.17); I² = 46%
Test for overall effect: Z = 3.94 (P < 0.0001)

Total (95% CI)			43			43	100.0%	-19.43 [-29.09, -9.77]		

Heterogeneity: Tau² = 23.20; Chi² = 1.87, df = 1 (P = 0.17); I² = 46%
Test for overall effect: Z = 3.94 (P < 0.0001)
Test for subgroup differences: Not applicable

Risk of bias legend
(A) Random sequence generation (selection bias)
(B) Allocation concealment (selection bias)
(C) Blinding of outcome assessment (detection bias)
(D) Incomplete outcome data (attrition bias)
(E) Selective reporting (reporting bias)
(F) Other bias

Fig. 6 The effect of supervised early PR versus usual care on health-related quality of life at the end of treatment using the St. George's Respiratory Questionnaire

studies to assess HRQoL. Two studies were included and data from 86 participants were pooled in a meta-analysis evaluating HRQoL directly after end of early PR [31, 32] and showed a statistically and clinically significant improvement of 19.43 units on the SGRQ scale (95% CI: [– 29.09 to – 9.77]) in the early PR group compared with the usual care group (Fig. 6) with low heterogeneity. Our confidence in the effect estimate was downgraded due to unclear sequence generation, allocation concealment, blinding of assessors and incomplete outcome data (Table 2).

Four different studies provided data from 323 participants on the effect of early PR on HRQoL 3–12 months from baseline [33–36] and showed a statistically and clinically relevant improvement of 8.74 units on the SGRQ scale (95% CI: [– 12.02 to – 5.45]) in the early PR

group compared with the usual care group (Fig. 7). Subgroup analysis showed no difference in effect between trials with PR initiated during admission and after discharge (P = 0.49). Unclear sequence generation, allocation concealment, blinding and selective outcome reporting led to downgrading of the confidence in our effect estimates (Table 2).

Walking distance
The walking distance (6-Minute Walking Test (6MWT) or Shuttle Walking Test (SWT)) after the end of treatment was investigated in eight studies [28, 29, 31, 32, 36–39]. Pooling the results (early PR: N = 139; usual care: N = 135) from five trials using 6MWT yielded a statistically significant mean difference in walking distance of 76.89 m, favoring early PR (95% CI: [21.34 to

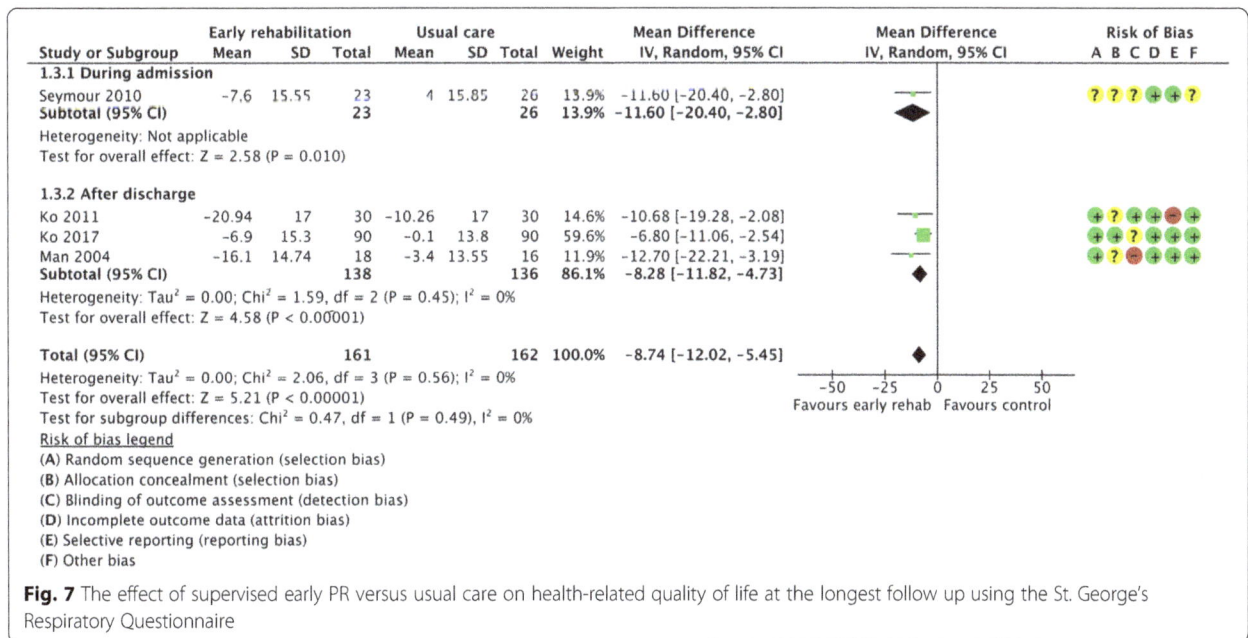

Study or Subgroup	Early rehabilitation			Usual care			Weight	Mean Difference IV, Random, 95% CI	Mean Difference IV, Random, 95% CI	Risk of Bias A B C D E F
	Mean	SD	Total	Mean	SD	Total				
1.3.1 During admission										
Seymour 2010	-7.6	15.55	23	4	15.85	26	13.9%	-11.60 [-20.40, -2.80]		? ? ? + + ?
Subtotal (95% CI)			23			26	13.9%	-11.60 [-20.40, -2.80]		

Heterogeneity: Not applicable
Test for overall effect: Z = 2.58 (P = 0.010)

1.3.2 After discharge										
Ko 2011	-20.94	17	30	-10.26	17	30	14.6%	-10.68 [-19.28, -2.08]		+ ? + + - +
Ko 2017	-6.9	15.3	90	-0.1	13.8	90	59.6%	-6.80 [-11.06, -2.54]		+ + ? + + +
Man 2004	-16.1	14.74	18	-3.4	13.55	16	11.9%	-12.70 [-22.21, -3.19]		+ ? + + + +
Subtotal (95% CI)			138			136	86.1%	-8.28 [-11.82, -4.73]		

Heterogeneity: Tau² = 0.00; Chi² = 1.59, df = 2 (P = 0.45); I² = 0%
Test for overall effect: Z = 4.58 (P < 0.00001)

Total (95% CI)			161			162	100.0%	-8.74 [-12.02, -5.45]		

Heterogeneity: Tau² = 0.00; Chi² = 2.06, df = 3 (P = 0.56); I² = 0%
Test for overall effect: Z = 5.21 (P < 0.00001)
Test for subgroup differences: Chi² = 0.47, df = 1 (P = 0.49), I² = 0%

Risk of bias legend
(A) Random sequence generation (selection bias)
(B) Allocation concealment (selection bias)
(C) Blinding of outcome assessment (detection bias)
(D) Incomplete outcome data (attrition bias)
(E) Selective reporting (reporting bias)
(F) Other bias

Fig. 7 The effect of supervised early PR versus usual care on health-related quality of life at the longest follow up using the St. George's Respiratory Questionnaire

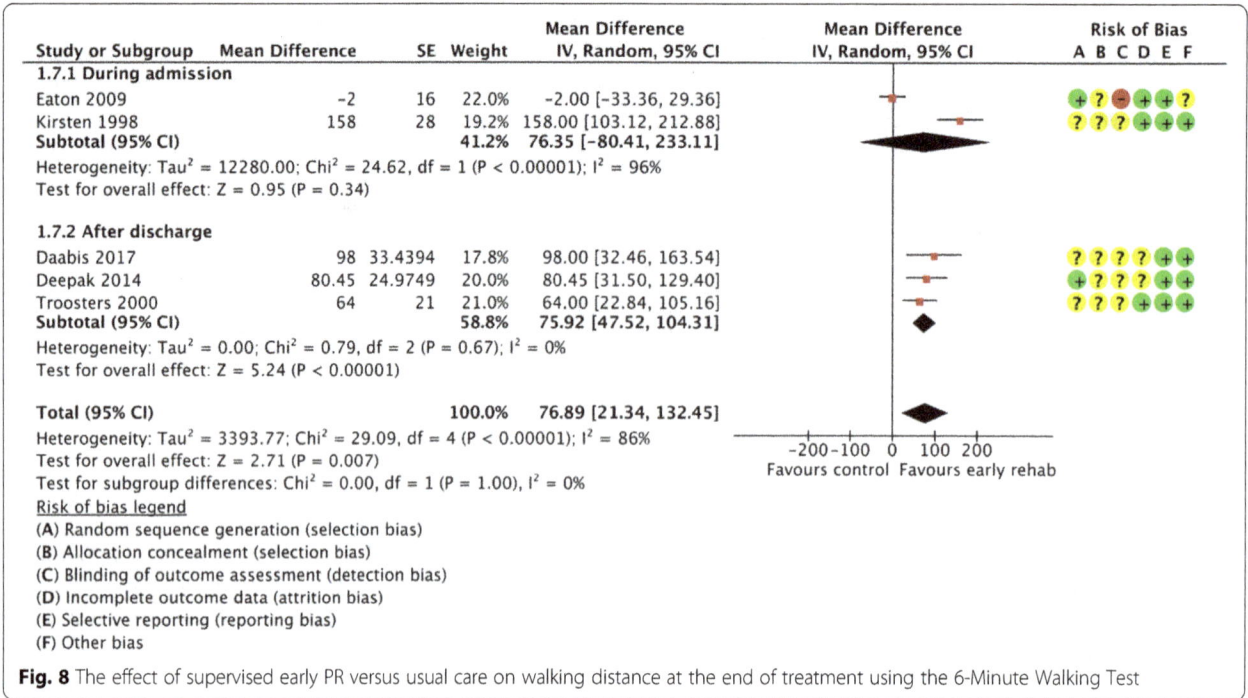

Fig. 8 The effect of supervised early PR versus usual care on walking distance at the end of treatment using the 6-Minute Walking Test

132.45]) with high heterogeneity (Fig. 8). The subgroup analysis showed no difference in the effect between PR initiated during admission and after discharge (*P* = 1.00). However, we found a significant within-group effect of early PR after discharge (Fig. 8). The quality of evidence was downgraded due to unclear sequence generation, allocation concealment, blinding of assessors and incomplete data together with high risk of inconsistency (Table 2). Three trials (early PR: *N* = 50; usual care: *N* = 45) used the

SWT to evaluate the walking distance after the end of treatment and showed a statistically significant mean difference in walking distance of 54.70 m, favoring early PR (95% CI: [30.83 to 78.57]). The subgroup analysis showed no difference in the effect between PR initiated during admission and after discharge (*P* = 0.40). However, we found a significant within-group effect of early PR during admission and after discharge (Fig. 9). The quality of evidence was downgraded due to unclear sequence generation, allocation

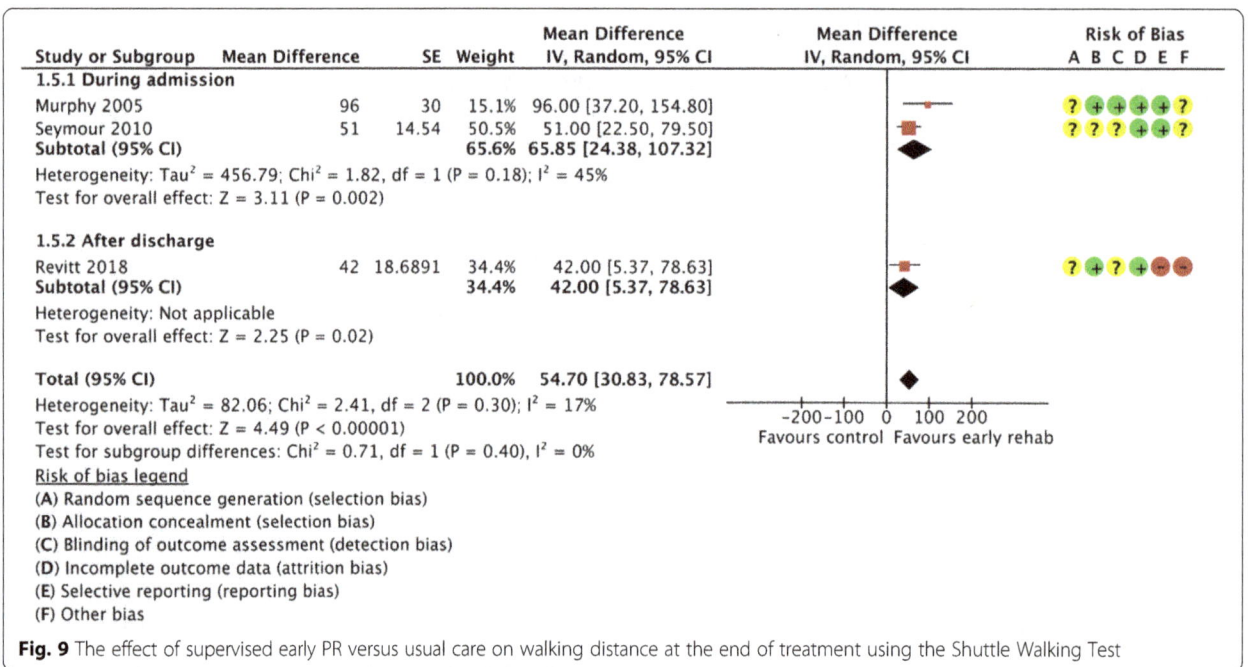

Fig. 9 The effect of supervised early PR versus usual care on walking distance at the end of treatment using the Shuttle Walking Test

Study or Subgroup	Mean Difference	SE	Weight	Mean Difference IV, Random, 95% CI	Mean Difference IV, Random, 95% CI	Risk of Bias A B C D E F
1.10.1 During admission						
Behnke 2000	215	28	36.0%	215.00 [160.12, 269.88]		? + + − ? ?
Subtotal (95% CI)			**36.0%**	**215.00 [160.12, 269.88]**		
Heterogeneity: Not applicable						
Test for overall effect: Z = 7.68 (P < 0.00001)						
1.10.2 After discharge						
Ko 2017	12.5	9.9134	37.4%	12.50 [−6.93, 31.93]		+ + ? + + +
Ko 2011	31	85	26.7%	31.00 [−135.60, 197.60]		+ ? + + − +
Subtotal (95% CI)			**64.0%**	**12.75 [−6.55, 32.05]**		
Heterogeneity: Tau² = 0.00; Chi² = 0.05, df = 1 (P = 0.83); I² = 0%						
Test for overall effect: Z = 1.29 (P = 0.20)						
Total (95% CI)			**100.0%**	**90.27 [−69.53, 250.08]**		
Heterogeneity: Tau² = 17697.85; Chi² = 46.48, df = 2 (P < 0.00001); I² = 96%						
Test for overall effect: Z = 1.11 (P = 0.27)						
Test for subgroup differences: Chi² = 46.43, df = 1 (P < 0.00001), I² = 97.8%						

−500 −250   0   250   500
Favours control   Favours early rehab

Risk of bias legend
(A) Random sequence generation (selection bias)
(B) Allocation concealment (selection bias)
(C) Blinding of outcome assessment (detection bias)
(D) Incomplete outcome data (attrition bias)
(E) Selective reporting (reporting bias)
(F) Other bias

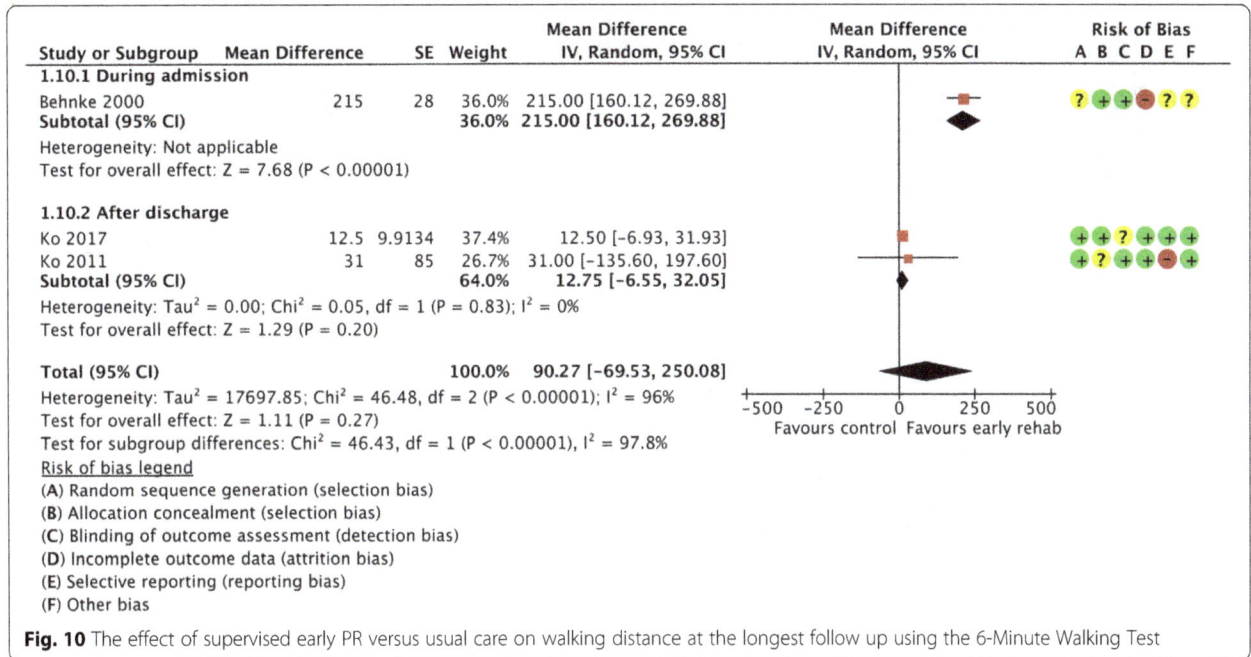

Fig. 10 The effect of supervised early PR versus usual care on walking distance at the longest follow up using the 6-Minute Walking Test

concealment, blinding of assessors, incomplete outcome together with selective outcome reporting (Table 2).

Three different studies provided data from 217 participants on the effect of early PR on walking distance assessed by 6MWT at 3–12 months from baseline [27, 33, 34] and showed no statistically, but a clinically relevant difference (mean difference: 90.27 m; 95% CI: [− 69.53 to 250.08]) with high heterogeneity (Fig. 10). Subgroup analysis showed a statistically significant difference between groups in favor of early PR during admission (P < 0.01) (Fig. 10). Due to unclear sequence generation, allocation concealment, blinding of assessors, incomplete data and

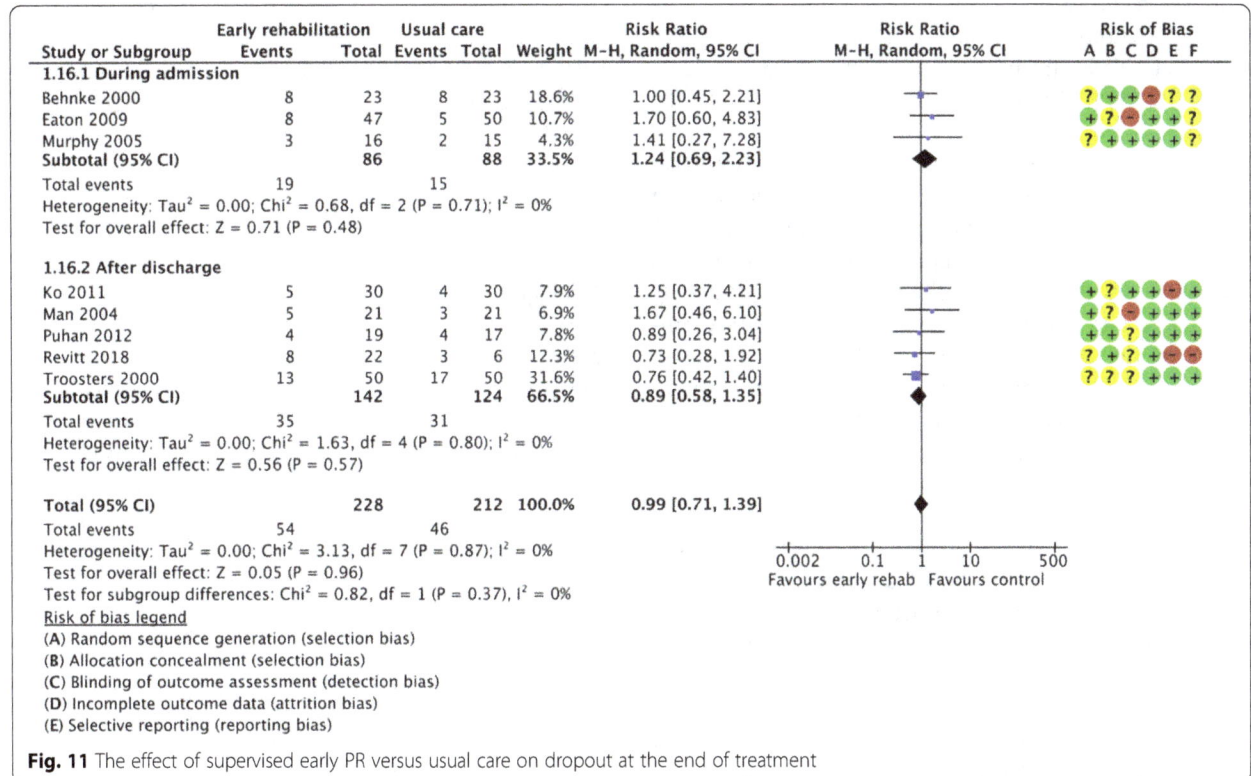

Study or Subgroup	Early rehabilitation Events	Total	Usual care Events	Total	Weight	Risk Ratio M–H, Random, 95% CI	Risk Ratio M–H, Random, 95% CI	Risk of Bias A B C D E F
1.16.1 During admission								
Behnke 2000	8	23	8	23	18.6%	1.00 [0.45, 2.21]		? + + − ? ?
Eaton 2009	8	47	5	50	10.7%	1.70 [0.60, 4.83]		+ ? − + + ?
Murphy 2005	3	16	2	15	4.3%	1.41 [0.27, 7.28]		? + + + + ?
Subtotal (95% CI)		86		88	33.5%	1.24 [0.69, 2.23]		
Total events	19		15					
Heterogeneity: Tau² = 0.00; Chi² = 0.68, df = 2 (P = 0.71); I² = 0%								
Test for overall effect: Z = 0.71 (P = 0.48)								
1.16.2 After discharge								
Ko 2011	5	30	4	30	7.9%	1.25 [0.37, 4.21]		+ ? + + − +
Man 2004	5	21	3	21	6.9%	1.67 [0.46, 6.10]		+ ? − + + +
Puhan 2012	4	19	4	17	7.8%	0.89 [0.26, 3.04]		+ + ? + + +
Revitt 2018	8	22	3	6	12.3%	0.73 [0.28, 1.92]		? + ? + − −
Troosters 2000	13	50	17	50	31.6%	0.76 [0.42, 1.40]		? ? ? + + +
Subtotal (95% CI)		142		124	66.5%	0.89 [0.58, 1.35]		
Total events	35		31					
Heterogeneity: Tau² = 0.00; Chi² = 1.63, df = 4 (P = 0.80); I² = 0%								
Test for overall effect: Z = 0.56 (P = 0.57)								
Total (95% CI)		228		212	100.0%	0.99 [0.71, 1.39]		
Total events	54		46					
Heterogeneity: Tau² = 0.00; Chi² = 3.13, df = 7 (P = 0.87); I² = 0%								
Test for overall effect: Z = 0.05 (P = 0.96)								
Test for subgroup differences: Chi² = 0.82, df = 1 (P = 0.37), I² = 0%								

0.002   0.1   1   10   500
Favours early rehab   Favours control

Risk of bias legend
(A) Random sequence generation (selection bias)
(B) Allocation concealment (selection bias)
(C) Blinding of outcome assessment (detection bias)
(D) Incomplete outcome data (attrition bias)
(E) Selective reporting (reporting bias)

Fig. 11 The effect of supervised early PR versus usual care on dropout at the end of treatment

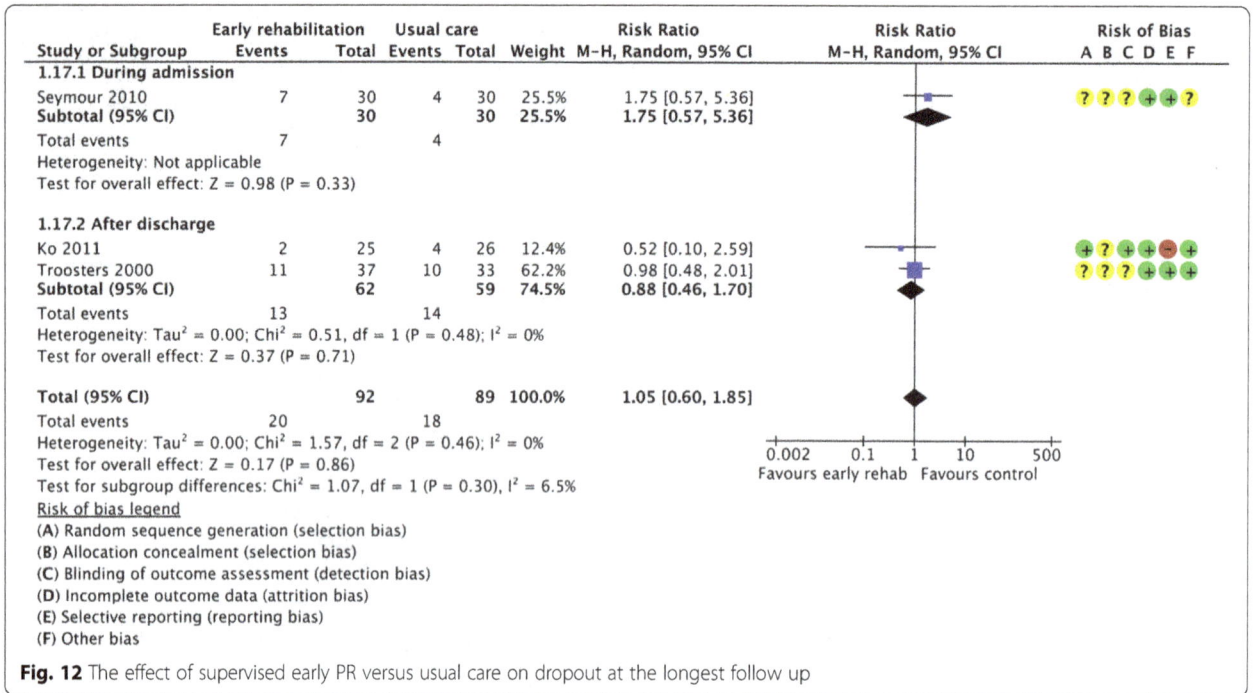

Study or Subgroup	Early rehabilitation Events	Total	Usual care Events	Total	Weight	Risk Ratio M–H, Random, 95% CI	Risk Ratio M–H, Random, 95% CI	Risk of Bias A B C D E F
1.17.1 During admission								
Seymour 2010	7	30	4	30	25.5%	1.75 [0.57, 5.36]		? ? ? + + ?
Subtotal (95% CI)		30		30	25.5%	1.75 [0.57, 5.36]		
Total events	7		4					
Heterogeneity: Not applicable								
Test for overall effect: Z = 0.98 (P = 0.33)								
1.17.2 After discharge								
Ko 2011	2	25	4	26	12.4%	0.52 [0.10, 2.59]		+ ? + + – +
Troosters 2000	11	37	10	33	62.2%	0.98 [0.48, 2.01]		? ? ? + + +
Subtotal (95% CI)		62		59	74.5%	0.88 [0.46, 1.70]		
Total events	13		14					
Heterogeneity: Tau² = 0.00; Chi² = 0.51, df = 1 (P = 0.48); I² = 0%								
Test for overall effect: Z = 0.37 (P = 0.71)								
Total (95% CI)		92		89	100.0%	1.05 [0.60, 1.85]		
Total events	20		18					
Heterogeneity: Tau² = 0.00; Chi² = 1.57, df = 2 (P = 0.46); I² = 0%								
Test for overall effect: Z = 0.17 (P = 0.86)								
Test for subgroup differences: Chi² = 1.07, df = 1 (P = 0.30), I² = 6.5%								

0.002   0.1   1   10   500
Favours early rehab   Favours control

Risk of bias legend
(A) Random sequence generation (selection bias)
(B) Allocation concealment (selection bias)
(C) Blinding of outcome assessment (detection bias)
(D) Incomplete outcome data (attrition bias)
(E) Selective reporting (reporting bias)
(F) Other bias

Fig. 12 The effect of supervised early PR versus usual care on dropout at the longest follow up

selective reporting together with high risk of inconsistency leading to high risk of imprecision the quality of evidence was downgraded (Table 2).

Drop-outs

The effect of early PR on the drop-out rate at the end of treatment was investigated in eight studies providing data from 440 randomized participants (early PR: $N = 228$; usual care: $N = 212$) [27, 28, 30, 34, 35, 37–39]. A total of 54 drop-outs were reported in the early PR group, whereas 46 drop-outs were reported in the usual care group, with no significant difference between groups (RR = 0.99 (95% CI: [0.71 to 1.39])) (Fig. 11). The subgroup analysis showed no difference in the effect between PR initiated during admission and after discharge ($P = 0.37$). Our confidence in the effect estimate was downgraded due to unclear sequence generation, allocation concealment, blinding of assessors and incomplete data outcome together with high risk of inconsistency (Table 2).

Three different studies provided data from 181 participants on the effect of early PR on drop-out at 3–18 months from baseline (early PR: $N = 92$; usual care: $N = 89$) [34, 36, 38]. A total of 20 drop-outs were reported in the early PR group, while 18 drop-outs were reported in the usual care group, with no difference between groups (RR = 1.05 (95% CI: [0.60 to 1.85])) (Fig. 12, Table 2). Subgroup analysis showed no difference in the effect between trials with PR initiated during admission and after discharge ($P = 0.30$; $I^2 = 6.5\%$) (Fig. 12).

None of the included studies reported results on the effect of early PR on ADL or the risk of falling.

Discussion

Summary of main findings

The present review summarized the evidence from 13 RCTs including 634 participants with an exacerbation of COPD and compared the use of early PR ($N = 322$) with usual care ($N = 312$). Subsequent meta-analysis showed that supervised early PR after acute exacerbation of COPD reduced mortality and number of days in hospital together with a reduction in COPD related hospital admissions and an improvement of HRQoL and exercise capacity (walking distance).

Mortality

We found that supervised early PR in patients with exacerbation of COPD reduced risk of mortality by ~ 42% compared with usual care. This finding was based on moderate quality of evidence due to methodological issues in the included studies and the relatively small numbers of participants. While similar conclusions have been reported in guidelines and systematic reviews in the past, results from a resent RCT by Greening et al. questioned the beneficial effects by reporting higher mortality in the early PR group [15–17]. In this study authors included patients with COPD related exacerbations during admission and instructed participants in the intervention group to be more physical active the next three months facilitated by technical devices [17]. In contrast, the majority of evidence favoring PR in stable

Table 2 GRADE Evidence Profile

Supervised early PR versus usual care for patients with acute exacerbation of COPD

Outcome Timeframe	Study results and measurements	Absolute effect estimates		Certainty in the effects estimates (Quality of evidence)	Plain text summary
		Usual care	Early PR		
Mortality End of treatment Critical	Relative risk 0.58 (CI 95% 0.35–0.98) Based on data from 319 patients (4 studies)	173 per 1.000	100 per 1.000	Moderate Due to serious risk of bias[a]	Early pulmonary rehabilitation probably decreases mortality at the end of treatment
		Difference: 73 fewer per 1.000 (CI 95% 112 fewer - 3 fewer)			
Mortality Longest follow-up Critical	Relative risk 0.55 (CI 95% 0.12–2.57) Based on data from 127 patients (3 studies)	63 per 1.000	35 per 1.000	Low Due to serious risk of bias and serious risk of imprecision[a,b]	Early pulmonary rehabilitation may decrease mortality slightly at the longest follow-up
		Difference: 28 fewer per 1.000 (CI 95% 55 fewer - 99 more)			
Days in hospital End of treatment Important	Measured by: Days Lower is better Based on data from 180 patients (1 study)	0.86 (mean)	4.59 (mean)	Moderate Due to serious imprecision[c]	Early pulmonary rehabilitation probably decreases days in hospital at the end of treatment
		Difference: MD 4.27 lower (CI 95% 6.85 lower - 1.69 lower)			
Days in hospital Longest follow-up Important					No studies were found that looked at number of days in hospital at the longest follow-up
Readmission due to exacerbation End of treatment Important					No studies were found that looked at readmission to hospital due to exacerbation at the end of treatment
Readmission due to exacerbation Longest follow-up Important	Rate ratio 0.47 (CI 95% 0.29–0.75) Based on data from 365 patients (6 studies)			Moderate Due to serious risk of bias[a,d]	Early pulmonary rehabilitation probably decreases readmission to hospital due to exacerbation at the longest follow-up
Health-related quality of life End of treatment Important	Measured by: SGRQ Lower is better Based on data from 86 patients (2 studies)	Difference: MD 19.43 lower (CI 95% 29.09 lower - 9.77 lower)		Low Due to serious risk of bias and serious risk of imprecision[a,c]	Early pulmonary rehabilitation may improve health-related quality of life at the end of treatment
Health-related quality of life Longest follow-up Important	Measured by: SGRQ Lower is better Based on data from 323 patients (4 studies)	Difference: MD 8.74 lower (CI 95% 12.02 lower - 5.45 lower)		Moderate Due to serious risk of bias[a,d]	Early pulmonary rehabilitation probably improves health-related quality of life at the longest follow-up
Exercise capacity End of treatment Important	Measured by: SWT (meters) Higher is better Based on data from 95 patients (3 studies)	Difference: MD 54.7 more (CI 95% 30.83 more - 78.57 more)		Moderate Due to serious risk of bias[a,d]	Early pulmonary rehabilitation probably increases exercise capacity at the end of treatment
Exercise capacity End of treatment Important	Measured by: 6MWT (meters) Higher is better Based on data from 274 patients (5 studies	Difference: MD 76.89 more (CI 95% 21.34 more - 132.45 more)		Low Due to serious risk of bias and serious inconsistency[a,d,e]	Early pulmonary rehabilitation probably increases exercise capacity at the end of treatment

Table 2 GRADE Evidence Profile *(Continued)*

Supervised early PR versus usual care for patients with acute exacerbation of COPD

Outcome Timeframe	Study results and measurements	Absolute effect estimates		Certainty in the effects estimates (Quality of evidence)	Plain text summary
		Usual care	Early PR		
Exercise capacity Longest follow-up Important	Measured by: SWT (meters) Higher is better Based on data from 2017 patients (3 studies)	Difference: MD 90.27 higher (CI 95% 69.53 lower - 250.08 higher)		Low Due to serious risk of bias and serious inconsistency leading to serious imprecision[a,b,d,e]	Early pulmonary rehabilitation may increase exercise capacity at the longest follow-up
Dropout rate End of treatment Important	Relative risk 0.99 (CI 95% 0.71–1.39) Based on data from 440 patients (8 studies)	217 per 1.000	215 per 1.000	Moderate Due to serious risk of bias[a,d]	Early pulmonary rehabilitation probably has little impact on the dropout rate at the end of treatment
		Difference: 2 fewer per 1.000 (CI 95% 63 fewer - 85 more)			
Dropout rate Longest follow-up Important	Relative risk 1.05 (CI 95% 0.6–1.85) Based on data from 181 patients (3 studies)	202 per 1.000	212 per 1.000	Moderate Due to serious risk of bias[a,d]	Early pulmonary rehabilitation probably has little impact on dropout at the longest follow-up
		Difference: 10 more per 1.000 (CI 95% 81 fewer - 172 more)			
Falls Longest follow-up Important					No studies were found that looked at falls at the longest follow-up
Activities of daily living End of treatment Important					No studies were found that looked at activities of daily living at the end of treatment
Activities of daily living Longest-follow-up Important					No studies were found that looked at activities of daily living at the longest follow-up

CI confidence interval, *COPD* chronic obstructive pulmonary disease, *MD* middle difference, *PR* pulmonary rehabilitation, *SGRQ* St. George's Respiratory Questionnaire, *SWT* Shuttle Walking Test, *6MWT* 6 min walking test
Quality of evidence. High quality: We are very confident that the true effect lies close to that of the estimate of the effect; Moderate quality: We are moderately confident in the effect estimate, the true effect is likely to be close to the estimate of the effect, but there is a possibility that it is substantially different; Low quality: Our confidence in the effect estimate is limited, the true effect may be substantially different from the estimate of the effect
[a]Risk of bias: Serious. Unclear/inadequate sequence generation and unclear/inadequate concealment of allocation during randomization process resulting in potential for selection bias
[b]Risk of imprecision: Serious. Wide confidence intervals
[c]Risk of imprecision: Serious. Low number of patients
[d]Risk of bias: Serious. Inadequate/unclear or lack of blinding of outcome assessors resulting in potential for detection bias
[e]Risk of inconsistency: Serious. The magnitude of statistical heterogeneity was high

COPD is based on supervised programs, and therefore we did not include Greening et al. in our review. However, to assess safety of early PR initiated during the hospital admission we performed a subgroup analysis showing no difference between groups rehabilitated during the admission and after discharge.

Results from this review differ from a previous review by Puhan et al. [14] who showed no statistically significant effect of early PR on mortality, but when the authors preformed a subgroup analysis, excluding results from Greening et al. [17], they did find a positive effect of early PR on mortality [14]. Moreover, the review by Puhan et al. [14] differs methodologically from the present review, as they included any inpatient and/or outpatient PR program with no criteria for the comprehensiveness or supervision of the rehabilitation program. We only included studies of supervised PR programs similar to what is offered to COPD patients in Denmark, which is based on the present large amount of evidence in favor of supervised PR in stable COPD. This might explain the lower heterogeneity and greater effects on mortality in the present review.

Hospital length of stay and readmissions

Moderate-quality evidence showed that supervised early PR significantly reduced the risk of COPD related hospital readmissions at the longest follow up with 53%. In addition, the number of days in hospital was reduced by an average of 4.27 days. Puhan et al. [14] have previously shown that PR significantly reduced the mean number of hospital admissions per participant from 1.6 to 0.9 during the year following after hospital admission for an acute exacerbation. Several explanations have been proposed for the substantial effect of PR on hospital readmission. The main reason is probably that hospitalization following an acute exacerbation of COPD leads to significant reductions in activity level [6]. It is well known that the recovery period after an acute exacerbation is long, even for patients with no subsequent exacerbations [40]. Thus, PR can be considered an effective intervention for reverting physical inactivity [41] and it has been shown that patients who achieved improvement in their daily physical activity level after an exacerbation of COPD experienced a ~ 50% reduction in risk of hospital readmission [42].

Health-related quality of life and exercise capacity

The primary result to support this, in the present review, are clinically relevant improvements in walking distance of respectively 76.89 m in 6 min walking distance (6MWD) and 54.70 m in shuttle walking distance (SWD) immediately after early PR and an improvement of 90.27 m in 6MWD at the longest follow up [43], which are in line with those results from Puhan et al. [14], showing an improvement of 62.38 m in 6MWD after early PR. Secondly, we found moderate quality of evidence supporting a clinically important improvement in HRQoL immediately after participation of 19.43 units on the SGRQ scale and an improvement of 8.74 units at the longest follow up. These effects on HRQoL exceeded the minimal clinically important difference (MCID) for the SGRQ (> 4-point improvement [44]), and the results are in line with previous studies showing a large effect of PR on HRQoL in stable patients with COPD [14]. Although statistically non-significant, the beneficial effects of early PR versus usual care on SGRQ at the longest follow up (8.74 units) in present review were close to those observed in stable COPD patients (6.89 units) [9]. In addition, the present review found a greater improvement in HRQoL at the end of treatment in patients with an exacerbation of COPD compared with stable COPD patients, which probably is due to the lower baseline during recovery from AECOPD.

Clinical application

We found no difference in drop-out rate between participants allocated to early PR compared with usual care. Thus, the effects were not driven solely by positive responders to PR, and secondly, the most severely affected patients will likely complete or drop-out to the same extent as usual care. As before mentioned, we did not include Greening et al. [17], since this study has been highly criticized for not offering a sufficiently extensive PR programs [45, 46], and interestingly, authors reported a high number of drop-outs. The participants in the rehabilitation group attended an average of 2.6 supervised sessions during hospital admission, followed by mainly unsupervised training after discharge, with a poor adherence to the home self-management exercise program (mean of 57.5) [17]. Nevertheless, these results suggest that it is important to assess how the PR is delivered. PR programs can differ in many aspects, which may influence their effectiveness. When assessing the extensiveness of the PR program; the number of exercise training sessions, frequency of exercise training, type of exercise training and supervision of training, as well as self-management, education and adherence to the PR program need to be considered [26].

In this review ten studies implemented an extensive PR program which mostly showed large and consistent effects on mortality, days in hospital, COPD related hospital readmissions, HRQoL, and walking distance. The PR programs were not exactly similar within the reviewed studies, but the majority provided either many training sessions (more than 16 sessions) [27, 29–31, 33, 34, 38], programs of long duration (> 12 weeks) [27, 38], or supported education [28, 30, 33, 35, 36]. Nevertheless, our results show that supervised early PR programs across studies with different protocols are effective in patients with COPD-related exacerbations.

Safety

Currently, the ideal timing of the onset of PR after AECOPD is highly debated. Based on low-quality of evidence, the ERS/ATS Task Force made a conditional recommendation against the initiation of PR during hospitalization since PR initiated during admission was found to increase mortality [18]. This conclusion seems based solely on results from Greening et al. [17], who reported a higher mortality in the unsupervised home-based rehabilitation group at 12 months compared with usual care group. The difference between groups however, was not related to the early rehabilitation intervention. Indeed, the per protocol analysis did not show a difference in mortality [17], suggesting that the participants who actually received the intervention were not accountable for the increased mortality [47]. We did not find any harms of early supervised PR across 13 RCTs, even when we isolated the subgroup that initiated PR during admission.

Conclusion

The results of the present review support the substantial and clinical important benefits of supervised early PR, indicating that this is an effective intervention with the purpose of reducing mortality following a hospitalization for AECOPD. Our meta-analysis shows that supervised PR during the recovery period after an AECOPD is superior to usual care in terms of improving prognosis, HRQoL and walking distance. Based on moderate to low quality of evidence, we conclude that supervised early PR reduces the risk of mortality, COPD-related hospital readmissions and the number of days in hospital, and lead to large and clinically relevant improvements in HRQoL and walking distance. Therefore, we recommend supervised PR to patients with COPD-related exacerbations. PR should be initiated during hospital admission or within 4 weeks after hospital discharge.

Abbreviations

1RM: One repetition maximum; 6MDT: 6-min walking test; 6MWD: 6-min walking distance; ADL: Activities of daily living; AECOPD: Acute exacerbation in chronic obstructive pulmonary disease; AGREE II: Appraisal of Guidelines for Research and Evaluation instrument version II; AMSTAR: A Measurement Tool to Asses Systematic Reviews; ATS: American Thoracic Society; BTS: British Thoracic Society; COPD: Chronic obstructive pulmonary disease; CT: Combined training; ERS: European Respiratory Society; ET: Endurance training; FEV_1: Forced expiratory volume in 1 s; GRADE: Grading of Recommendations Assessment, Development and Evaluation; HR_{max}: Maximum heart rate; HRQoL: Health-related quality of life; I^2: I-square; MCID: Minimal clinically important difference; MD: Mean difference; PICO: Population, intervention, comparison and outcomes; PR: Pulmonary rehabilitation; RCT: Randomized controlled trials; Reps: Repetitions; RT: Resistance training; SGRQ: St. George's Respiratory Questionnaire; SMD: Standardized mean difference; SWD: Shuttle walking distance; SWT: Shuttle walking test; VO_{2max}: Maximal oxygen uptake; W_{max}: Maximal work load in Watts

Acknowledgments

Birgitte Holm Petersen and Kirsten Birkefoss, search specialists at the Danish Health Authority, are acknowledged for their contributions.

Funding

This study was initiated and financed by the Danish Health Authority. The writhing of the article was supported by the Centre of Inflammation and Metabolism and the Centre for Physical Activity Research, Rigshospitalet, University of Copenhagen, Denmark.

Authors' contributions

All authors contributed to the conception, design, interpretation, drafting, revising and final approval of the manuscript. CKR, UWI, NSG and LMK selected the manuscripts for analysis. CKR, HEC and BT performed the data extraction and the meta-analysis.

Competing interests

The authors declare that they have no competing interests.

Author details

[1]The Centre of Inflammation and Metabolism and the Centre for Physical Activity Research, Rigshospitalet, University of Copenhagen, Blegdamsvej 9, DK-2100 Copenhagen, Denmark. [2]Danish Health Authority, Copenhagen, Denmark. [3]Department of Respiratory Medicine, Copenhagen University Hospital, Hvidovre, Denmark. [4]Department of Clinical Medicine, University of Copenhagen, Copenhagen, Denmark. [5]Department of Physiotherapy, Copenhagen University Hospital, Hvidovre, Denmark. [6]Department of Pulmonary and Infectious Diseases, Copenhagen University Hospital, Nordsjælland, Hillerød, Denmark. [7]The Department of the Elderly and Disabled, Odense Municipality, Odense, Denmark. [8]Department of Gastroenterology, Center for Nutrition and Bowel Disease, Aalborg University Hospital, Aalborg, Denmark. [9]Unit for Psychooncology and Health Psychology, Aarhus University Hospital and Aarhus University, Aarhus, Denmark. [10]Department of Public Health, Section of Social Medicine, University of Copenhagen, Copenhagen, Denmark. [11]Medical Department O, Respiratory Section, Herlev and Gentofte Hospital, Herlev, Denmark.

References

1. Rosenberg SR, Kalhan R, Mannino DM. Epidemiology of chronic obstructive pulmonary disease: prevalence, morbidity, mortality, and risk factors. Semin Respir Crit Care Med. 2015;36(4):457–69.
2. Halpin DM, Miravitlles M, Metzdorf N, Celli B. Impact and prevention of severe exacerbations of COPD: a review of the evidence. Int J Chron Obstruct Pulmon Dis. 2017;12:2891–908.
3. Singanayagam A, Schembri A, Chalmers JD. Predictors of mortality in hospitalized adults with acute exacerbation of chronic obstructive pulmonary disease. Ann Am Thorac Soc. 2013;10(2):81–9.
4. Goto T, Faridi MK, Gibo K, Toh S, Hanania NA, Camargo CA Jr, et al. Trends in 30-day readmission rates after COPD hospitalization, 2006-2012. Respir Med. 2017;130:92–7.
5. Eriksen N, Vestbo J. Management and survival of patients admitted with an exacerbation of COPD: comparison of two Danish patient cohorts. Clin Respir J. 2010;4(4):208–14.
6. Pitta F, Troosters T, Probst VS, Spruit MA, Decramer M, Gosselink R. Physical activity and hospitalization for exacerbation of COPD. Chest. 2006;129(3):536–44.
7. Donaldson GC, Wilkinson TM, Hurst JR, Perera WR, Wedzicha JA, et al. Exacerbations and time spent outdoors in chronic obstructive pulmonary disease. Am J Respir Crit Care Med. 2005;171(5):446–52.
8. Seidel D, Cheung A, Suh ES, Raste Y, Atakhorrami M, Spruit MA. Physical inactivity and risk of hospitalisation for chronic obstructive pulmonary disease. Int J Tuberc Lung Dis. 2012;16(8):1015–9.
9. McCarthy B, Casey D, Devane D, Murphy K, Murphy E, Lacasse Y, et al. Pulmonary rehabilitation for chronic obstructive pulmonary disease. Cochrane Database Syst Rev. 2015;2:CD003793.
10. Spruit MA, Singh SJ, Garvey C, ZuWallack R, Nici L, Rochester C, et al. An official American Thoracic Society/European Respiratory Society statement: key concepts and advances in pulmonary rehabilitation. Am J Respir Crit Care Med. 2013;188(8):e13–64.
11. Iepsen UW, Jørgensen KJ, Ringbaek T, Hansen H, Skrubbeltrang C, Lange P. A systematic review of resistance training versus endurance training in COPD. J Cardiopulm Rehabil Prev. 2015;35(3):163–72.
12. Iepsen UW, Jørgensen KJ, Ringbæk T, Hansen H, Skrubbeltrang C, Lange P. A combination of resistance and endurance training increases leg muscle strength in COPD: an evidence-based recommendation based on systematic review with meta-analysis. Chron Respir Dis. 2015;12(2):132–42.
13. Ringbaek T, Brondum E, Martinez G, Thogersen J, Lange P. Long-term effects of 1-year maintenance training on physical functioning and health status in patients with COPD: a randomized controlled study. J Cardiopulm Rehabil Prev. 2010;30(1):47–52.
14. Puhan MA, Gimeno-Santos E, Cates CJ, Troosters T. Pulmonary rehabilitation following exacerbations of chronic obstructive pulmonary disease. Cochrane Database Syst Rev. 2016;12:CD005305.
15. Puhan MA, Gimeno-Santos E, Scharplatz M, Troosters T, Walters EH, Steurer J. Pulmonary rehabilitation following exacerbations of chronic obstructive pulmonary disease. Cochrane Database Syst Rev. 2011;10:CD005305.
16. National Institute for Health and Clinical Excellence: Guidance. Chronic Obstructive Pulmonary Disease: Management of Chronic Obstructive Pulmonary Disease in Adults in Primary and Secondary Care: National Clinical Guideline Centre; 2010.
17. Greening NJ, Williams JEA, Hussain SF, Harvey-Dunstan TC, Bankart MJ, Chaplin EJ, et al. An early rehabilitation intervention to enhance recovery during hospital admission for an exacerbation of chronic respiratory disease: randomised controlled trial. BMJ. 2014;349:g4315.

18. Wedzicha JA, Miravitlles M, Hurst JR, Calverley PM, Albert RK, Anzueto A, et al. Management of COPD exacerbations: a European Respiratory Society/ American Thoracic Society guideline. Eur Respir J. 2017;49(3).

19. The Grading of Recommendations Assessment, Development and Evaluation (GRADE) Working Group. [Online] http://www. gradeworkinggroup.org. Accessed 28 Nov 2017.

20. Guyatt GH, Oxman AD, Kunz R, Atkins D, Brozek J, Vist G, et al. GRADE guidelines: 2. Framing the question and deciding on important outcomes. J Clin Epidemiol. 2011;64(4):395–400.

21. COPD Working Group. Pulmonary rehabilitation for patients with chronic pulmonary disease (COPD): an evidence-based analysis. Ont Health Technol Assess Ser. 2012;12(6):1–75.

22. Higgins JPT, Green S (editors). Cochrane Handbook for Systematic Reviews of Interventions Version 5.1.0 [updated March 2011]. The Cochrane Collaboration. 2011. Availble from http://handbook.cochrane.org. Accessed 28 Nov 2017.

23. Review Manager (RevMan) [Computer program]. Version 5.3. Copenhagen: The Nordic Cochrane Centre, The Cochrane Collaboration; 2014.

24. Guyatt GH, Oxman AD, Kunz R, Woodcock J, Brozek J, Helfand M, et al. GRADE guidelines: 7. Rating the quality of evidence--inconsistency. J Clin Epidemiol. 2011;64(12):1294–302.

25. Balshem H, Helfand M, Schünemann HJ, Oxman AD, Kunz R, Brozek J, et al. GRADE guidelines: 3. Rating the quality of evidence. J Clin Epidemiol. 2011; 64(4):401–6.

26. Bolton CE, Bevan-Smith EF, Blakey JD, Crowe P, Elkin SL, Garrod R, et al. British Thoracic Society guideline on pulmonary rehabilitation in adults. Thorax. 2013;68(Suppl 2):ii1–30.

27. Behnke M, Taube C, Kirsten D, Lehnigk B, Jörres RA, Magnussen H, et al. Home-based exercise is capable of preserving hospital-based improvements in severe chronic obstructive pulmonary disease. Respir Med. 2000;94(12): 1184–91.

28. Eaton T, Young P, Fergusson W, Moodie L, Zeng I, O'Kane F, et al. Does early pulmonary rehabilitation reduce acute health-care utilization in COPD patients admitted with an exacerbation? A randomized controlled study. Respirology. 2009;14(2):230–8.

29. Kirsten DK, Taube C, Lehnigk B, Jörres RA, Magnussen H, et al. Exercise training improves recovery in patients with COPD after an acute exacerbation. Respir Med. 1998;92(10):1191–8.

30. Puhan MA, Spaar A, Frey M, Turk A, Brändli O, Ritscher D, et al. Early versus late pulmonary rehabilitation in chronic obstructive pulmonary disease patients with acute exacerbations: a randomized trial. Respiration. 2012; 83(6):499–506.

31. Daabis R, Hassan M, Zidan M. Endurance and strength training in pulmonary rehabilitation for COPD patients. Egypt J Chest Dis Tuberc. 2017; 66(2):231–6.

32. Deepak TH, Mohapatra PR, Janmeja AK, Sood P, Gupta M. Outcome of pulmonary rehabilitation in patients after acute exacerbation of chronic obstructive pulmonary disease. Indian J Chest Dis Allied Sci. 2014;56(1):7–12.

33. Ko FW, Cheung NK, Rainer TH, Lum C, Wong I, Hui DS. Comprehensive care programme for patients with chronic obstructive pulmonary disease: a randomised controlled trial. Thorax. 2017;72(2):122–8.

34. Ko FW, Dai DL, Ngai J, Tung A, Ng S, Lai K, et al. Effect of early pulmonary rehabilitation on health care utilization and health status in patients hospitalized with acute exacerbations of COPD. Respirology. 2011;16(4):617–24.

35. Man WD, Polkey MI, Donaldson N, Gray BJ, Moxham J. Community pulmonary rehabilitation after hospitalisation for acute exacerbations of chronic obstructive pulmonary disease: randomised controlled study. BMJ. 2004;329(7476):1209.

36. Seymour JM, Moore L, Jolley CJ, Ward K, Creasey J, Steier JS, et al. Outpatient pulmonary rehabilitation following acute exacerbations of COPD. Thorax. 2010;65(5):423–8.

37. Revitt O, Sewell L, Singh S. Early versus delayed pulmonary rehabilitation: a randomized controlled trial - can we do it? Chron Respir Dis. 2018. https:// doi.org/10.1177/1479972318757469.

38. Troosters T, Grosselink R, Decramer M. Short- and long-term effects of outpatient rehabilitation in patients with chronic obstructive pulmonary disease: a randomized trial. Am J Med. 2000;109(3):207 12.

39. Murphy N, Bell C, Costello RW. Extending a home from hospital care programme for COPD exacerbations to include pulmonary rehabilitation. Respir Med. 2005;99(10):1297–302.

40. Spencer S, Jones PW. Time course of recovery of health status following an infective exacerbation of chronic bronchitis. Thorax. 2003;58(7):589–93.

41. Troosters T, Gosselink R, Janssens W, Decramer M. Exercise training and pulmonary rehabilitation: new insights and remaining challenges. Eur Respir Rev. 2010;19(115):24–9.

42. Garcia-Aymerich J, Farrero E, Félez MA, Izquierdo J, Marrades RM, Antó JM. Risk factors of readmission to hospital for a COPD exacerbation: a prospective study. Thorax. 2003;58(2):100–5.

43. ATS Committee on Proficiency Standards for Clinical Pulmonary Function Laboratories. ATS statement: guidelines for the six-minute walk test. Am J Respir Crit Care Med. 2002;166(1):111–7.

44. Jones PW. Interpreting thresholds for a clinically significant change in health status in asthma and COPD. Eur Respir J. 2002;19(3):398–404.

45. Hopkinson NS. What is and what is not post exacerbation pulmonary rehabilitation? BMJ. 2014;349:g4315.

46. Spruit MA, Rochester CL, Pitta F, Goldstein R, Troosters T, Nici L, et al. A 6-week, home-based, unsupervised exercise training program is not effective in patients with chronic respiratory disease directly following a hospital admission. BMJ. 2014;g4315:349.

47. Wilson KC, Krishnan JA, Sliwinski P, Criner GJ, Miravitlles M, Hurst JR. et al. Pulmonary rehabilitation for patients with COPD during and after an exacerbation-related hospitalisation: back to the future? Eur Respir J. 2018; 51(1).

16

Role of medical Thoracoscopy in the Management of Multiloculated Empyema

Kamran Khan Sumalani[1*], Nadeem Ahmed Rizvi[1] and Asif Asghar[2]

Abstract

Background: The treatment of early pleural empyema depends on the treatment of ongoing infection by antimicrobial therapy along with thoracocentesis. In complicated empyema this treatment does not work and lung will not expand until removal of adhesions. The objective of the current study is to analyze the experience of management of multiloculated, exudative and fibrinopurulent empyema through rigid medical thoracoscopy under local anaesthesia and to explore new ways to manage the entity.

Methods: This is a descriptive case series in which 160 patients were recruited through non-probability convenient sampling, from department of pulmonology, Jinnah postgraduate medical centre, Karachi, from September 2014 to August 2016. All patients underwent medical thoracoscopy under local anesthesia. Written Informed consent was taken from the study participants. Ethical approval was obtained from Ethical Review Committee of the hospital. Patients age > 70 years, those with multiple organ failure and bleeding disorders were excluded.

Results: Out of 160 patients, 108 (67.50%) were male and 52 (32.5%) were female with mean age 25.37 years (range 16 to 70 years). Out of total, 102 (63.7%) had tuberculous empyema, while pleural biopsy of 58 (36.3%) patients was suggestive of non-tuberculous empyema. Final evolution through chest x-ray revealed complete resolution in 92 (57.5%), partial resolution in 58 (36.25%) patients. 9 (5.6%) developed persistent air leak while 1 (0.6%) patient expired due to urosepsis.

Conclusion: Medical Thoracoscopy under local anesthesia is a safe, efficient and cost effective intervention for management of complicated empyema, particularly in resource constraint settings.

Keywords: Thoracoscopy, Empyema pleural, Tuberculosis, Inflammation, Video-assisted thoracoscopic surgery

Background

Pleural empyema is defined as pus accumulation in the pleural space; it is associated with significant morbidity and mortality in adults and children [1]. It can be subdivided into three stages: Stage 1: exudative which is freely moving pleural fluid, Stage 2: fibrino-purulent in which fibrin deposits on the pleural surfaces with a turbid, viscous fluid which has a tendency to loculate, and Stage 3: organizing which is characterized by fibrous thickening of the visceral pleura leading ultimately to a trapped lung by fibrous adhesions on pleura. [2, 3].

Ultrasound chest outperforms CT scan chest in visualizing septations and loculations within empyema.

Diaphragmatic movement can be visualized in real-time which is reduced in heavily septated effusions or fibrothorax [4].

The visualization of these radiological features is useful in practice as the therapeutic approach clearly differs even when clinical trials to guide treatment are still lacking [5]. However, medical thoracoscopy is a least invasive procedure that provides access to the pleural space using a combination of visualizing and working instruments.

The term thoracoscopy is confusing because it refers to both the medical and surgical procedures. To avoid confusion, some authors suggest that medical thoracoscopy should be referred to as pleuroscopy. The term thoracoscopy may be used exclusively for the surgical thoracoscopic procedure [6, 7]. Advances in medicine and medical instruments, thoracoscopy has now become

* Correspondence: drkamrankn@hotmail.com
[1]Department of Chest Medicine, Jinnah Postgraduate Medical Centre, Karachi 75400, Pakistan
Full list of author information is available at the end of the article

a routine procedure in the management of the disease of the chest including pleura.

In empyema, medical thoracoscopy is a drainage procedure, midway between tube thoracostomy and video-assisted thoracoscopic surgery (VATS), which is efficient, significantly cheaper and prevents from surgical thoracoscopy under general anaesthesia. It is important that it is performed in the start of disease and is particularly advisable for frail patients at high risk of surgery [8].

No local data is available on this subject. Thus, we planned to conduct this study to report our experience about the effectiveness and safety of medical thoracoscopy in multiloculated, exudative and fibrinopurulent empyema confirmed by chest ultrasonography and CT scan. (Fig. 1).

Methods

This was a case series in which 160 out of 199 patients with empyema were recruited from department of pulmonology, Jinnah Postgraduate Medical Centre, Karachi Pakistan from September 2014 to August 2016. This study was performed in accordance with the Declaration of Helsinki. This human study was approved by Ethical review committee Jinnah postgraduate medical center, Karachi. All adult participants provided written informed consent to participate in this study.

All patients underwent chest radiography and CT scan chest for confirmation of the disease. Ultrasonography of chest was done in all patients to localize the effusion, assess the echogenicity, diaphragmatic motility and presence of septations and loculations. For ultrasonographic chest examination convex transducer with frequency of 3.5–5 MHz was used and the examination was performed by a group of pulmonologists of the department who had received specific training and performed the examination on regular basis.

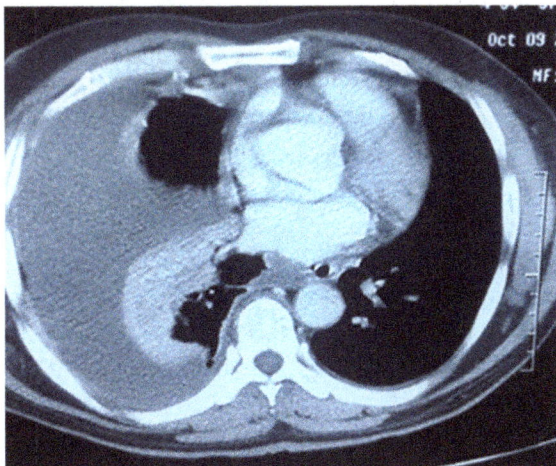

Fig. 1 CT scan of the chest showing loculated empyema

Inclusion criteria

- Prolong presentation of empyema (> 30 days)
- No response to antibiotics therapy
- Failure of complete drainage by tube thoracostomy
- Multi-septated, multi-loculated empyema as evidenced by ultrasonography

Exclusion criteria

- Age more than 70 years
- Consent not given for the procedure
- Bleeding disorders
- Multi-organ failure
- Hemodynamic instability
- Simple empyema, without septations and loculations
- Organized stage 3 empyema as evident on chest CT scan or ultrasound
- Terminally ill patients

Out of 199, thirty nine patients were excluded as 12 did not give consent for the procedure, 2 had acute myocardial infarction, 10 were hemodynamically unstable, and 11 patients had organized empyema. 4 patients did not meet the age criteria of the study so were excluded.

Thoracoscopy was performed in a dedicated endoscopic suite with facilities of ultrasonography. The procedure was fully informed to the patient. Prior to the procedure intercostal nerve block was given at paravertebral area in multiple adjacent intercostal spaces. Local anesthetic is administered with a syringe facing upwards at an angle of 20° to approach the neurovascular bundle at the lower border of the rib. After confirmation by aspiration of blood, 3–5 mL of local anesthetic (1% solution of lidocaine, total 30 - 50 mg) is administered. The whole procedure is repeated for other levels of intercostal blockade needed.

Patient placed in a lateral decubitus position with empyema side up and arm above the head. Vitals and oxygen saturation were continuously monitored during the procedure. The incision site was anesthetized locally and adequate analgesia and conscious sedation was achieved so that patient can tolerate the procedure while maintaining cardiorespiratory functions. Lidocaine with adrenaline 3 mL of 1% solution (not exceeding 4.5 mg/kg) was used for local anesthesia. Drugs used for analgesia and sedation were nalbuphine in a dose of 0.3–3 mg/kg IV over 10–15 min, and midazolam 0.5–1 mg IV given over 2 min, not exceeding 2.5 mg/dose.

Single port was made using 10 mm trocar under direct ultrasound guidance. Optical telescope at 0° was inserted into the pleural cavity for video inspection. Fibrinous septa were removed with forceps, (Fig. 2a and b)

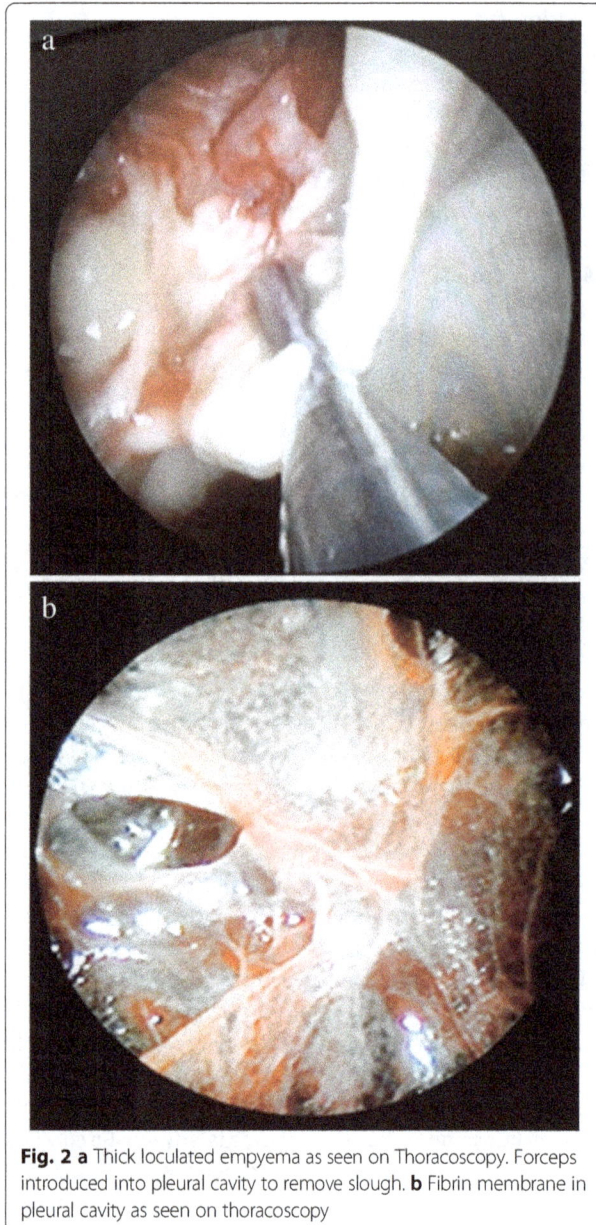

Fig. 2 a Thick loculated empyema as seen on Thoracoscopy. Forceps introduced into pleural cavity to remove slough. **b** Fibrin membrane in pleural cavity as seen on thoracoscopy

while in case of thick debris and adhesions a second port was made to introduce large forceps.

Multiple targeted biopsies were also taken from the parietal pleura. At the end single or dual (28–32 Fr) chest tube(s) were placed in the cavity and attached to under-water seal with a suction pressure of – 20 cmH$_2$O. Patients were encouraged to use incentive spirometer and early mobilization with the help of training stairs and bicycle ergometers.

All patients received broad spectrum 3rd generation cephalosporins after the procedure. Antibiotics were changed later on if needed on the basis of pleural fluid culture and sensitivity results. Patients diagnosed as having tuberculous empyema were treated with anti-tuberculous

therapy. After successful procedure average time for chest tube removal was 7–25 days.

Complete resolution was labelled when opacity on chest radiograph was reduced to less than one-third of the hemithorax, and partial resolution was labelled when it was more than one-third of the hemithorax.

Treatment success included both complete and partial resolution cases. It was defined as radiologic confirmation of successful pleural drainage with no recurrence and hence no need for further treatment i.e. subsequent tube thoracostomies or surgical interventions and objective evidence of resolution of sepsis (improvement in temperature and clinical condition and decreasing inflammatory markers, total white cell count and serum C-reactive protein) at the time of discharge from hospital.

Statistical analysis

Data was analysed on Statistical analysis software package (SPSS) version 21. Mean, frequencies and percentages were calculated for quantitative data. Chi-square test was used and $P < 0.05$ was considered significant with confidence interval taken as 95%.

Results

A total of 160 patients with multi-loculated empyema were included in the study. Males were 108 (67.5%) and females 52 (32.5%) with the mean age of the study participants was 25.37 years (range: 19–60 years). The etiology of empyema as confirmed by thoracoscopic pleural biopsy as shown in table 1 and Fig. 3a and b.

As shown in Fig. 4, follow-up chest radiograph shows complete resolution in 92 (57.5%) and partial resolution in 58 (36.25%) patients with no further intervention.

Treatment success of 93.75% was achieved. A total of 2 complications were observed after the procedure; 9 (5.6%) of the patients developed persistent air leak and required surgical intervention and only one death was reported on 4th day post-procedure due to urosepsis. Comparison of chest X-rays before and after the procedure is shown in Fig. 5.

Table 1 Etiology of empyema as confirmed by thoracoscopic pleural biopsy

Etiology	n (%)
Tuberculosis	102/160 (63.7)
Non-tuberculous	58/160 (36.36)
Acute on chronic inflammation	26/58 (16.25)
Malignancy(Adenocarcinoma)	20/58 (12.5)
Non-specific inflammation	12/58 (7.5)

n is the number of cases. Percentage is shown in parenthesis

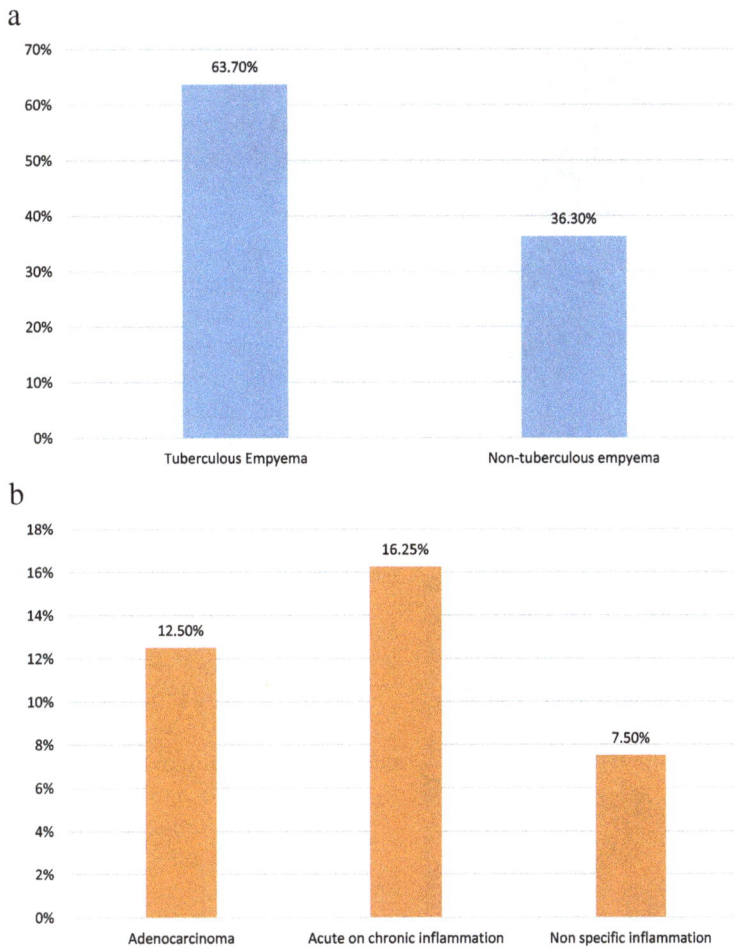

Fig. 3 **a** Etiology of empyema as confirmed by thoracoscopic pleural biopsy **b**: Etiology of non-tuberculous empyema as confirmed by thoracoscopic pleural biopsy

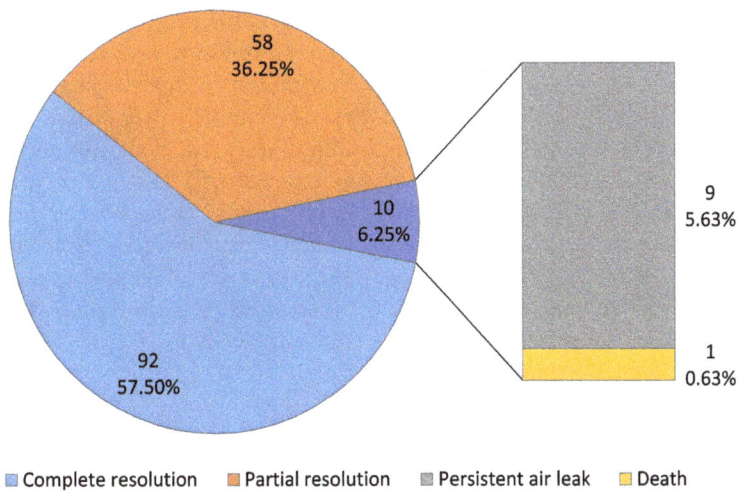

Fig. 4 Outcome of radiograph resolution

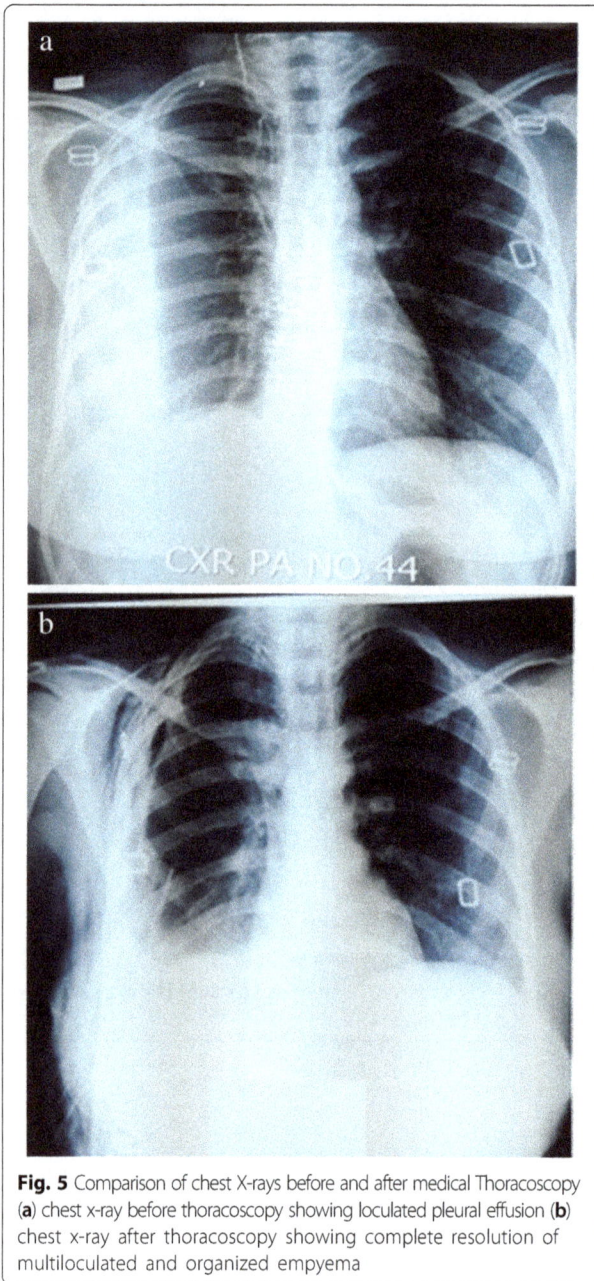

Fig. 5 Comparison of chest X-rays before and after medical Thoracoscopy (**a**) chest x-ray before thoracoscopy showing loculated pleural effusion (**b**) chest x-ray after thoracoscopy showing complete resolution of multiloculated and organized empyema

Discussion

In our study we assessed the efficacy and safety of rigid medical thoracoscopy in cases of multi-loculated empyema stratified by chest ultrasonography. Treatment success rate with rigid medical thoracoscopy was found to be 93.75%. This included both complete and partial resolution cases. It was defined as radiologic confirmation of successful pleural drainage with no recurrence and hence no need for further treatment i.e. later tube thoracostomies or surgical procedures and sign of resolution of sepsis like decrement in total leukocyte count, serum C-reactive protein and fever at the time of

discharge from hospital, i.e. after 7–25 days. The remaining 6.25% cases were labelled as treatment failure who required further surgical intervention.

Medical thoracoscopy is at the stage of its inception in Pakistan and there are only few centers scattered in the country doing this procedure, while the use of this minimally invasive procedure was introduced in 1910 in Europe to diagnose and treat pleural diseases [4, 9, 10].

The technique is similar to chest tube insertion with advantage that the pleural space can be visualized, biopsies can be taken, multiple loculations can be converted into a single communicating cavity and adequate drainage of fluid and thick fibrinous debris can be removed. The main advantage of medical thoracoscopy over VATS (video assisted thoracoscopy) is that it is less invasive, cheap procedure which can be done in an endoscopic suite and is better tolerated in frail patients who are under high risk with general anesthesia and tracheal intubation [11].

We did not use intrapleural fibrinolytic agents before or after the intervention in our cases due to high cost of some drugs and unavailability of others in the country. But as compared to failure rate (29%) of a large trial [11] using streptokinase and tube thoracostomy, the failure rate of medical thoracoscopy was only 6.25% in our study, 9 patients had persistent air leak which needed further surgical interventions and there was one death due to urosepsis. The most common cause of exudative pleural effusion/empyema in Pakistan is tuberculosis. [12] This is consistent with our study where we found tuberculosis to be the culprit in 63.3% of the empyema patients.

In countries where tuberculosis is endemic, it is very important to differentiate between the two most common causes of exudative pleural effusion that are malignancy and tuberculosis, as their treatment and prognosis vary. It is a common practice in resource limited settings to start empiric anti-tuberculous therapy (ATT) in all patients with empyema, if the effusion fails to respond to regimen only then alternate diagnosis is considered. However, if malignant pleural effusion (MPE) is treated as tuberculosis it would not only become the source of unnecessary delay but also affects them with the adverse reaction of ATT [13]. YU Xiang et.al in their study conducted on 430 cases of tuberculous pleural effusion, confirmed that medical thoracoscopy is a safe and efficacious way of managing multiloculted and organized tuberculous pleural effusion [14]. It is reported in literature that in 26 to 54% of cases pleural thickening of 10 mm or more can cause symptoms in patients with tuberculous empyema [15]. So it is vital to re-expand the trapped lung and decrease residual pleural thickening.

Many terms have been used for rigid medical Thoracoscopy in literature, like video-assisted Thoracoscopy medical (VAT-M), non-intubated VATS, pleuroscopy (local anesthesia) or simply medical thoracoscopy. We have used the term medical Thoracoscopy in our article to avoid confusion with VATS as there is much debate between pulmonologists and thoracic surgeons on this subject.

One noteworthy feature of the approach to empyema is the liaison between pulmonologists and thoracic surgeons. These two specialties ought to share patients with clinical quandaries as pulmonologists need the surgical back-up and likewise thoracic surgeons would benefit from the availability of a keen clinician.

Conclusion

Medical thoracoscopy in early management of multiloculated pleural empyema is perhaps a valuable intervention in underdeveloped countries where facilities of thoracic surgery are scant. All lymphocytic predominant pleural effusions are not tuberculosis. Medical thoracoscopy is also beneficial in timely diagnosis of tuberculous empyema and discriminating it from pyogenic empyema in countries with high burden of tuberculosis.

This is case series on management of empyema by medical thoracoscopy and further prospective studies are needed on the long term follow up of the cases.

Abbreviations
ATT: Anti-tuberculous therapy; CT scan: Computed tomography scan; Fr: French unit; MHz: Mega hertz; MPE: Malignant pleural effusion; SPSS: Statistical analysis software package; VATS: Video-assissted thoracoscopic surgery

Acknowledgements
Not applicable.

Funding
None.

Authors' contributions
KKS: Designed, data acquisition, analysis and drafted the manuscript. NAR: Conceived, designed and drafted the manuscript. AA: Designed, analysed and reviewed the manuscript. KKS, NAR, AA gave final approval of the version to be published and agree to be accountable for all aspects of the work.All authors read and approved the final manuscript.

Competing interests
The authors declare that they have no competing interests.

Author details
[1]Department of Chest Medicine, Jinnah Postgraduate Medical Centre, Karachi 75400, Pakistan. [2]Department of Thoracic Surgery, Combined Military Hospital, Peshawar, Pakistan.

References
1. Yu H. Management of Pleural Effusion, empyema, and lung abscess. Semin Interv Radiol. 2011;28(1):75–86.
2. Ahmed AE, Yacoub TE. Empyema Thoracis. Clin Med Insights Circ Respir Pulm Med. 2010;4:1–8.
3. Light RW. Parapneumonic effusions and empyema. Proc Am Thorac Soc. 2006;3(1):75–80.
4. Brutsche MH, Tassi GF, Györik S, Gökcimen M, Renard C, Marchetti GP, Tschopp JM. Treatment of Sonographically stratified Multiloculated thoracic empyema by medical Thoracoscopy. Chest. 2005;128(5):3303–9.
5. Tassi G, Marchetti G, Pinelli V, Chiari S. Practical management of pleural empyema. Monaldi Arch Chest Dis. 2016;73(3):124–9.
6. Loddenkemper R, Mathur P, Lee P, Noppen M. History and clinical use of thoracoscopy/pleuroscopy in respiratory medicine. Breathe. 2011;8(2):144–55.
7. Shojaee S, Lee HJ. Thoracoscopy: medical versus surgical-in the management of pleural diseases. J Thorac Dis. 2015;7(4):339–51.
8. Tassi GF, Davies RJ, Noppen M. Advanced techniques in medical thoracoscopy. Eur Respir J. 2006;28(5):1051–9.
9. Cafiero F. Jacobaeus operation during parapneumothoracic empyema. Minerva Med. 1954;45(72):553–7.
10. Diacon AH, Brutsche MH, Solèr M. Accuracy of pleural puncture sites: a prospective comparison of clinical examination with ultrasound. Chest. 2003;123(2):436–41.
11. Kern L, Robert J, Brutsche M. Management of Parapneumonic Effusion and Empyema: medical Thoracoscopy and surgical approach. Respiration. 2011; 82(2):193–6.
12. Maskell NA, Davies CWH, Nunn AJ, Hedley EL, Gleeson FV, Miller R, Gabe R, Rees GL, Peto TEA, Woodhead MA, Lane DJ, Darbyshire JH, Davies RJO. U.K. controlled trial of Intrapleural streptokinase for pleural infection. N Engl J Med. 2005;352(9):865–74.
13. Rehan M, Alam MT, Aurangzeb M, Imran K, Farrukh SZ, Masroor M, Kumar P. The frequency of various diseases in patients presenting with pleural effusion. Gomal J Med Sci. 2013;11:78–83.
14. Maturu VN, Dhooria S, Bal A, Singh N, Aggarwal AN, Gupta D, Behera D, Agarwal R. Role of medical thoracoscopy and closed-blind pleural biopsy in undiagnosed exudative pleural effusions: a single-center experience of 348 patients. J Bronchology Interv Pulmonol. 2015;22(2):121–9.
15. Lai YF, Chao TY, Wang YH, et al. Pigtail drainage in the treatment of tuberculous pleural effusions: a randomised study. Thorax. 2003;58:149–51.

17

Degree of control of patients with chronic obstructive pulmonary disease in Spain: SINCON study

Adolfo Baloira[1]*[iD], José Miguel Rodriguez Gonzalez-Moro[2], Estefanía Sanjuán[3], Juan Antonio Trigueros[4] and Ricard Casamor[5]

Abstract

Background: Disease control is an important objective of COPD management. The SINCON study evaluated the level of control in terms of respiratory symptoms and exacerbations in Spanish patients with COPD for ≥2 years.

Methods: SINCON was a descriptive, cross-sectional, multicenter study that assessed degree of control using a combined index comprising COPD assessment test (CAT), modified Medical Research Council dyspnea scale (mMRC), and number of moderate/severe exacerbations in the last year. Based on this score, patients were categorized as "well controlled" or "poorly controlled". Degree of control was also assessed relative to patient phenotype, setting (primary care [PC] vs respiratory care [RC]), and impact of treatment on morning symptoms.

Results: Of the 481 patients (PC: 307, RC: 174) analyzed, COPD was poorly controlled in 63.2%. Some differences were found between clinical settings: PC patients were more poorly controlled (PC: 66.4% vs RC: 57.5%; $P = 0.06$) and had higher CAT score (PC: 17.9 vs RC: 15.5; $P < 0.05$), and higher rate of moderate/severe exacerbations during previous year (PC: 1.5 vs RC: 1.1; $P < 0.05$), while dyspnea degree was similar in both settings. Regarding phenotypes, non-exacerbators demonstrated better control vs exacerbators. Morning symptoms score improved between waking and 3 h after bronchodilator treatment ($P < 0.05$), with greater improvements in PC patients (PC: − 6.5 vs RC: − 5.0 points; $P < 0.05$).

Conclusions: Most COPD patients were poorly controlled with some differences observed between PC and RC settings and between patient phenotypes. Our index may be easily used in PC settings to optimize COPD treatment.

Keywords: COPD, Disease control, CAT, mMRC, Exacerbations

Background

Chronic obstructive pulmonary disease (COPD) is usually characterized as having a progressive clinical course, interrupted by more or less frequent exacerbations over time. The speed of lung function loss may vary greatly and seem mildly impacted by the available treatments, as observed in the UPLIFT study [1]. The key objectives of treatment are to decrease symptoms, improve quality of life (QoL) and prevent exacerbations and, therefore, the definition of control of the disease should include these clinical variables. COPD Assessment Test (CAT) is

a simple questionnaire developed to know how the disease affects the patient's life. CAT has been validated in different studies, being one the most important tools for the GOLD strategy [2–4]. Due to its simplicity, it can be easily used in the daily clinic. Dyspnea is possibly the most important symptom in patients with COPD. The modified Medical Research Council (mMRC) scale is an easy way to know the limitations that the patient presents due to dyspnea. It is included in the GOLD guidelines along with the CAT questionnaire, but both are not equivalent [5]. It is widely used in clinical trials and correlates with different clinical variables in COPD, being a better predictor of mortality than FEV1 [6]. In general, its use is recommended in the follow-up of patients.

* Correspondence: adolfo.baloira.villar@sergas.es
[1]Hospital de Montecelo, Mourente, s/n, 36071 Pontevedra, Spain

Bronchodilators are the cornerstone in the long-term treatment of stable COPD, as recognized in the various guidelines and recommendations [7], while inhaled corticosteroids (ICS) may also play a relevant role in certain patients [8]. Given the progressive nature of the disease, the therapeutic strategy should be a progressive combination of drugs, depending on clinical variables (symptoms, exacerbations, and lung function), but adequate measuring tools are not always well established. The objective should be to achieve a good degree of disease control. However, it is not easy to define control in a specific patient with a disease that is as variable in its clinical manifestations as COPD. The term "control" (well-controlled or poorly controlled patient) should refer to both the clinical situation at a certain time and the risk of worsening or death in the relatively near future [9]. Since COPD has various levels of severity, the patient's degree of control will be greatly influenced by the level of severity, since, unlike asthma, it is not possible to fully reverse bronchial obstruction or the underlying inflammation.

A key aspect of control is to define the clinical phenotype of the patient. Guía Española de la EPOC (GesEPOC) was the first guideline to classify COPD per clinical phenotypes and recommend treatments accordingly [10]. Exacerbations are a crucial aspect of COPD progression, and influence QoL, lung function loss and mortality risk [11, 12]. Several studies have shown a positive effect of different available treatments on reduction of exacerbations [13–15]. In light of the current knowledge, clinical guidelines have created simple therapeutic algorithms for easy application in clinical practice, which should allow for better control of patients with COPD. Using a British database, an international group tried different approaches to evaluate the control of patients, using either clinical aspects or the CAT questionnaire, with different thresholds. The results were different, as expected, depending on the criteria used, but in all cases, worse control was associated with a greater probability of having an exacerbation [16]. More recently, the same group has conducted a study with the aim to validate this concept of control. This study found that an exacerbation in the three previous months and a high score in questionnaires of dyspnea and quality of life were associated to classify the patient as poorly controlled [17].

There is little information on the degree of control of patients with COPD, applying easy-to-use indexes in daily clinical practice. The main objective of the SINCON study was to assess the degree of control of COPD patients in Spain, taking into account the symptoms and exacerbations, the most important variables associated with the concept of control according to available data. As secondary objectives, we assessed the degree of control related to patient phenotype or level of care (primary care [PC] physicians vs respiratory care [RC] specialists) and the impact of treatment on morning symptoms.

Methods

SINCON was a descriptive, cross-sectional, multicenter study with representation from all the Spanish geography. In order to obtain a representative sample of the Spanish population, the number of patients was limited to a maximum of 5 for each PC doctor and 10 in the case of RC. Obviously, PC could not include patients who were also followed by pulmonologists This study was conducted in accordance with the ICH Harmonised Tripartite Guidelines for Good Clinical Practice, with applicable local regulations (including the European Directive 2001/83/EC and U.S. Code of Federal Regulations Part 21), and with the ethical principles established in the Declaration of Helsinki. The study protocol, including de informed consent, was reviewed and approved by the Institutional Review Board of Complejo Hospitalario de Toledo (23 December 2014, protocol number 156). All patients signed the informed consent before being included in the study. To minimize screening bias, patients were recruited consecutively from among those who attended the outpatient clinic, met the inclusion and exclusion criteria, and signed the informed consent. Inclusion criteria were age > 40 years, COPD diagnosis for ≥2 years (post-bronchodilator forced expiratory volume in 1 s [FEV_1] < 80% of the theoretical value and FEV_1/forced vital capacity [FVC] ratio < 0.7 measured in scheduled visit), no exacerbations in the last 3 months, able to follow the study protocol and willing to sign the informed consent. Patients with symptomatic systemic diseases, respiratory conditions other than COPD, serious diseases with a life expectancy of < 1 year, or unable to respond to the questionnaires were excluded.

The primary objective of the study was to assess the degree of control of COPD. For this purpose, we created a combined index that included three variables: COPD Assessment Test (CAT), modified Medical Research Council dyspnea scale (mMRC) and number of moderate/severe exacerbations in the previous year. An exacerbation was considered as moderate when it required treatment with systemic corticosteroids and/or antibiotics and as severe when the patient visited a hospital, with emergency room stay of at least 12 h or hospital admission. The assignment of scores to each of these variables is described in Table 1. The degree of control was defined by the sum of scores, establishing the four groups: optimal control (0 points), suboptimal control (1 point), poor control (2 points), and very poor control (3 points). To better summarize the outcomes, patients with optimal or suboptimal control were considered

Table 1 Assignment of scores to individual clinical variables

Clinical Variable	Value	Score
mMRC	0,1	0
	2,3,4	1
CAT	< 10	0
	≥ 10	1
Exacerbations in the previous year	none or one with no hospitalization	0
	more than one or one with hospitalization	1

CAT COPD assessment test, *mMRC* modified Medical Research Council dyspnea scale

Table 2 Characteristics of patients

Characteristic	Evaluable COPD patients (N = 481)
Sex, male, n (%)	392 (81.5)
Age, years, mean (SD)	67.7 ± 10.0
Body mass index, kg/m^2	27.9 ± 4.6
FEV$_1$, % theoretical	59.4 ± 19.4
FEV$_1$/FVC ratio	0.6 ± 0.2
Current smokers, n (%)	179 (37.2)
Former smokers, n (%)	302 (62.8)
Tobacco exposure, pack-years	39.8 ± 22.4
Time since COPD diagnosis, years	9.3 ± 7.1

Data are presented as mean ± SD unless specified otherwise
COPD Chronic obstructive pulmonary disease, *FEV$_1$* forced expiratory volume in 1 s, *FVC* forced vital capacity, *SD* standard deviation

"well controlled" and patients with poor and very poor control were considered "poorly controlled".

In order to assess morning symptoms and the impact of treatment on these symptoms, a patient-reported outcome questionnaire previously validated was used [18]. Patients completed the first part when they woke up at home and the second part, 3 h after the administration of bronchodilator medication, at the doctor's office. The score for each part varied between 0 and 60; the higher the score, the higher the severity of the morning symptoms. The following variables were also included: age, sex, body mass index, smoking status, comorbidities, time since COPD diagnosis, phenotype as per GesEPOC guidelines (assessed by local investigator), lung function with post-bronchodilator spirometry, treatment for the last 3 months and history of exacerbations in the previous year. All data were collected in a single visit.

Statistical analysis
A sample size of 700 patients was calculated, which corresponded to 0.14% of the total COPD population diagnosed in Spain for a margin of error of ±3.70% [19]. Continuous variables were expressed as mean and 95% confidence interval (CI), and qualitative variables as absolute and relative frequency. Differences in the degree of control per phenotype were analyzed using the chi-square or Fisher's exact test depending on the sample. The significance level was set to $P < 0.05$.

Results
A total of 100 PC centers and 33 RC departments participated. Initially, 584 patients were enrolled; 103 patients were excluded as they did not satisfy inclusion/exclusion criteria or did not complete the information required. The analysis sample comprised 481 patients (18.5% female) with a mean (± SD) age of 67 (± 10) years (Table 2). Of the total patients analyzed, 307 and 174 patients were monitored in PC and RC settings, respectively. The mean (± SD) exposure to tobacco was 39.8 (± 22.4) pack-years and 62.8% of patients were former

smokers. The mean (± SD) time since COPD diagnosis to the visit was 9.3 (± 7.1) years. The mean (± SD) FEV$_1$ was 59% (± 19%) of the theoretical value, and the mean (± SD) FEV$_1$/FVC ratio was 0.58 (± 0.14). The majority of patients had dyspnea grade 2–4 (moderate-to-very severe) (Fig. 1), both in PC and RC settings. The mean CAT score was 17.0 (95% CI, 16.3–17.8), which was slightly lower in patients from RC departments (PC: 17.9 vs RC: 15.0; $P < 0.05$). A significant correlation was observed between FEV$_1$ and dyspnea grade ($P < 0.0001$) (Fig. 2), between dyspnea and CAT score ($P < 0.0001$) and between FEV$_1$ and CAT score ($P = 0.0133$) (Fig. 3).

In terms of exacerbations, 58.6% of patients had at least one moderate or severe exacerbation during the previous year (Table 3). PC patients showed a significantly higher frequency of moderate exacerbations per patient during the previous year, compared with RC patients (PC: 1.3 vs RC: 0.8; $P < 0.05$). The rate of severe

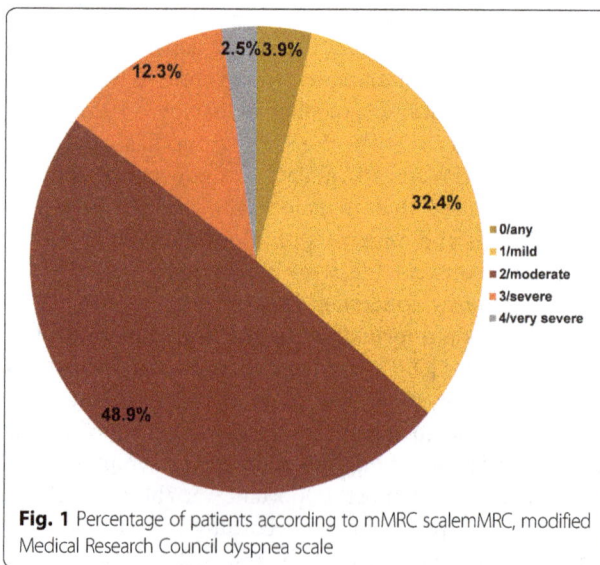

Fig. 1 Percentage of patients according to mMRC scalemMRC, modified Medical Research Council dyspnea scale

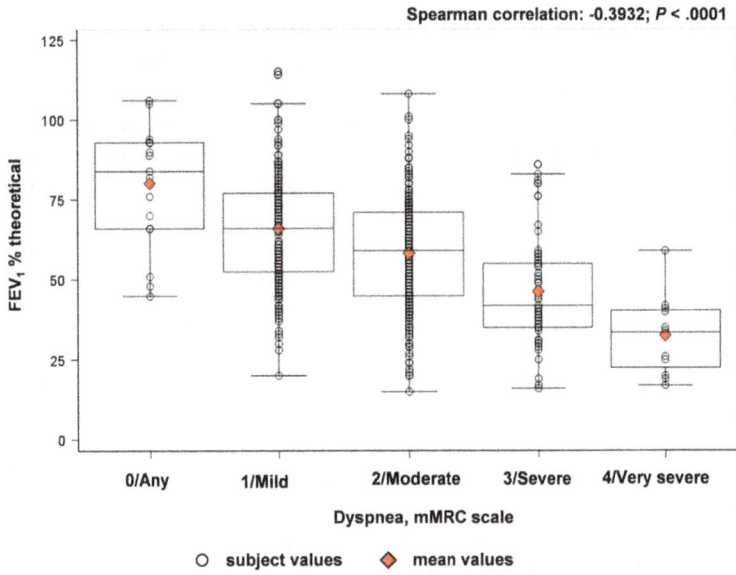

Fig. 2 Correlation between pulmonary function (FEV₁) and dyspneaFEV₁, forced expiratory volume in 1 s; mMRC, modified Medical Research Council dyspnea scale

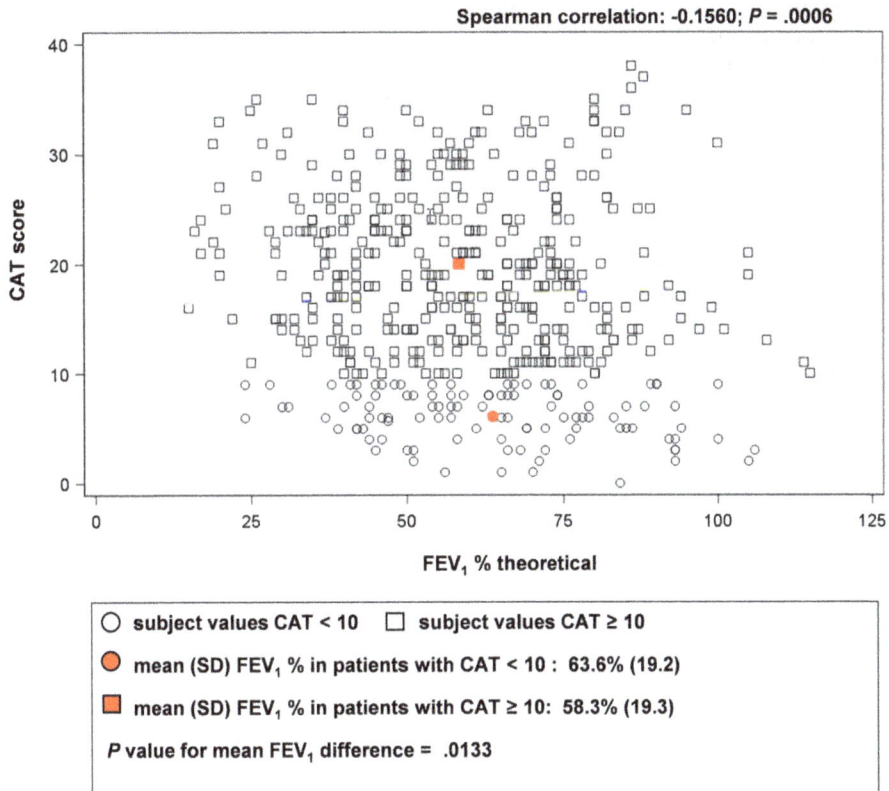

Fig. 3 Correlation between CAT and pulmonary function (FEV₁)CAT, COPD assessment test; FEV₁, forced expiratory volume in 1 s; SD, standard deviation

Table 3 Recorded Exacerbations in Previous Year

	PC (N = 307)	RC (N = 174)	Total (N = 481)
Moderate exacerbations, n (%)	188 (61.2%)	82 (47.1%)	270 (56.1%)
Rate[a], mean (95% CI)	1.3 (1.1–1.5)	0.8 (0.6–0.9)	1.1 (1.0–1.2)
Severe exacerbations, n (%)	39 (12.7%)	33 (18.9%)	72 (14.9%)
Rate[a], mean (95% CI)	0.2 (0.1–0.2)	0.3 (0.2–0.4)	0.2 (0.2–0.3)
Moderate/Severe exacerbations, n (%)	191 (62.2%)	91 (52.3%)	282 (58.6%)
Rate[a], mean (95% CI)	1.5 (1.3–1.7)	1.1 (0.8–1.3)	1.3 (1.2–1.5)

[a]events/patient/year
CI confidence interval, PC primary care, RC respiratory care

exacerbations was low, with a tendency to be more frequent in RC patients, although the difference did not achieve statistical significance (PC: 0.2 vs RC: 0.3; P = 0.91). Based on clinical phenotypes, 46% of patients were classified as non-exacerbators, 13.7% as exacerbators with emphysema, 28.3% as exacerbators with chronic bronchitis, and 10.6% as asthma-COPD overlap phenotype. In seven cases, the phenotype could not be established.

Analysis of the degree of control showed that 14 and 23% of patients achieved optimal and suboptimal control, respectively, with the remaining 63% of patients being poorly controlled, in accordance with the definition proposed (Table 4). A slightly higher proportion of patients in PC vs RC were poorly controlled, though this difference was not statistically significant (PC: 66.5% vs RC: 57.5%; P = 0.06). Significant differences were observed depending on clinical phenotype: non-exacerbating patients showed poor control in 41.6% of cases, while a higher percentage of exacerbating patients with chronic bronchitis (86.0%) and emphysema (87.9%) had poor control (non-exacerbating vs exacerbating; P < 0.0001). Patients in good control received more often dual bronchodilation than a long-acting β_2-agonist (LABA)/ICS combination (good control percentage of treatments, DBD: 72.5% vs LABA/ICS: 45.0%; P < 0.05). Patients with bad control were treated with ICS more frequently in RC than in PC (63,2% vs 31.5% respectively, P < 0.01).

Table 4 Degree of Control of COPD Patients

Degree	PC (N = 307)	RC (N = 174)	Total (N = 481)
0: Optimal, n (%)	32 (10.4)	33 (18.9)	65 (13.5)
1: Suboptimal, n (%)	71 (23.1)	41 (23.5)	112 (23.2)
2: Poor, n (%)	106 (34.5)	58 (33.3)	164 (34.1)
3: Very Poor, n (%)	98 (31.9)	42 (24.1)	140 (29.1)

COPD chronic obstructive pulmonary disease, PC primary care, RC respiratory care
Although there was a trend to a better degree of control in RC, the differences did not reach statistical significance

In terms of morning symptoms and changes after bronchodilator treatment (Table 5), the mean score in the patient-reported outcome questionnaire decreased significantly (indicating symptom improvement) between waking and the evaluation performed after 3 h at the clinic (mean improvement: – 6.5; 95% CI, – 7.1– – 4.1 points; P < 0.05). In patients from PC this improvement was – 7.3 (– 8.2– – 6.5) points, while in patients from RC it was – 5.0 (95% CI, – 5.9– – 4.1) points. This improvement occurred regardless of GOLD stage. Patients in stages B and D, most symptomatic, obviously had a worse score in the PRO questionnaire. Patients treated with LABA/LAMA showed a greater improvement than those treated with a LABA/ICS or with a long-acting muscarinic antagonist (LAMA) alone (LABA/LAMA: – 7.4; 95% CI, – 8.4– – 6.5 vs LABA/ICS: – 6.2; 95% CI, – 7.3– – 5.0 vs LAMA: – 5.5; 95% CI, – 6.4– – 4.6) but without reaching statistical significance (p = 0.06) (Table 6).

Discussion

The concept of control in a disease such as COPD is difficult to define and quantify, as there is usually a progressive lung function loss that seems to be only mildly modified by current treatments. In this study, we used three variables that constitute the central axis of the clinical manifestations of COPD: dyspnea, QoL and exacerbations. Considering the impact of these variables on patients, achieving optimal control seems to be a major challenge. Some factors that appear to influence the proportion of patients who achieve good control include phenotype, lung function and, to a lesser degree, the level of care in the setting where the patient is seen (PC vs RC).

Concept of control

In the absence of a well-established definition for COPD control, we developed and used an index that included some of the parameters most related to the impact of

Table 5 PRO questionnaire according to 2015 and 2017 GOLD stage

	GOLD	Patients N 475	Waking (SD)	3 h after treatment (SD)
GOLD 2015	A	57	6.61 (9.44)	4.21 (8,68)
	B	154	18.46 (12.81)	11.46 (9.83)
	C	25	5.84 (5.20)	3.34 (3.19)
	D	239	21.51 (13.37)	13.61 (10.25)
GOLD 20017	A	70	6.47 (8.73)	4.18 (7.91)
	B	225	18.27 (12.45)	11.56 (9.53)
	C	12	5.83 (5.92)	2.33 (3.36)
	D	168	23.05 (13.75)	14.52 (10.66)

Significant differences (p < 0.01) in all cases before and after treatment. There were no differences between GOLD 2015 and GOLD 2017

Table 6 PRO questionnaire according to treatment

Long-acting COPD treatment	Waking	3 h after treatment	Difference between both evaluations
LABA/LAMA	19.9 (18.8, 21.8)	12.3 (10.9,13.7)	−7.4 (− 8.4,-6.5)
LABA/ICS	18.0 (15.8, 20.1)	11.9 (10.1,13.6)	−6.2 (−7.3,-5.0)
LAMA	16.6 (14.7,18.5)	11.1 (9.6,12.7)	−5.5 (−6.4,-4.6)

All values mean (95% CI). Difference between LABA / LAMA and LAMA with a trend to statistical significance (p = 0.06)

the disease, based both on the symptoms perceived by the patient and on the prognosis. Lung function has traditionally been a key aspect in the management of COPD patients; however, it has some drawbacks.

1. The references used to measure the lung function allow some differences that, in many cases, exceed the efficacy outcomes obtained in clinical trials [20]
2. Lung function has significant intra-patient variations, thus an isolated value may be mildly significant
3. Even though there is a certain correlation between lung function and dyspnea or QoL, there is a significant dispersion of results
4. It has not yet been proven that the available drugs slow the loss of lung function. Therefore, it is difficult to justify lung function as a parameter when trying to assess the degree of control of COPD patients. It is obviously more difficult to achieve an adequate control in patients with severely impaired lung function than in those with mild obstruction. However, since the primary objective of the study was to obtain a global view of the degree of control in a set of patients from Spain, we chose not to include lung function in our index.

Quality of life and dyspnea: Do we have appropriate tools to measure them?

Quality of life and symptoms are two key aspects when designing a definition of control in patients with COPD. Due to their subjective nature, they are difficult to measure. The mMRC dyspnea scale and the CAT questionnaire are two semi-quantitative tools used in clinical trials and in clinical practice. They have proven to be effective in terms of prognosis and are sensitive to the effect of different drugs used in COPD treatment [21]. The Global Initiative for Chronic Obstructive Lung Disease (GOLD) strategy document recommends either of these tools to assess the patients' symptoms; however, these tools actually explore different aspects of the disease and their degree of consistency varies greatly [22]. CAT has an acceptable correlation with the GOLD classification [23]. It is difficult to determine a strict cut-off point to define a good/poor score, since in reality these scales or questionnaires are inaccurate in their limits and rather work as a continuum. Therefore, it seemed

appropriate to use both when creating an index to assess the patients' control. Good control was defined in our index considering the cut-off values that GOLD recommends to classify a low-symptom patient, both for the mMRC scale and the CAT questionnaire, but obviously this is debatable.

Controversial aspects in exacerbations

Exacerbations are another key aspect of COPD progression with a significant impact on the patient's QoL and prognosis. However, there are some issues related to exacerbations. They are not easy to define, and the classification of severity is mainly based on subjective criteria. Therefore, it is likely that the assessment of whether or not there is an exacerbation and the degree of severity are influenced by the investigator. Given the nature of our study, these limitations are impossible to avoid. Another aspect is that there are different types of exacerbations not adequately profiled. Even though all exacerbations affect patients in some way, we only included moderate/severe exacerbations in our index for degree of control, given the difficulty to properly diagnose mild exacerbations in a retrospective view. Most of the participating centers had an electronic medical record, which allowed having a reliable information.

Level of control

Our definition of good control included two groups: optimal and suboptimal. Taking into consideration the fact that the drugs available for COPD treatment do not normalize the clinical situation in a vast majority of patients, we deemed it more realistic and practical to declare "good control" when the values associated with poor prognosis or with high impact on QoL and symptoms were not present, i.e. when mMRC score was < 2, CAT score was < 10 and a maximum of one moderate exacerbation occurred in the previous year. Available evidence suggests that under these circumstances the patient is reasonably controlled, both in terms of symptoms and prognosis [21, 22]. The percentage of patients who reached this degree of good control in our study was 36%, indicating that approximately two-third of patients had a clinical situation that did not meet the minimal requirements. Small differences were observed between PC and RC settings.

Comparison of our results with previous studies

There are few publications with similar characteristics to our research. A recently conducted study from a database in the United Kingdom proposed three ways to measure the degree of control for a period of 3 months: stability, clinical symptoms or CAT score. Results varied depending on the method used and the level of severity established by the body mass index, airflow obstruction, dyspnea, and exacerbations index (BODEx), which did not achieve a wide acceptance in clinical practice. Among patients with mild/moderate severity (90% of the total), 21.5% were well controlled based on a CAT score < 10; however, only 4.5% were well controlled based on clinical criteria. In the severe/very severe group, none of the patients achieved an adequate control per clinical criteria, while 8.5% of patients achieved adequate control based on a CAT score < 20 [16]. This study is completely different from ours, both in its design and in its objectives. If patients are previously classified according to the degree of severity of the disease, which implies including some of the criteria used to estimate the degree of control, the results can be predicted in a certain way. The aim of our study was to have an overview of the degree of control of patients with COPD in Spain in a sample that was quantitatively representative of the entire geography. The other study, published more recently by the same group, used largely the same parameters that we defined in our study [17]. An interesting finding was that changing the cut-off point of severity in the BODEx index (5 to 3) the percentage of well-controlled patients did not vary significantly, which supports the use of a simple index such as the one we used in our study.

Our results, together with the above findings, reinforce the fact that we are far from obtaining satisfactory rates of good control in COPD patients, regardless of the method used to measure it.

Level of control PC vs RC

In our study, a slightly higher percentage of patients from RC were well-controlled compared to the PC setting, although no statistical significance was achieved. Even though the most severe patients are usually seen in RC settings, it is likely that other variables, including adherence to treatment, may have influenced this result. It is a field that should be explored in subsequent studies.

COPD phenotypes and level of control

Patients with exacerbating phenotype were observed to be more often poorly controlled, as was expected based on our definition of good control. Patients with asthma-COPD overlap phenotype showed a degree of control intermediate between exacerbators and non-exacerbators. This was expected as, though they are known to have some exacerbations, patients with this phenotype also show a good response to treatment with inhaled corticosteroids [24]. A limitation to this analysis comes from the fact that each investigator assigned their patients' phenotype, which may imply differences in criteria.

Level of control according to treatment

A better degree of control was observed in patients treated with DBD compared with patients treated with a LABA/ICS combination, with greater differences in the RC setting. Obviously, this information has limited value due to the observational nature of our study This finding is not surprising because different studies have shown that the combination of LAMA/LABA is in general the most effective treatment to control the symptoms. Regarding exacerbations, the evidence seems to indicate that the most potent combinations of long-acting bronchodilators outweigh the association of LABA/ICS [15]. Another interesting finding is that in PC 13% of patients with very poor control were treated with a LABA/ICS combination only, even though all the guidelines recommend using LAMA/LABA together with ICS if the patient is a frequent exacerbator. This did not happen in any patient in RC. It is clear that we are still far from using correctly the available treatments.

Effect of treatment on morning symptoms

Similar results were observed when evaluating the variations in morning symptoms. As expected, patients using a combination of two long-acting bronchodilators achieved a more intense improvement than with any other treatment; however, the clinical relevance of these findings needs to be confirmed in adequate studies. An interesting finding is that there was significant clinical improvement in all stages of GOLD, without differences when applying GOLD 2015 or GOLD 2017. Although this study is not designed for it, these data could support the early use of long-acting bronchodilators even in patients who perceive few symptoms.

Conclusions

To conclude, we created and tested a simple index to measure the level of control in COPD, built in accordance with the well-accepted guidelines. In our research we observed a very high percentage of COPD patients who do not achieve an adequate control of their disease. We found no significant differences between patients seen in PC and RC settings. The regular use of an index such as the one presented in this work may help improve the disease control and optimize the treatment, as it includes the most relevant variables related to the clinical situation and the risk for the patients. In addition, the index is easily usable in primary care clinics.

Abbreviations

BODEx: Body mass index, airways obstruction, dyspnea, exacerbations; CAT: COPD assessment test; CI: Confidence interval; COPD: Chronic obstructive pulmonary disease; DBD: Dual bronchodilation; FEV_1: Forced expiratory volume in 1 s; FVC: Forced vital capacity; GesEPOC: Guía Española de la EPOC; GOLD: Global Initiative for Chronic Obstructive Lung Disease; ICS: Inhaled corticosteroids; LABA: Long-acting β_2-agonist; LAMA: Long-acting muscarinic antagonist; mMRC: Modified Medical Research Council dyspnea scale; PC: Primary care; QoL: Quality of life; RC: Respiratory care; SD: Standard deviation

Acknowledgements
The authors thank all the investigators from both primary care and respiratory care clinics for their participation in the study.

Funding
The research was funded by Novartis Farmacutica SA, Barcelona, Spain. Novartis provided general funding for the study, including statistical analysis and medical writing for the first draft of the manuscript.

Prior abstract publication/presentations
Part of this article has been presented as abstracts at the Spanish Society of Pneumology and Thoracic Surgery Congress (SEPAR), June 2–5, 2017, Madrid, Spain and the European Respiratory Society Annual Congress (ERS), September 9–13, 2017, Milan, Italy.

Authors' contributions
ABV takes responsibility for the content of this article, including data and analysis. ABV, JMRG-M, ES, JAT, RC have contributed substantially to the design, conduct and analysis of the study. The manuscript draft was written and revised based on inputs from all the authors, who also provided their consent and approval for the final version and the submission of this manuscript.

Competing interests
AB has participated as a consultant in meetings sponsored by Novartis, Boehringer Ingelheim, GSK, Astra, Esteve Laboratories and TEVA and has received grants from GSK, Novartis, Boehringer Ingelheim and Esteve Laboratories. JMRG-M has received consultancy and speaker fees from Boehringer-Ingelheim, Novartis, Rovi and GSK. ES has received speaker fees from Chiesi, Novartis, Pfizer; consultancy fees from Novartis, Almirall, GSK, Orion; sponsorship to travel to scientific meetings from Chiesi, Teva, Rovi, Mundipharma and Boehringer. JAT has received consultancy and speaker fees from AstraZeneca, Boehringer Ingelheim, Teva, Menarini and Novartis. RC is a full time employee of Novartis Farmaceutica SA.

Author details
[1]Hospital de Montecelo, Mourente, s/n, 36071 Pontevedra, Spain. [2]Hospital Universitario Príncipe de Asturias, Alcalá de Henares, Madrid, Spain. [3]CAP María Bernades, Viladecans, Barcelona, Spain. [4]Centro de Salud Menasalbas, Toledo, Spain. [5]Novartis Farmacéutica S.A, Barcelona, Spain.

References
1. Tashkin DP, Celli B, Senn S, Burkhart D, Kesten S, Menjoqe S, et al. A 4-year trlal of tiotropium in chronic obstructive pulmonary disease. N Engl J Med. 2008;359(15):1543–54.
2. Jones PW, Tabberer M, Chen WH. Creating scenarios of the impact of COPD and their relationship to COPD assessment test (CAT™) scores. BMC Pulm Med. 2011;11:42.
3. Miravitlles M, García-Sidro P, Fernández-Nistal A, Buendía MJ, Espinosa de Los Monteros MJ, Esquinas C, et al. The chronic obstructive pulmonary disease assessment test improves the predictive value of previous exacerbations for poor outcomes in COPD. Int J Chron Obstruct Pulmon Dis. 2015;10:2571–9.
4. Gupta N, Pinto LM, Morogan A, Bourbeau J. The COPD assessment test: a systematic review. Eur Respir J. 2014;44(4):873–84.
5. Jones PW, Adamek L, Nadeau G, Banik N. Comparisons of health status scores with MRC grades in COPD: implications for the GOLD 2011 classification. Eur Respir J. 2013;42(3):647–54.
6. Nishimura K, Izumi T, Tsukino M, Oga T. Dyspnea is a better predictor of 5-year survival than airway obstruction in patients with COPD. Chest. 2002; 121(5):1434–40.
7. Miravitlles M, Soler-Cataluña JJ, Calle M, Molina J, Almagro P, Quintano JA, et al. Spanish guideline for COPD (GesEPOC). Updated 2014. Arch Bronconeumol. 2014;50(Suppl1):1 16.
8. Yang IA, Clarke MS, Sim EH, Fong KM. Inhaled corticosteroids for stable chronic obstructive pulmonary disease. Cochrane Database Syst Rev. 2012;7:CD002991.
9. Soler-Cataluña JJ, Alcázar Navarrete B, Miravitlles M. The concept of control of COPD in clinical practice. Int J Chron Obstruct Pulmon Dis. 2014;9:1397–405.
10. Miravitlles M, Soler-Cataluña JJ, Calle M, Molina J, Almagro P, Quintano JA, et al. Spanish COPD guidelines (GesEPOC): pharmacological treatment of stable COPD. Arch Bronconeumol. 2012;48(7):247–57.
11. Martin AL, Marvel J, Fahrbach K, Cadarette SM, Wilcox TK, Donohue JF. The association of lung function and St. George's respiratory questionnaire with exacerbations in COPD: a systematic literature review and regression analysis. Respir Res. 2016;17:40.
12. Soler-Cataluña JJ, Martínez-García MA, Román Sánchez P, Salcedo E, Navarro M, Ochando R. Severe acute exacerbations and mortality in patients with chronic obstructive pulmonary disease. Thorax. 2005;60(11):925–31.
13. Wedzicha JA, Calverley PM, Seemungal TA, Hagan G, Ansari Z, Stockley RA, et al. The prevention of chronic obstructive pulmonary disease exacerbations by salmeterol/fluticasone propionate or tiotropium bromide. Am J Respir Crit Care Med. 2008;177(1):19–26.
14. Anzueto A, Ferguson GT, Feldman G, Chinsky K, Seibert A, Emmett A, et al. Effect of fluticasone propionate/salmeterol (250/50) on COPD exacerbations and impact on patient outcomes. COPD. 2009;6(5):320–9.
15. Wedzicha JA, Banerji D, Chapman KR, Vestbo J, Roche N, Ayers RT, et al. Indacaterol-glycopyrronium versus salmeterol-fluticasone for COPD. N Engl J Med. 2016;374(23):2222–34.
16. Nibber A, Chisholm A, Soler-Cataluña JJ, Alcazar B, Price D, et al. Validating the concept of COPD control: a real-world cohort study from the United Kingdom. COPD. 2017;14:504–12.
17. Miravitlles M, Sliwinski P, Rhee CK, Costello RW, Carter V, Tan J, et al. Evaluation of criteria for clinical control in a prospective, international, multicenter study of patients with COPD. Respir Med. 2018;136:8–14. https://doi.org/10.1016/j.rmed.2018.01.019 Epub 2018 Jan 31.
18. Kulich K, Keininger DL, Tiplady B, Banerji D. Symptoms and impact of COPD assessed by an electronic diary in patients with moderate-to-severe COPD: psychometric results from the SHINE study. Int J Chron Obstruct Pulmon Dis. 2015;10:79–94.
19. Encuesta Nacional de Salud 2011/2012. Available from: https://www.msssi. gob.es/estadEstudios/estadisticas/encuestaNacional/encuestaNac2011/ informesMonograficos/Act_fis_desc_ocio.4.pdf
20. García-Río F, Calle M, Burgos F, Casan P, Del Campo F, Galdiz JB, et al. Spirometry. Spanish Society of Pulmonology and Thoracic Surgery (SEPAR) Arch Bronconeumol. 2013;49(9):388–401.
21. Casanova C, Marin JM, Martinez-Gonzalez C, de Lucas-Ramos P, Mir-Viladrich I, Cosio B, et al. Differential effect of modified Medical Research Council dyspnea, COPD assessment test, and clinical COPD questionnaire for symptoms evaluation within the new GOLD staging and mortality in COPD. Chest. 2015;148(1):159 68.
22. Karloh M, Fleig Mayer A, Maurici R, Pizzichini MM, Jones PW, Pizzichini E. The COPD assessment test: what do we know so far?: a systematic review and meta-analysis about clinical outcomes prediction and classification of patients into GOLD stages. Chest. 2016;149(2):413–25.
23. Lopez-Campos JL, Fernandez-Villar A, Calero-Acuña C, Represas-Represas C, Lopez-Ramírez C, Fernández VL, et al. Evaluation of the COPD assessment test and GOLD patient types: a cross-sectional analysis. Int J Chron Obstruct Pulmon Dis. 2015;10:975–84.
24. Ekerljung L, Mincheva R, Hagstad S, Bjerg A, Telg G, Stratelis G, et al. Prevalence, clinical characteristics and morbidity of the asthma-COPD overlap in a general population sample. J Asthma. 2017;55:1–9.

18

National survey: current prevalence and characteristics of home mechanical ventilation in Hungary

Luca Valko*[iD], Szabolcs Baglyas, Janos Gal and Andras Lorx

Abstract

Background: Home mechanical ventilation is an established treatment for chronic respiratory failure resulting in improved survival and quality of life. Technological advancement, evolving health care reimbursement systems and newly implemented national guidelines result in increased utilization worldwide. Prevalence shows great geographical variations and data on East-Central European practice has been scarce to date. The aim of the current study was to evaluate prevalence and characteristics of home mechanical ventilation in Hungary.

Methods: We conducted a nationwide study using an online survey focusing on patients receiving ventilatory support at home. The survey focused on characterization of the site (affiliation, type), experience with home mechanical ventilation, number of patients treated, indication for home mechanical ventilation (disease type), description of home mechanical ventilation (invasive/noninvasive, ventilation hours, duration of ventilation) and description of the care provided (type of follow up visits, hospitalization need, reimbursement).

Results: Our survey uncovered a total of 384 patients amounting to a prevalence of 3.9/100,000 in Hungary. 10.4% of patients received invasive, while 89.6% received noninvasive ventilation. The most frequent diagnosis was central hypopnea syndromes (60%), while pulmonary (20%), neuromuscular (11%) and chest wall disorders (7%) were less frequent indications. Daily ventilation need was less than 8 h in 74.2%, between 8 and 16 h in 15.4% and more than 16 h in 10.4% of patients reported. When comparing sites with a limited (< 50 patients) versus substantial (> 50 patients) case number, we found the former had significantly higher ratio of neuromuscular conditions, were more likely to ventilate invasively, with more than 16 h/day ventilation need and were more likely to provide home visits and readmit patients ($p < 0,001$).

Conclusions: Our results show a reasonable current estimate and characterization of home mechanical ventilation practice in Hungary. Although a growing practice can be assumed, current prevalence is still markedly reduced compared to international data reported, the duality of current data hinting to a possible gap in diagnosis and care for more dependent patients. This points to the importance of establishing home mechanical ventilation centers, where increased experience will enable state of the art care to more dependent patients as well, increasing overall prevalence.

Keywords: Home mechanical ventilation, Chronic respiratory failure, Home care

* Correspondence: valko.luca@med.semmelweis-univ.hu
Department of Anesthesiology and Intensive Therapy, Semmelweis University, 1082 Üllői út 78B, Budapest, Hungary

Background

Home mechanical ventilation (HMV) is an established mode of treatment in patients with chronic respiratory failure, resulting in increased survival in several different patient groups [1–3] as well as improved quality of life and reduced hospitalization rates [4]. Use of HMV differs greatly in different parts of the world, with prevalence ranging from 2.9/100,000 in Hong Kong [5], 10.5 in Sweden [6], to 9.9–12.0 in Australia and New Zealand [7] and 12.9 in Canada [8]. The most comprehensive survey of HMV practice to date has been the Eurovent survey, although the survey mainly focused on western- and central European centers and showed a markedly reduced rate of use in the one East-Central European country reviewed (0.1 versus 6.6 overall prevalence) [9].

Since the Eurovent survey, use of this technique has been more widespread, aided by better health care reimbursement systems, improving technological supply and other advancements such as telemonitoring [10]. Many countries have created national registries, implemented national guidelines and established large HMV centers [6]. New indications have been gaining ground, with obesity hypoventilation syndrome and chronic obstructive pulmonary disease supplying an increased demand for long term mechanical ventilation [5, 7, 11].

As a result of this, current prevalence of HMV is expected to be greater than those described in the Eurovent study, even in the countries where the practice was not widespread in the last decade and organization is still lacking compared to the aforementioned nations. Poland, the only country representing the East-Central European region in the Eurovent survey reported an astonishing 116-fold increase in the number of patients treated from 2000 to 2010, with diversifying indication groups and increased prevalence of the use of noninvasive interfaces [12].

There has been no published data on HMV in Hungary, although the practice has been established since the 1990's and has been increasingly used in recent years with the emergence of noninvasive respiratory units and increased use of noninvasive ventilation [13]. Extrapolation from the overall European prevalence of HMV from the Eurovent study would estimate about 650 patients in Hungary, not accounting for further possible increase by evolving indication guidelines, better diagnostics and improved patient recruitment.

National guidelines for HMV in the pediatric population have recently been published [14], likely improving diagnostics and care for these patients. The current Hungarian medical reimbursement system permits HMV for patients approved by the Committee of College of Health, but there are currently no assigned HMV centers.

The aim of the current study was to evaluate prevalence of home mechanical ventilation in Hungary and describe its characteristics to better aid future development of home mechanical ventilation practice in the country.

Methods

We conducted a nationwide study in Hungary using an online survey focusing on patients receiving ventilatory support through a bilevel pressure or volume device with or without internal batteries at home under the care of a prescribing physician. Representatives of intensive care units, pulmonology centers and pediatric centers were invited to participate in the survey. Questions of the survey included characterization of the site (type of unit, yearly patient number), experience with home mechanical ventilation, number of patients treated, indication for home mechanical ventilation (disease type), description of home mechanical ventilation (invasive/noninvasive, ventilation hours, duration of ventilation) and description of the care provided (type of follow up visits, hospitalization need, reimbursement).

The study was approved by the research ethics board of Semmelweis University. Participation was voluntary and consent was implied by response to the survey. Surveys were sent out via email to all identified sites, followed by an email reminder and a telephone reminder. Survey responses were collected from March 2018 to July 2018 via an online survey program (Google Forms, Google LLC, Mountain View, United States). Sites not submitting an answer by the end of the study period were recontacted through telephone and were asked to identify the reason for non-responder status as A ("missed deadline or did not wish to submit data") or B ("had no relevant information to share"). Returned surveys were analyzed anonymously. Data was summarized for all sites. Data are presented as median (interquartile range) for continuous and as percentages for categorical values. Relationships between sites and therapy characteristics were analyzed by Chi-squared test. Analyses were conducted using Sigma-Plot 12 (Systat Software, San Jose, United States). 2018 Hungarian population data was obtained from the Hungarian Central Statistical Office [15].

Results

Comprehensive results of the survey are provided as Additional file 1.

Survey response rate

Overall 117 potential sites were contacted to participate in the survey. Initial response rate was 33.3% (39 sites). Telephone recontact of the sites after the initial study period showed that 91% (71) of the initially non-responder sites had no relevant information to share, while 9% (7 sites) missed the initial deadline or did not wish to participate in the survey. 47.2% (17) of sites that responded reported to actively oversee home mechanical patients, while 25% (9) provide care if needed, 13.9% (5) direct patients to other sites with more established practice. 11.1% (4) sites reported no need for HMV in any of their practice, while 11.1% (4) reported a need with inability to provide HMV. Out of the sites that responded, 72.2% (26) was aware of a HMV center, while 28.8% (10) was not. A HMV protocol was used in only 19.4% (7) sites.

Prevalence

Overall, the 17 sites reported 384 patients receiving home mechanical ventilation, corresponding to an overall prevalence of 3.9/100.000 for home mechanical ventilation in Hungary. When looking at number of patients treated by sites, we found that 93.2% of patients were treated by four sites that had a patient number of > 50. When comparing sites with substantial case number (> 50 patients) to sites with limited case number (< 50 patients), we found that sites with a substantial case number had a significantly higher patient number (87.5(58.5;122.5) vs. 1(1;2.75); $p = 0.002$) and were more likely to be pulmonology affiliated (75% versus 0%, $p = 0.003$). Sites with a limited patient number were more likely to be intensive care unit affiliated (84.6% vs. 25%, $p = 0.003$) Table 1.

Mode of ventilation

Out of the 384 patients, 10.4% (40) received invasive, while 89.6% (344) received noninvasive ventilation. Noninvasive ventilation was used more commonly by sites with substantial case number (95.6% vs. 7.7%, $p = 0.001$), whereas invasive ventilation was the predominant mode in sites with limited case number (92.3% vs. 4.5%, $p < 0.001$) (Fig. 1).

Indication for home mechanical ventilation

Possible indications for home mechanical ventilation need were identified as the following: central hypopnea syndromes (central alveolar hypoventilation syndrome, obesity hypoventilation syndrome); pulmonary diseases (chronic obstructive pulmonary disease, fibrosis); neuromuscular diseases (amyotrophic lateral sclerosis, systemic muscular atrophies, myasthenia, trauma related paralysis) and chest wall disorders (scoliosis, etc.) Fig. 2.

When observing the indications for sites with a substantial versus limited case number we found that most common diagnosis was central hypopnea in sites with substantial case number (62.3%) whereas neurological

Table 1 Distribution of responding sites involved in HMV

	Intensive care unit affiliated	Pulmonology affiliated	Pediatric affiliated
Number of responding sites involved in HMV	12	3	2
Number of patients treated	70	306	8

disease was the most frequent indication in sites with a limited case number (80%) ($p < 0.001$).

Characteristics of home mechanical ventilation

Daily ventilation need was less than 8 h in 74.2%, between 8 and 16 h in 15.4% and more than 16 h in 10.4% of patients reported to be receiving HMV. We found that increased hours of ventilation (> 16 h/day) was more common in patients treated by a site with limited case number (80% vs. 5.6%, $p < 0.001$).

Duration of home mechanical ventilation was less than 6 months in 3.6%, 6–12 months in 9.5%, 1–5 years in 50.1%, 5–10 years in 32% and more than 10 years in 4,7% of patients reported. Distribution of duration of ventilation did not differ significantly in sites with larger versus sites with limited case number ($p = 0,111$), although there was a trend that showed a longer duration with patients treated in sites with limited experience.

Characteristics of care provided

Follow up of patients treated with home mechanical ventilation was provided during home visits in 13.4% of cases reported, while ambulatory follow up was provided in 86.6% of cases. Home visits were more frequent at sites with limited case number compared to sites with a substantial case number (96.2% vs. 7.2%, $p < 0.001$).

Readmission rates were low overall in reported cases, with readmission needed more than twice a year in 12.6%, once a year in 4.2% and less rarely than once a year in 4.8% of reported cases. 78.4% of reported cases had no reported readmissions. When comparing sites with limited and substantial case numbers, readmission was more frequent in the former (82.9% vs. 15%, $p < 0.001$).

88.2% of sites treating home mechanical ventilation patients reported using additional devices to aid secretion elimination. Since most sites were ones treating a limited number of invasively ventilated patients, the most common reported secretion elimination method was endotracheal suction provided by 76.5% of sites, while a cough assisting device (11.8%) or both methods (11.8%) were reported to be provided by less sites (11.8 and 11.8% respectively). Notedly, cough assisting devices were only used by sites with substantial experience.

Reimbursement for HMV was either daily government reimbursement (26.4%) or initial government aid (73.5%) provided in most reported cases. Daily government reimbursement was used more frequently by sites with limited case number versus those with substantial case number (92.3% vs. 32.3%, $p < 0.001$).

Discussion

The present study is the first comprehensive data on the use of home mechanical ventilation in Hungary. The results of our current survey show an overall prevalence of

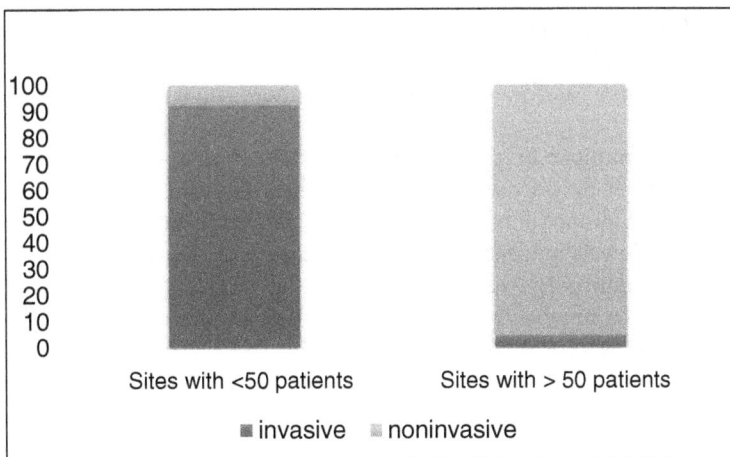

Fig. 1 Distribution of mode of ventilation. Y axis shows percentage of patients. First column shows data from sites that care for less than 50 patients, the second column shows data from units that care for more than 50 patients. Dark shading shows patients ventilated invasively, lighter shading shows patients ventilated noninvasively.

3.9/100,000 in Hungary, with noninvasive ventilation as the most common mode of ventilation and most reported cases initiated in the last 5 years, proving the fact that HMV in Hungary has been an increasing practice in recent years. Still, the current prevalence is markedly lower than other parts of the world and even the overall prevalence of HMV in Europe identified by the Eurovent survey in 2003.

As there is no established registry for HMV and currently no assigned centers are in operation, we aimed to contact all sites possibly managing patients with failed weaning situations (intensive care units) or chronic respiratory failure patients and complex sleep related breathing disorders (pulmonology and pediatric centers). The low initial response rate of the sites contacted were thought to be indicative of the practice of home

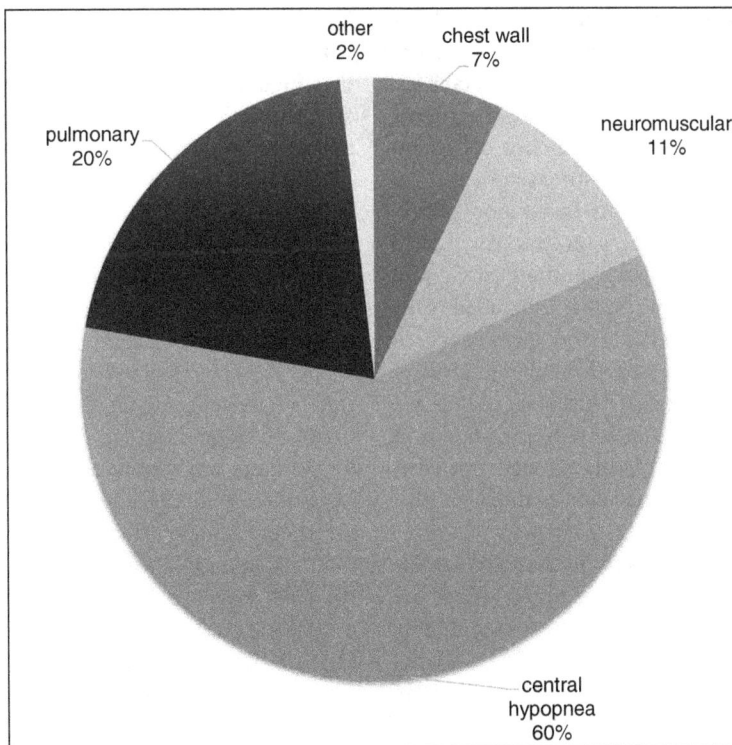

Fig. 2 Pie chart of prevalence of indications for home mechanical ventilation

mechanical ventilation being limited to a number of sites in the country. This was verified by repeated phone contact of the non-responder sites, as 91% of nonresponding sites cited "no relevant data to share" as the reason for not completing the form.

The validity of the uncovered number of patients is further supported by reimbursement data acquired from the Hungarian National Health Insurance Fund as well as mechanical ventilator distribution data acquired from the top three distributors in the country (personal communication). As per the HNHIF, the number of patients who received active daily reimbursement for home mechanical ventilation was 97 for the month of February 2018, while an additional 102 patients were estimated to be alive who received initial government aid during the past 10 years and were not transferred to active daily reimbursement (data acquired through personal correspondence). This reimbursement data approximates a total of 199 patients receiving home mechanical ventilation in Hungary, but does not account for patients acquiring ventilators through alternative financing.

Distributor data identified a total of 244 ventilators purchased in the 10 years preceding the study period, not accounting for other potential distributors or ventilators acquired from abroad. These two alternative sources of data both provide a similar, albeit lower number of patients compared to the number uncovered by our survey, pointing to the fact that some of the patients reported in our cohort might not meet the criteria for home mechanical ventilation but rather a sleep aid device for sleep apnea, which is regarded as a different group in both reimbursement and distribution databases. Overall, this data corroborates the number of patients uncovered by our survey. More precise data collection would be possible with a national registry system.

Previous data published shows an increasing prevalence of HMV in many countries across the world [6, 11, 12, 16–18], but data is scarce on the East-Central European region. The Eurovent survey included only Poland from this region, showing a low prevalence of HMV, with patients usually treated through an invasive interface and because of a neuromuscular indication. Since then, Poland showed a remarkable improvement in patient recruitment and quality of care as well as prevalence of HMV, aided by newly established national recommendations [19].

Current practice in Hungary is still limited and can be described as two toned: intensive care units taking the burden of acutely admitted decompensated, highly ventilator dependent chronic respiratory failure patients and newly established noninvasive ventilation centers equipped with sleep labs prescribing therapy to less ventilator dependent patients but without regulated follow up. Our current results prove this duality, as the small number of sites with substantial patient numbers were significantly more likely to be pulmonology affiliated than the sites with limited patient numbers, as these were more likely to be intensive care unit affiliated.

Out of the 17 sites providing care for patients in need of home mechanical ventilation, only 4 had a patient number of more than 50 and only one unit provided care for both invasively and noninvasively ventilated patients with home visits as standard follow up care, meeting the theoretical criteria for home mechanical ventilation centers.

The relatively high ratio (89.6%) of patients receiving HMV through a noninvasive interface, is similar to recent prevalence data published from around the world [7, 8, 12], although noninvasive ventilation for home use seems to be limited to a small number of sites in Hungary.

When examining indications for HMV in Hungary, the most frequent diagnosis was central hypopnea syndromes (60%), whereas pulmonary (20%), neurological (11%) and chest wall disorder (7%) was a less frequent indication. The relative high percentage of central hypopnea cases might be due to the increased awareness of complicated sleep apnea and obesity hypoventilation syndromes and it is in par with recent data from England [20] as well as Australia and New Zealand [7].

Ventilator dependence was examined in our survey. Reported cases received ventilation mostly in less than 8 h per day, which points to the Hungarian HMV population being less ventilator dependent. Those cases with increased daily ventilation need were reported by sites with a limited case number, proving our initial theory that high ventilator dependent patients are usually initiated through an intensive care unit due to acute decompensation of chronic respiratory failure.

Quality of care of HMV patients depends on follow up visits, airway clearance methods and can be accurately described by the frequency of hospital readmissions. Our current survey on Hungarian home mechanically ventilated patients shows infrequent hospital readmission need with follow ups provided by mostly ambulatory visits. Airway clearance techniques utilized were less state of the art, mostly done by deep suctioning in patients receiving invasive mechanical ventilation, supplied by the large number of sites caring for a limited number of invasively ventilated patients. Only 23.6% of sites provided cough assisting devices for patients if needed, despite recommendations for their use in patients with reduced peak cough flows [21].

Reimbursement for home mechanical ventilation in Hungary has been reformed in 2013, with eligible patients receiving a daily funding supplied to the treatment site. Spending of funds, including choice of ventilator type, interface type and additional airway clearance devices is left to the discretion of the physician in charge of treatment, permitting a personalized treatment plan tailored to the need of the specific patient. Before 2013, government funding was available only as an initial aid in helping to obtain equipment for home mechanical ventilation often resulting in patients needing to take part in reimbursement or servicing of their equipment. Our current survey results show that despite a newer, more flexible reimbursement, the most frequently used reimbursement was still initial government aid used in 73.5% of reported cases.

When comparing sites with a limited versus larger case number, we found a clear difference. Sites caring for a limited number of patients usually managed 1 to 7 patients, were more likely to treat patients with neuromuscular indications through invasive mode, with patients requiring more than 16 h/day ventilation, home visits and more frequent readmissions. This data points to a possible gap in home mechanical ventilation provision, as patients that are more ventilator dependent but might be managed with noninvasive ventilation seem to be missing from current practice, despite recent data proving that even highly dependent, previously tracheostomized patients might be managed with continuous noninvasive ventilation [22].

The reasons for this missing group of patients can be as follows: lack of diagnosis or untimely diagnosis, misdiagnosis of patients with chronic respiratory failure and insufficient quality of care.

Lack of diagnosis or untimely diagnosis is especially prominent for patients with neuromuscular diseases, restrictive chest wall diseases and chronic obstructive pulmonary disease, when late diagnosis often results in acute hospitalization, at which point initiation of home mechanical ventilation is more difficult and results in a worse outcome [23]. Misdiagnosis of patients with chronic respiratory failure usually affects central hypoventilation syndrome patients, as these conditions are often misdiagnosed as chronic right heart failure or as simple obstructive sleep apnea, when patients only receive oxygen therapy or CPAP therapy. Our current study did not include sleep labs, nor focused on patients prescribed only long-term oxygen therapy or CPAP machines as ventilatory support, although in some of these patients HMV might be indicated with more precise work up. This points to the importance of the implementation of national guidelines on the subject. Lastly, even with timely and adequate diagnosis, insufficient care and follow up can result in worsened outcome for patients with HMV, resulting in seemingly diminished prevalence. According to our study in Hungary, so far only one established center exists that provides > 16 h/day ventilation through a noninvasive interface for the majority of its patients, state of the art secretion management devices and has a steadily growing patient number since its establishment in 2014 at Semmelweis University (data shown in supplements).

These described reasons are the most likely explanation for the still reduced prevalence of home mechanical ventilation in Hungary compared to other countries. Attempts to better identify and recruit these patients for HMV rest on establishing a system with a nationally approved adult HMV guideline, at least one center with sufficient diagnostic and follow up infrastructure and a national registry to follow care of patients already under treatment, all of which are currently evolving projects at Semmelweis University.

The main limitation of our current study is that data collection was done through a voluntary basis, possibly leading to some misidentified and some not identified cases. Overall response rate was quite low, which can be explained by the wide range of sites contacted in order to identify sites with limited patient number and experience. Another limitation of the study is that survey identification of patients and treatment characteristics is less reliable, although most published prevalence data are based on surveys conducted with similar methodology.

Conclusion

In conclusion, our results, despite a low response rate of the survey, are the first in the country to describe current practice and based on the limited patient numbers of most responding sites, show a reasonable current estimate and characterization of home mechanical ventilation in Hungary. Although a growing practice can be assumed, current prevalence of home mechanical ventilation is still markedly reduced compared to international data reported. Our results show that currently sites with large case numbers are mainly focused on noninvasive ventilation for less ventilator dependent cases, whereas invasive interfaces are used for dependent patients with mostly neuromuscular diseases, pointing to a possible gap in diagnosis and care for more dependent patients. This points to the importance of establishing home mechanical ventilation centers, where increased experience will enable state of the art care to more dependent patients as well, increasing overall prevalence.

Abbreviations

CPAP: Continuous positive airway pressure; HMV: Home mechanical ventilation; HNHIF: Hungarian National Health Insurance Fund

Acknowledgements

Borbala Kozma contributed to word processing.

Funding

No external funding was utilized during this study.

Authors' contributions
LV, SB and AL designed the survey, summarized responses, analyzed and interpreted the data. LV, AL and JG contributed to the writing of the manuscript. All authors read and approved the final manuscript.

Authors' information
JG is the head of the Department of Anesthesiology and Intensive Therapy at Semmelweis University, overseeing the Semmelweis University Home Mechanical Ventilation Program, headed by AL. LV and SB have been involved with the Program since its establishment in 2014.

Competing interests
The authors declare that they have no competing interests.

References
1. Hodgson LE, Murphy PB. Update on clinical trials in home mechanical ventilation. J Thor Dis. 2016;8:255–67.
2. van den Bergen JC, Ginjaar HB, van Essen AJ, Pangalila R, de Groot IJ, Wijkstra PJ, et al. Forty-five years of Duchenne muscular dystrophy in the Netherlands. J Neuromusc Dis. 2014;1:99–109.
3. Kohnlein T, Windisch W, Kohler D, Drabik A, Geiseler J, Hartl S, et al. Non-invasive positive pressure ventilation for the treatment of severe stable chronic obstructive pulmonary disease: a prospective, multicentre, randomised, controlled clinical trial. Lancet Respir Med. 2014;2:698–705.
4. MacIntyre EJ, Asadi L, McKim DA, Bagshaw SM. Clinical outcomes associated with home mechanical ventilation: a systematic review. Can Respir J. 2016; 2016:6547180.
5. Chu CM, Yu WC, Tam CM, Lam CW, Hui DS, Lai CK. Home mechanical ventilation in Hong Kong. Eur Respir J. 2004;23:136–41.
6. Laub M, Berg S, Midgren B. Home mechanical ventilation in Sweden--inequalities within a homogenous health care system. Respir Med. 2004; 98:38–42.
7. Garner DJ, Berlowitz DJ, Douglas J, Harkness N, Howard M, McArdle N, et al. Home mechanical ventilation in Australia and New Zealand. Eur Respir J. 2013;41:39–45.
8. Rose L, McKim DA, Katz SL, Leasa D, Nonoyama M, Pedersen C, et al. Home mechanical ventilation in Canada: a national survey. Respir Care. 2015;60:695–704.
9. Lloyd-Owen SJ, Donaldson GC, Ambrosino N, Escarabill J, Farre R, Fauroux B, et al. Patterns of home mechanical ventilation use in Europe: results from the Eurovent survey. Eur Resp J. 2005;25:1025–31.
10. Ambrosino N, Vitacca M, Dreher M, Isetta V, Montserrat JM, Tonia T, et al. Tele-monitoring of ventilator-dependent patients: a European Respiratory Society statement. Eur Respir J. 2016;48:648–63.
11. Janssens JP, Derivaz S, Breitenstein E, De Muralt B, Fitting JW, Chevrolet JC, Rochat T. Changing patterns in long-term noninvasive ventilation: a 7-year prospective study in the Geneva Lake area. Chest. 2003;123:67–79.
12. Nasilowski J, Wachulski M, Trznadel W, Andrzejewski W, Migdal M, Drozd W, et al. The evolution of home mechanical ventilation in Poland between 2000 and 2010. Respir Care. 2015;60:577–85.
13. Lorx A, Bartusek D, Losonczy G, Gal J. Non-invasive respiratory unit in the Hungarian health care system. Orv Hetil. 2012;153:918–21.
14. National Health Guidelines. Home noninvasive and invasive mechanical ventilation for children. Egészségügyi Közlöny. 2017; EüK 3.
15. Hungarian Central Statistical Office. https://www.ksh.hu/docs/hun/xstadat/xstadat_eves/i_wnt001b.html. Accessed on 20 July 2018.
16. Tan GP, McArdle N, Dhaliwal SS, Douglas J, Rea CS, Singh B. Patterns of use, survival and prognostic factors in patients receiving home mechanical ventilation in Western Australia: a single Centre historical cohort study. Chron Respir Dis. 2018;15(4):356–64.
17. Povitz M, Rose L, Shariff SZ, Leonard S, Welk B, Jenkyn KB, et al. Home mechanical ventilation: a 12-year population-based retrospective cohort study. Respir Care. 2018;63:380–7.
18. Goodwin S, Smith H, Langton Hewer S, Fleming P, Henderson AJ, Hilliard T, Fraser J. Increasing prevalence of domiciliary ventilation: changes in service demand and provision in the south west of the UK. Eur J Pediatr. 2011;170:1187–92.
19. Nasilowski J, Szkulmowski Z, Migdal M, Andrzejewski W, Drozd W, Czajkowska-Malinowska M, et al. Prevalence of home mechanical ventilation in Poland. Pneumonol Alergol Pol. 2010;78:392–8.
20. Mandal S, Suh E, Davies M, Smith I, Maher TM, Elliott MW, et al. Provision of home mechanical ventilation and sleep services for England survey. Thorax. 2013;68:880–1.
21. McKim DA, Road J, Avendano M, Abdool S, Cote F, Duguid N, et al. Home mechanical ventilation: a Canadian thoracic society clinical practice guideline. Can Respir J. 2011;18:197–215.
22. Bach JR, Goncalves MR, Hamdani I, Winck JC. Extubation of patients with neuromuscular weakness: a new management paradigm. Chest. 2010;137:1033–9.
23. Duiverman ML, Bladder G, Meinesz AF, Wijkstra PJ. Home mechanical ventilatory support in patients with restrictive ventilatory disorders: a 48-year experience. Respir Med. 2006;100:56–65.

19

Efficacy of 1, 5, and 20 mg oral sildenafil in the treatment of adults with pulmonary arterial hypertension

Carmine Dario Vizza[1*], B. K. S. Sastry[2], Zeenat Safdar[3], Lutz Harnisch[4], Xiang Gao[5], Min Zhang[6], Manisha Lamba[5] and Zhi-Cheng Jing[7]

Abstract

Background: In a previous study, 6-minute walk distance (6MWD) improvement with sildenafil was not dose dependent at the 3 doses tested (20, 40, and 80 mg 3 times daily [TID]). This study assessed whether lower doses were less effective than the approved 20-mg TID dosage.

Methods: Treatment-naive patients with pulmonary arterial hypertension were randomized to 12 weeks of double-blind sildenafil 1, 5, or 20 mg TID; 12 weeks of open-label sildenafil 20 mg TID followed. Changes from baseline in 6-minute walk distance (6MWD) for sildenafil 1 or 5 mg versus 20 mg TID were compared using a Williams test. Hemodynamics, functional class, and biomarkers were assessed.

Results: The study was prematurely terminated for non-safety reasons, with 129 of 219 planned patients treated. At week 12, 6MWD change from baseline was significantly greater for sildenafil 20 versus 1 mg ($P = 0.011$) but not versus 5 mg. At week 24, 6MWD increases from baseline were larger in those initially randomized to 20 versus 5 or 1 mg (74 vs 50 and 47 m, respectively). At week 12, changes in hemodynamic parameters were generally small and variable between treatment groups; odds ratios for improvement in functional class were not statistically significantly different. Improvements in B-type natriuretic peptide levels were significantly greater with sildenafil 20 versus 1 but not 5 mg.

Conclusions: Sildenafil 20 mg TID appeared to be more effective than 1 mg TID for improving 6MWD; sildenafil 5 mg TID appeared to have similar clinical and hemodynamic effects as 20 mg TID.

Keywords: Sildenafil, Clinical trial, Pulmonary hypertension, Exercise test, Echocardiography, Dose

Background

Pulmonary arterial hypertension (PAH) is a fatal disease in which increasing pulmonary vascular resistance ultimately culminates in right ventricular failure and death [1, 2]. The phosphodiesterase type 5 (PDE5) inhibitor sildenafil is approved to treat adult patients with PAH [2]; pediatric use is approved in the European Union.

In the 12-week, randomized, double-blind, SUPER-1 study [3], statistically significant improvements in 6-minute walk distance (6MWD) were observed with sildenafil versus placebo in treatment-naive patients at all 3 tested doses (20, 40, and 80 mg 3 times daily [TID]); improvements were similar among groups and did not appear to be dose related. However, hemodynamic parameters, including mean pulmonary arterial pressure (mPAP), cardiac index, and pulmonary vascular resistance index (PVRI), appeared to improve dose dependently with sildenafil treatment. Sildenafil 20 mg TID appeared to reach the plateau of the

* Correspondence: dario.vizza@gmail.com; dario.vizza@uniroma1.it
[1]Department of Cardiovascular and Respiratory Disease, University of Rome La Sapienza, Viale del Policlinico 155, 00161 Rome, Italy
Full list of author information is available at the end of the article

dose-response curve for 6MWD [3] and was confirmed by subsequent population pharmacokinetic and pharmacodynamic analysis [4].

This study was conducted to fulfill a postapproval commitment from the US Food and Drug Administration (FDA) to further explore the sildenafil dose-response curve. This multinational, randomized, double-blind study investigated whether low doses of sildenafil (1 and 5 mg TID) were less effective in adult patients with PAH than the currently approved 20-mg TID dose.

However, before completion of this low-dose study, results from another randomized, double-blind, placebo-controlled study (PACES-1) became available that supported approval of a clinical worsening indication by the FDA [5]. PACES-1 evaluated oral sildenafil in patients with PAH who were receiving stable epoprostenol therapy [6]. In PACES-1, ≥75% of patients were titrated from sildenafil 20 mg TID, received during the first 4 weeks, to sildenafil 40 mg TID at week 4, and then to sildenafil 80 mg TID at week 8 (and were maintained on this dose, as patients tolerated). After 16 weeks, 6MWD, hemodynamic parameters, and functional class improved. There was a significant delay in time to clinical worsening (TTCW) [6], defined as death, lung transplantation, hospitalization due to PAH, initiation of bosentan therapy, or clinical deterioration requiring a change in epoprostenol therapy, with sildenafil compared with placebo. The effect was apparent by week 4, when all patients were receiving sildenafil 20 mg TID ($P = 0.0074$) [4].

Following approval of the clinical worsening indication in the United States in 2009, the FDA released Pfizer from the postapproval commitment to conduct a low-dose study. The study was subsequently terminated (June 2010) based on the recommendation of the data monitoring committee (DMC) because sildenafil 20 mg TID had been shown to reduce time to clinical worsening in PACES-1 and also acknowledging that with recruitment issues the study was unlikely to meet original enrollment targets. Accumulated results are presented here.

Methods
Study design
Patients were stratified by baseline 6MWD (<325 or ≥325 m) and PAH etiology and randomly assigned 1:1:1 to receive 12 weeks of treatment with sildenafil 1, 5, or 20 mg TID, respectively, during the double-blind phase of the study (Fig. 1). Patients who completed the double-blind phase were eligible for a 12-week, open-label extension in which they received sildenafil 20 mg TID. Patients who withdrew during the study were to be followed up for safety assessments 30 days after the last treatment date.

The primary objective of the study was to demonstrate a dose response for 6MWD for 1, 5, and 20 mg TID oral

sildenafil. The hypothesis was that there is a dose that is significantly less effective than sildenafil 20 mg TID.

Secondary objectives included assessment of the safety and tolerability of low-dose sildenafil during the 12 weeks of treatment in patients with PAH and evaluation of the effects of sildenafil on perceived PAH-progression biomarkers (B-type natriuretic peptide [BNP]/pro-BNP levels and tricuspid annular plane systolic excursion [TAPSE]). The study protocol and amendments were reviewed and approved by the Institutional Review Board and/or Independent Ethics Committee at each participating center (Additional file 1); informed consent was obtained from all patients.

Patients
Patients were aged >18 years with idiopathic or heritable PAH or PAH associated with connective tissue disease or surgical repair (≥5 years before enrollment) of atrial septal defect, ventricular septal defect, patent ductus arteriosus, or aorto-pulmonary window and 6MWD 100 to 450 m. PAH, defined as mPAP ≥25 mmHg and pulmonary artery wedge pressure ≤15 mmHg at rest (or a left ventricular end diastolic pressure <14 mmHg and absence of mitral stenosis on echocardiography), was confirmed by right heart catheterization (RHC) within 12 weeks before randomization. Patients had to be on stable (≥30 days before RHC) doses of background medication.

Patients were excluded for use of PAH-specific therapy, including prostacyclin, PDE5 inhibitors, and endothelin-receptor antagonists (ETRAs); nitrates or nitric oxide donors; protease inhibitors, such as ritonavir and saquinavir; ketoconazole, itraconazole, or other strong cytochrome P450 (CYP) 3A4 inhibitors; and alpha blockers. Patients previously receiving any of these drugs must have stopped use for ≥1 month before screening. Concomitant medications were to remain stable throughout the treatment phase of the study; patients withdrew if they required additional PAH-specific therapy.

Assessments
Six-minute walk distance was assessed at baseline (day 1) and at weeks 4, 8, 12, 16, 20, and 24 as close to sildenafil trough levels as possible (ie, just before dosing and ≥4 h after the last scheduled dose). Borg dyspnea score was assessed at the end of the 6MWD evaluation. Hemodynamic status was assessed at baseline and week 12, using RHC. World Health Organization functional class was assessed at baseline; weeks 4, 8, 12, and 24; and follow-up.

Time to clinical worsening was assessed during the double-blind phase. Clinical worsening was defined as death, lung transplantation, hospitalization attributable

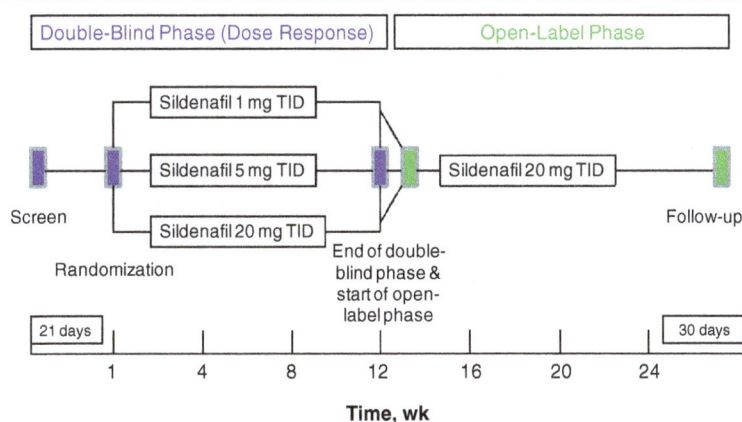

Fig. 1 Study design. Legend: TID = 3 times daily

to pulmonary hypertension, or initiation of prostacyclin or ETRA therapy.

Blood samples for determination of BNP/pro-BNP levels were collected at baseline and at weeks 1, 4, 8, 12, 16, 20, and 24. Echocardiography for TAPSE was performed at baseline and at weeks 4, 8, 12, and 24. A 2-dimensional Doppler examination was performed using an apical 4-chamber view. TAPSE index was measured as the total displacement of the tricuspid annulus (cm) from end diastole to end systole, with values representing the average TAPSE of 3 to 5 beats.

For pharmacokinetic analysis, blood samples were collected at the baseline visit (between 15 min and 3 h, >3 and 6 h, and >6 and 8 h postdose), week 1 (immediately after BNP/pro-BNP sampling), weeks 4 and 8 (immediately before 6MWD), and week 12 (between 15 min and 3 h and between >3 and 6 h postdose, immediately before 6MWD, between >6 and 8 h postdose, and during RHC assessment).

Adverse events (AEs) were monitored throughout the study. Laboratory testing and physical examinations were performed at screening, baseline, and weeks 4, 8, and 12.

Dose selection

The relationship between 6MWD and sildenafil exposure could not be modeled because 6MWD had reached a plateau across all SUPER-1 dose groups [3]. Therefore, the relationship between PVRI and exposure was used to select doses predicting exposures from the population pharmacokinetic/pharmacodynamic model. The average sildenafil plasma concentration required to achieve 50% effect (EC_{50}) on PVRI was approximately 3 ng/mL; at a 20-ng/mL concentration, sildenafil appeared to have a 90% maximal effect (EC_{90}) on PVRI [4]. Therefore, after receipt of 20 mg TID, sildenafil concentrations were anticipated to be > EC_{90} for the entire 8-hour dosing interval; for 5 mg TID, above EC_{50} for the entire 8-hour dosing interval but < EC_{90} for most of the interval; and

for 1 mg TID, sildenafil concentrations were anticipated to be at approximately EC_{50}.

Pharmacokinetic modeling

Population modeling characterized sildenafil pharmacokinetics; available sildenafil concentrations from all patients across all visits were merged to develop a nonlinear mixed effects model (NONMEM®, version 7.2; ICON Development Solutions, Ellicott City, MD). Estimation was performed for underlying pharmacokinetic parameters affecting the concentration-time profile. Only covariates that were previously reported to affect pharmacokinetic parameters [5] were tested in the model. To test for appropriateness, a visual predictive check was performed by calculating the median and 90% prediction interval from 500 simulations of the resulting population pharmacokinetic model.

Statistical analysis

The estimated sample size was based on the primary endpoint and was determined using simulations. Assuming a treatment effect of 30 m for sildenafil 20 versus 1 mg TID, with a standard deviation of 60 m [3], 70 patients per group were required to detect a difference between treatments with 80% power at a 1-sided significance level of 2.5%. Allowing for 4% postrandomization nonevaluability, approximately 219 patients (73 per group) were required to be randomized.

For the primary endpoint, statistical significance was assessed with a 1-sided Williams trend test on the intent-to-treat (ITT) population; the ITT population consisted of randomized patients who received ≥1 dose of study medication. The highest noneffective dose (ie, the highest dose that is statistically significantly different from sildenafil 20 mg) was determined. Missing values were replaced according to the last observation carried forward (LOCF) in the primary analysis and via multiple imputation for sensitivity analyses.

Additionally, changes in the primary endpoint were modeled by analysis of covariance (ANCOVA) with randomized treatment, baseline 6MWD, and etiology as stratification factors. Pairwise treatment group differences were estimated. In the open-label phase, changes to week 24 (LOCF) were analyzed using this ANCOVA model (but also including week 12 [LOCF] in the model) if there was a nonmissing post–week-12 assessment.

Secondary endpoints (including hemodynamic parameters) were assessed in the ITT population using LOCF; covariates for each analysis included baseline value as well as the randomization strata of baseline 6MWD and etiology. Methods for LOCF, time to clinical worsening (TTCW), and Borg assessments are described in Additional file 2. For secondary endpoints, statistical significance was assessed based on nominal P values (<0.05; 2-sided) without adjustment for multiplicity.

Results

The study was conducted at 34 centers in Europe, Asia, Russia, the United States, and Brazil. Of the planned 219 patients, 169 were screened, 130 were randomized, and 129 were treated (1 patient [sildenafil 1 mg] did not meet entry criteria). Treated patients were mostly female and mostly Asian; baseline cardiac index was significantly higher in the sildenafil 20-mg group versus the 1- and 5-mg groups ($P = 0.0328$ and 0.0030, respectively; Table 1).

Patient disposition is shown in Fig. 2. Two patients died during the double-blind phase (pneumonia [1 mg TID; death was the reason for discontinuation] and acute exacerbation of idiopathic pulmonary fibrosis [5 mg TID; patient was enrolled in error and received 4 days of treatment]), neither of which was considered to be treatment related; no deaths were reported in the open-label phase (Fig. 2).

Sildenafil concentration

Overall, 129 patients provided 1068 sildenafil concentrations. A 1-compartment pharmacokinetic model adequately described the sparse data. From this model, the estimated apparent clearance was 43.9 (95% CI, 39.3–48.6) L/h, the apparent volume of distribution was 458 (95% CI, 393–523) L, and the absorption rate constant was 2.16 (95% CI, 1.48–2.84) h^{-1}. Coadministration of weak or moderate CYP3A4 inhibitors ($n = 12$ patients/110 samples) reduced CL/F by 40.4% (95% CI, 19.2%–61.6%). The model supported dose proportionality of exposures.

The limit of quantification of the pharmacokinetic assay was 1 ng/mL; 134 samples were below the limit of quantification (BLQ). The majority of BLQ samples (approximately 75%) were measured at the 1-mg TID sildenafil dose, but had little effect on the population pharmacokinetic parameter estimates.

Figure 3 represents the sildenafil concentration data. Because a small accumulation existed between the first (at baseline visit) and subsequent doses, only concentrations after the second and subsequent doses are shown (for data including baseline visit, see Additional file 3). Concentrations after concomitant administration of CYP3A4 inhibitors were adjusted for the estimated effect. Visual inspection of observed concentration distribution across each dose indicated consistency of the observed data with the model. In particular, in the 8 h after drug administration, most of the determinations in the 1-mg TID group had a concentration below 3 ng/mL, whereas in the 5-mg TID and 20-mg TID groups, most of the determinations had a concentration above 3 ng/mL, which is the average sildenafil plasma concentration required to achieve 50% effect (EC$_{50}$) on PVRI [4]. An exploratory assessment (see Additional files 4 and 5) of the relationship between 6MWD, PVR, and steady-state concentrations revealed a significant relationship for 6MWD, whereas only a small trend could be seen for PVR across the concentration range observed (Additional files 6 and 7).

Six-minute walk distance

At week 12, compared with baseline, the increase in 6MWD was of a magnitude consistent with estimates of clinical significance [7, 8] in 5- and 20-mg TID groups and smaller although statistically significant in the 1-mg TID group. Among dose groups, the mean change in 6MWD from baseline was statistically significantly different only for the sildenafil 20- versus 1-mg group (Fig. 4a).

Analysis of change from baseline in 6MWD at week 12 showed a statistically significant ($P = 0.011$) difference between sildenafil 1 mg and 20 mg, but not sildenafil 5 mg and 20 mg (Table 2). The results were confirmed by an analysis of variance; the mean treatment difference between sildenafil 20 mg and 1 mg was 23 (3–43) m and between 20 mg and 5 mg was −3 (−23 to 17) m ($P = 0.02$ and 0.76, respectively).

Patients with baseline 6MWD <325 m at baseline had greater increases in 6MWD after sildenafil treatment than patients with baseline 6MWD ≥325 m (Fig. 4b).

Differences in 6MWD between Asian and non-Asian patients were noted for sildenafil 1 mg but not for 5 mg or 20 mg (Fig. 5a and b); the number of non-Asian patients was small.

During the open-label period (weeks 12 to 24), in which all patients received sildenafil 20 mg TID, patients who received sildenafil 1 mg TID during the double-blind phase (weeks 0 to 12) had a larger increase in 6MWD than patients who received sildenafil 5 mg TID (mean change, 31 vs 6 m, respectively); the magnitude of change was similar between patients who received sildenafil 1 mg and 20 mg TID in the double-blind phase (mean change, 31 vs 26 m; Fig. 4a).

Table 1 Baseline Patient Demographic and Clinical Characteristics

Baseline Characteristic	Sildenafil Dose, TID		
	1 mg (n = 41)	5 mg (n = 43)	20 mg (n = 45)
Women, n (%)	28 (68)	33 (77)	26 (58)
Age, y	42.5 (16.5)	44.4 (17.4)	46.4 (17.7)
Range	18–77	18–78	20–88
Race, n (%)			
White	11 (27)	11 (26)	14 (31)
Black	2 (5)	2 (5)	1 (2)
Asian	27 (66)	30 (70)	30 (67)
Other	1 (2)	0	0
Height, cm	159.0 (11.3)	160.2 (10.7)	160.7 (8.7)
Range	130.0–181.6	129.0–189.0	147.0–181.0
Weight, kg	61.7 (17.0)	63.1 (19.7)	61.4 (15.7)
Range	32.0–117.0	26.5–126.1	35.0–100.0
BMI, kg/m^2	24.3 (5.6)	24.3 (6.6)	23.8 (6.2)
Range	15.6–35.8	13.3–42.1	15.6–38.6
WHO functional class, n (%)			
I	0	1 (2.3)	3 (6.7)
II	25 (61.0)	22 (51.2)	27 (60.0)
III	16 (39.0)	16 (37.2)	13 (28.9)
IV	0	1 (2.3)	0
Missing	0	3 (7.0)	2 (4.4)
Etiology, n (%)			
Idiopathic	30 (73)	31 (72)	34 (76)
Mean duration (range) since diagnosis, y	1.1 (0–6.7)	0.7 (0–6.5)	0.9 (0–14.9)
Associated with CTD	6 (15)	8 (19)	5 (11)
Mean duration (range) since diagnosis, y	0.6 (0–2.3)	0.4 (0–1.8)	0.4 (0–1.9)
Associated with surgical repair	5 (12)	4 (9)	6 (13)
Mean duration (range) since diagnosis, y	5.9 (0.3–14.2)	3.5 (0–7.3)	4.5 (0–15.7)
6MWD, m[a]	347.5 (67.3)	347.7 (73.4)	340.4 (76.3)
Range	167.5–441.5	109.0–455.0	114.0–429.0
Heart rate, bpm[b]	83.6 (17.2)	78.9 (16.4)	80.1 (15.0)
Range	48–122	42–113	53–110
RAP, mmHg[c]	10.5 (5.1)	10.1 (6.1)	8.4 (4.7)
Range	4.0–20.0	2.0–23.0	2.0–27.0
mPAP, mmHg[c]	57.2 (21.9)	55.4 (19.7)	51.1 (21.4)
Range	25.0–110.0	26.3–117.0	25.0–106.0
Cardiac index, L/min/m^2[d]	2.1 (0.7)	2.3 (0.6)	2.8 (1.2)
Range	1.0–3.5	1.0–3.8	1.1–5.9
PVR, Wood units[e]	15.7 (9.9)	13.2 (8.3)	11.7 (9.1)
Range	3–43	3–48	2–35

Table 1 Baseline Patient Demographic and Clinical Characteristics *(Continued)*

MVO$_2$, %[f]	63.4 (10.5)	63.0 (9.6)	64.3 (14.5)
Range	41–82	42–77	31–90
TAPSE index[g]	1.25 (0.62)	1.2 (0.71)	1.36 (0.83)
Range	0.1–2.6	0.1–2.5	0.2–2.8
Borg dyspnea score[h]	2.9 (2.5)	3.1 (1.9)	2.8 (2.1)
Range	0–10	0–8	0–9

All values are presented as mean (SD) unless stated otherwise
6MWD 6-minute walk distance, *BMI* body mass index, *bpm* beats per minute, *CTD* connective tissue disease, *mPAP* mean pulmonary arterial pressure, *MVO$_2$* mixed venous oxygen saturation, *PVR* pulmonary vascular resistance, *RAP* right atrial pressure, *TAPSE* tricuspid annular plane systolic excursion, *TID* 3 times daily, *WHO* World Health Organization
[a]n = 2 and 3 patients missing a baseline assessment in sildenafil 5- and 20-mg groups, respectively
[b]n = 33, 32, and 33 patients contributing data in sildenafil 1-, 5-, and 20-mg groups, respectively
[c]n = 33, 33, and 34 patients contributing data in sildenafil 1-, 5-, and 20-mg groups, respectively
[d]n = 33, 33, and 32 patients contributing data in sildenafil 1-, 5-, and 20-mg groups, respectively
[e]n = 33, 32, and 32 patients contributing data in sildenafil 1-, 5-, and 20-mg groups, respectively
[f]n = 33, 28, and 31 patients contributing data in sildenafil 1-, 5-, and 20-mg groups, respectively
[g]n = 40 for all sildenafil groups
[h]n = 41, 40, and 42 patients contributing data in sildenafil 1-, 5-, and 20-mg groups, respectively

Secondary and tertiary evaluations
Hemodynamics
Compared with baseline, there was a trend toward reduction in pulmonary vascular resistance (PVR) at week 12 in all groups; the mean reduction was statistically significantly different from 0 only in the 20-mg TID group (ie, 95% CIs do not include 0). There were no statistically significant differences among treatment groups for change in PVR (Table 3). Changes at week 12 in the additional hemodynamic parameters were generally small and variable between groups.

Functional class and clinical worsening
Most patients in each treatment group remained in the same functional class from baseline to week 12; the same was true through week 24 (Table 4). Odds ratios (ORs) showed no significant differences for functional class between sildenafil 20 mg and the 5-mg (OR, 1.08 [95% CI, 0.35–3.32]; $P = 0.897$) or 1-mg (OR, 1.55 [95% CI, 0.50–7.78]; $P = 0.448$) dose at week 12. Similarly, there were no differences between sildenafil 20 mg and the 5-mg (OR, 1.31 [95% CI, 0.42–4.05]; $P = 0.639$) or 1-mg (OR, 0.93 [95% CI, 0.30–2.91]; $P = 0.899$) dose at week 24. Four patients (sildenafil 1 mg and 5 mg, $n = 1$ each; sildenafil 20 mg, $n = 2$) reported events defined as clinical worsening (initiation of ETRA therapy [sildenafil 5-mg patient] and hospitalization due to PAH [all others]).

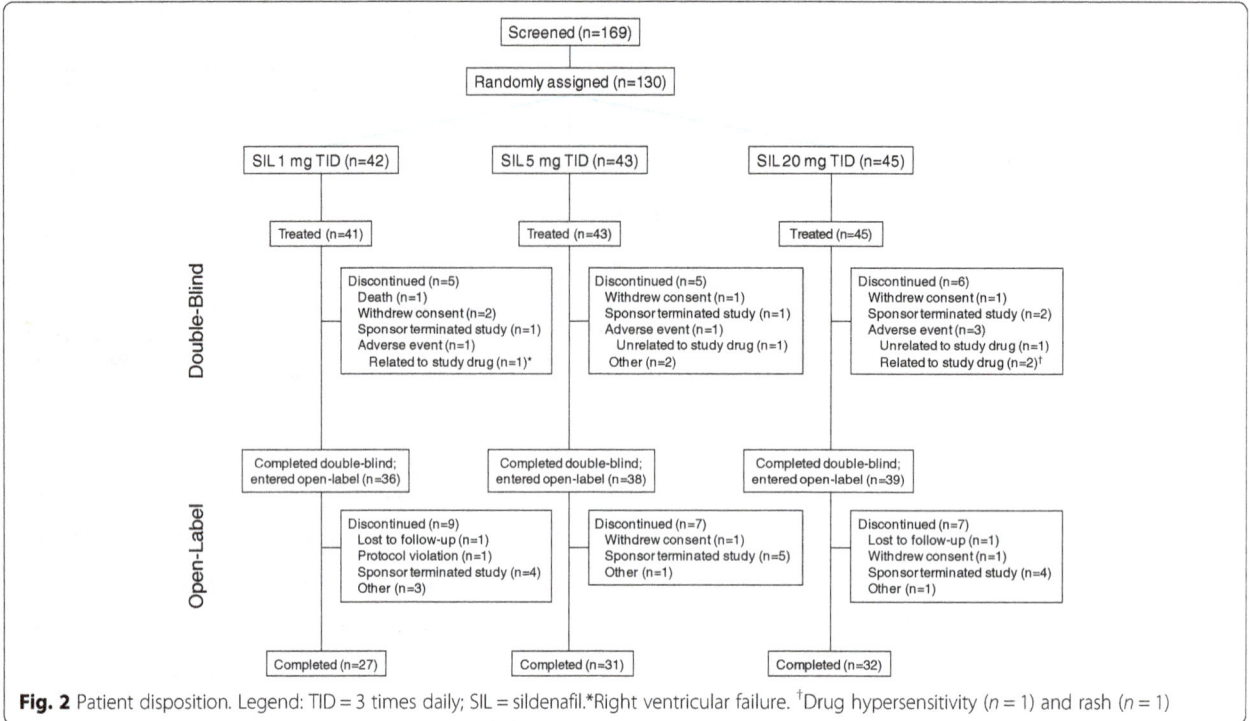

Fig. 2 Patient disposition. Legend: TID = 3 times daily; SIL = sildenafil.*Right ventricular failure. †Drug hypersensitivity (*n* = 1) and rash (*n* = 1)

Neurohormones

Decreases from baseline in BNP occurred in all groups at week 12; the response was dose related (Fig. 6a). The sildenafil 20-mg group was statistically significantly (*P* = 0.005) different from the 1-mg but not the 5-mg group (*P* = 0.496). At week 24, changes from baseline for sildenafil 20 mg were not significantly different among groups.

Pro-BNP decreases occurred in all groups at week 12 and were dose related (Fig. 6b). Differences were significant when sildenafil 20 mg was compared with 1 but not

5 mg (*P* = 0.009 and 0.414, respectively). At week 24, changes from baseline were not significantly different among groups.

Echocardiography

There was a trend toward a mean increase in TAPSE in all groups, but there were no statistically significant differences in mean TAPSE index among groups (mean [95% CI] increases of 0.14 [0.02–0.26], 0.17 [0.06–0.28], and 0.04 [−0.08 to 0.16] cm for sildenafil 1, 5, and 20 mg TID, respectively, at week 12 [LOCF] and 0.21

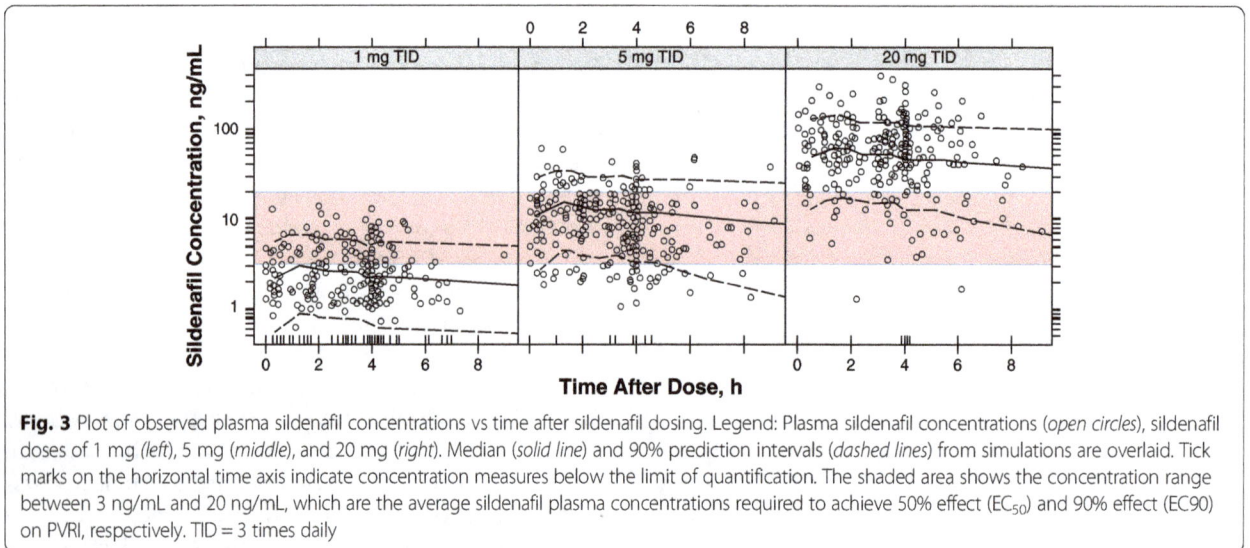

Fig. 3 Plot of observed plasma sildenafil concentrations vs time after sildenafil dosing. Legend: Plasma sildenafil concentrations (*open circles*), sildenafil doses of 1 mg (*left*), 5 mg (*middle*), and 20 mg (*right*). Median (*solid line*) and 90% prediction intervals (*dashed lines*) from simulations are overlaid. Tick marks on the horizontal time axis indicate concentration measures below the limit of quantification. The shaded area shows the concentration range between 3 ng/mL and 20 ng/mL, which are the average sildenafil plasma concentrations required to achieve 50% effect (EC$_{50}$) and 90% effect (EC90) on PVRI, respectively. TID = 3 times daily

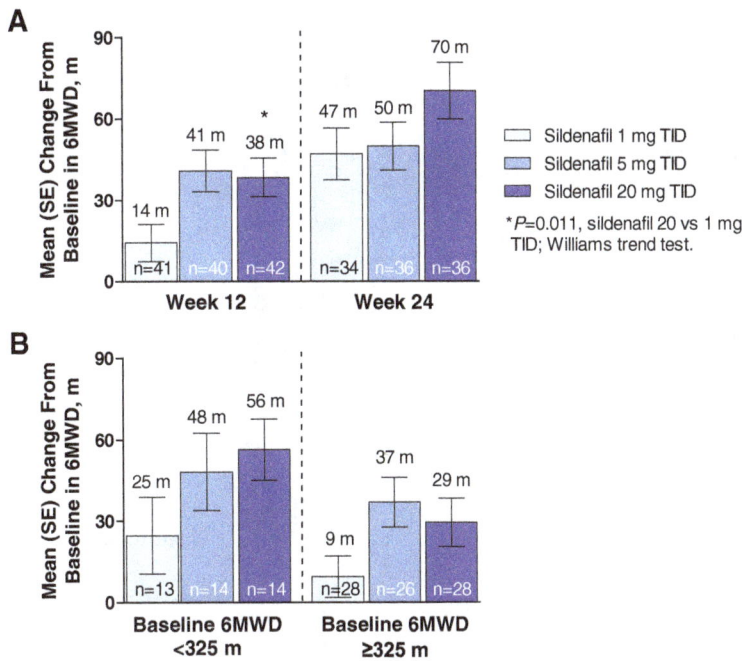

Fig. 4 Mean change from baseline in 6MWD. Legend: Mean (SE) overall change from double-blind baseline in 6MWD in double-blind (week 12) and open-label (week 24) phases of the study (**a**), and change from baseline to week 12 in 6MWD by baseline 6MWD (**b**). All patients received sildenafil 20 mg TID in the open-label phase of the study (weeks 13–24). 6MWD = 6-minute walk distance; TID = 3 times daily

[0.06–0.37], 0.40 [0.19–0.61], and 0.15 [−0.09 to 0.39] at week 24 [LOCF]).

Borg dyspnea score

Borg dyspnea scores trended toward reduction in all groups (mean [95% CI] changes of −0.28 [−0.76 to 0.20], −0.89 [−1.35 to −0.43], and −0.43 [−0.94 to 0.08] for sildenafil 1, 5, and 20 mg TID, respectively, at week 12

Table 2 Change From Baseline[a] in 6MWD at Week 12 (LOCF) Williams Trend Test

Value	Sildenafil Dose, TID		
	1 mg (n = 41)	5 mg (n = 43)	20 mg (n = 45)
Least squares mean	14.21	40.75	38.36
MLE mean[b]	14.21	39.52	39.52
Mean difference[c]	24.15	−1.17	—
Williams statistic	2.37	−0.11	—
97.5% lower confidence limit	3.37	−21.48	—
P value[d]	0.011	0.545	—

6MWD 6-minute walk distance, LOCF last observation carried forward, MLE maximum likelihood estimation, TID 3 times daily

[a]Baseline is the average of the screening and day 1 values
[b]MLE mean is defined as least squares mean if it satisfies descending response relationship for descending doses; if descending relationship does not hold, MLE mean is defined as weighted mean of adjacent least squares means
[c]Mean difference was calculated as the least squares mean for sildenafil 20 mg minus the MLE mean for sildenafil lower dose
[d]From directional test vs 20 mg TID

[LOCF] and −1.10 [−1.75 to −0.46], −1.07 [−1.55 to −0.58], and −0.28 [−0.75 to 0.20] at week 24 [LOCF]), with no significant differences between sildenafil 1- and 5-mg TID groups compared with sildenafil 20 mg TID.

Correlations among parameters

Baseline 6MWD was weakly correlated with BNP ($r = -0.19$; $P = 0.0393$) and pro-BNP ($r = -0.22$; $P = 0.0145$). The change in 6MWD at week 12 was also weakly correlated with changes at week 12 in BNP ($r = -0.18$; $P = 0.0499$) and pro-BNP ($r = -0.22$; $P = 0.0193$).

Adverse events

The overall number of AEs and numbers of patients reporting AEs were similar between treatment groups in the double-blind and open-label portions of the study; treatment-related AEs (number of AEs and patients reporting AEs) increased with increasing dose (Table 5). Sildenafil was generally well tolerated, with most AEs being mild or moderate in severity. Dyspnea was the most common AE reported in both phases of the study; headache was the most common treatment-related AE (Table 5). No patients discontinued as a result of abnormal laboratory test results, and there was no evidence of dose-related increase in laboratory test abnormalities with increasing sildenafil dose.

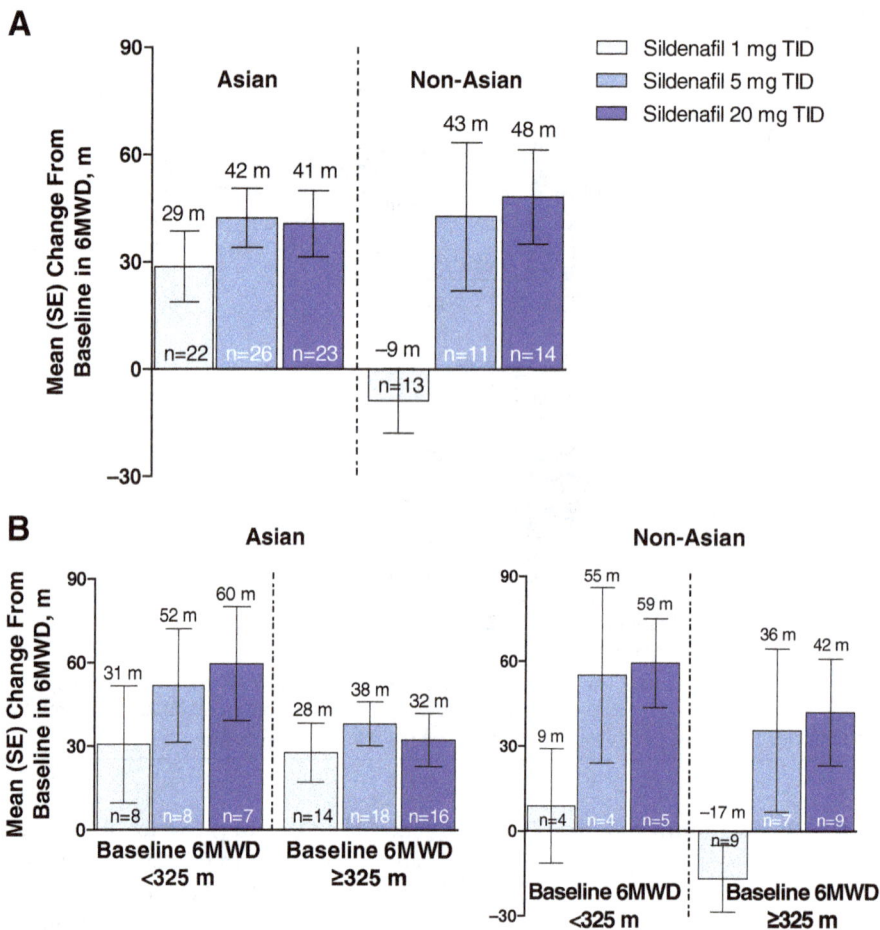

Fig. 5 Mean change from baseline in 6MWD assessed by race. Legend: Mean (SE) overall change from double-blind baseline in 6MWD in the double-blind (week 12) phase of the study (**a**) and change from baseline to week 12 in 6MWD by baseline 6MWD (**b**) assessed by race (Asian vs non-Asian). 6MWD = 6-minute walk distance; TID = 3 times daily

Discussion

Sildenafil is one of the most widely used drugs in the treatment of PAH. The dose of 20 mg TID was approved based on the results of the SUPER-1 study which demonstrated that Sildenafil 20 mg TID appeared to reach the plateau of the dose-response curve for 6MWD, despite the larger hemodynamic effects seen with the highest dosage (80 mg TID). These results raise the question as to whether a lower dosage could have a similar effect on 6MWD compared to the approved dose. This aspect was addressed in the present study.

We found a significant increase from baseline in 6MWD at 12 weeks with all sildenafil doses; however, only at higher doses (5 and 20 mg TID) was the improvement of a magnitude considered to be clinically relevant (~40 m) [7, 8]. In the absence of a placebo control arm, the small non-clinically significant increase in 6MWD in the 1 mg TID group in the double blind phase should be interpreted with caution as being a treatment effect as it is possible that this improvement could be seen as a "placebo effect" due to participation in an RCT.

Among dose groups, the change in 6MWD from baseline was significant only with sildenafil 20 mg TID compared with sildenafil 1 mg TID. A Williams trend test confirmed that sildenafil 1 mg TID was the only dose statistically inferior to the approved dose of 20 mg TID. Generally, patients had greater improvements in hemodynamic parameters with sildenafil 20 mg TID versus 1 mg TID; however, these improvements were not statistically significantly different. Significant differences were observed between sildenafil 1 mg TID and 20 mg TID for neurohormones at week 12.

There were no statistically significant differences between sildenafil 20 and 5 mg TID in 6MWD, hemodynamics, or changes in functional class.

Results from pharmacokinetic modeling showed that the observed exposure with sildenafil 1 mg TID was slightly below EC_{50} for maximal PVR change, the observed exposure with sildenafil 5 mg TID was above

Table 3 Adjusted Change From Baseline in Hemodynamic Parameters at Week 12

Baseline Characteristic	Sildenafil Dose, TID		
	1 mg	5 mg	20 mg
Heart rate			
n	33	32	33
LS mean (95% CI), bpm	3.4 (−1.1 to 7.9)	−0.7 (−5.2 to 3.7)	−5.0 (−9.3 to −0.8)
P value vs 20 mg TID	0.0019	0.1066	—
RAP			
n	33	33	34
LS mean (95% CI), mmHg	−0.5 (−2.3 to 1.2)	−0.8 (−2.5 to 0.9)	−1.7 (−3.3 to 0)
P value vs 20 mg TID	0.2741	0.4098	—
mPAP			
n	33	33	34
LS mean (95% CI), mmHg	−0.1 (−4.0 to 3.7)	−2.2 (−5.9 to 1.5)	−2.6 (−6.2 to 0.9)
P value vs 20 mg TID	0.2776	0.8458	—
Cardiac index			
n	32	31	30
LS mean (95% CI), L/min/m^2	0.1 (−0.2 to 0.3)	0.1 (−0.1 to 0.4)	0.1 (−0.2 to 0.3)
P value vs 20 mg TID	0.9023	0.7590	—
PVR			
n	32	31	30
LS mean (95% CI), Wood units	−1.2 (−3.3 to 0.9)	−2.0 (−4.1 to 0)	−2.4 (−4.3 to −0.4)
P value vs 20 mg TID	0.3694	0.8010	—
PVRI			
n	32	31	30
LS mean (95% CI), Wood units*m^2	−1.7 (−4.9 to 1.5)	−3.1 (−6.2 to 0)	−3.5 (−6.4 to −0.5)
P value vs 20 mg TID	0.3868	0.8628	—
MVO$_2$			
n	33	28	31
LS mean (95% CI), %	1.5 (−2.2 to 5.2)	3.0 (−0.8 to 6.7)	3.0 (−0.4 to 6.4)
P value vs 20 mg TID	0.4918	0.9791	—

bpm beats per minute, LS least squares, mPAP mean pulmonary arterial pressure, MVO$_2$ mixed venous oxygen saturation, PVR pulmonary vascular resistance, PVRI PVR index, RAP right atrial pressure, TID 3 times daily

Table 4 Change From Baseline to Weeks 12 and 24 in Functional Class (LOCF)

Change, n (%)	Sildenafil Dose, TID					
	Double-Blind Phase (Week 12)			Open-Label Phase (Week 24)		
	1 mg (n = 41)	5 mg (n = 43)	20 mg (n = 45)	1 mg (n = 41)	5 mg (n = 43)	20 mg (n = 45)
Worsened 2 classes	0	0	0	0	0	1 (2)
Worsened 1 class	1 (2)	3 (7)	2 (4)	0	3 (7)	1 (2)
No change	35 (85)	27 (63)	35 (78)	23 (56)	19 (44)	22 (49)
Improved 1 class	4 (10)	10 (23)	6 (13)	11 (27)	13 (30)	11 (24)
Improved 2 classes	1 (2)	0	0	1 (2)	1 (2)	1 (2)
Missing	0	3 (7)	2 (4)	6 (15)	7 (16)	9 (20)

LOCF last observation carried forward, TID 3 times daily

A

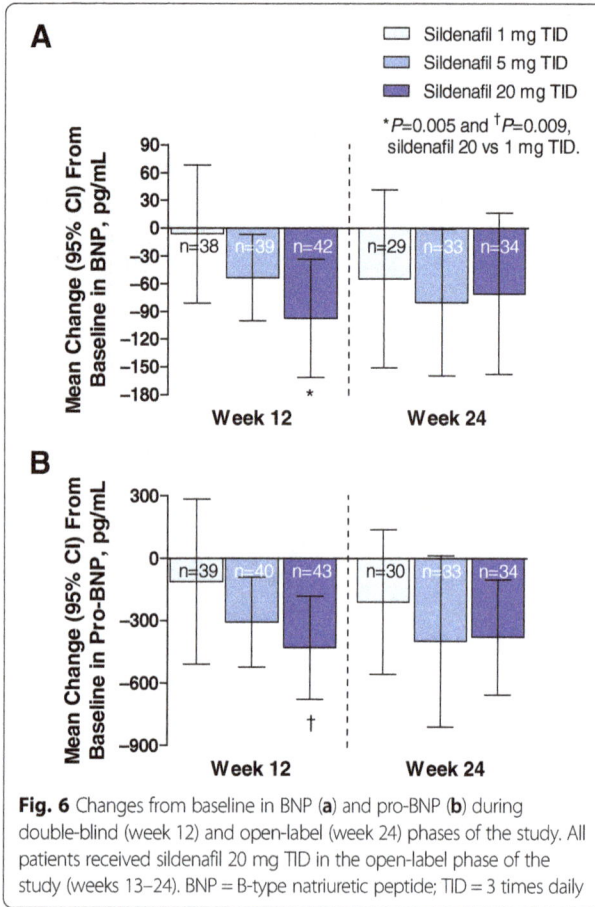

Sildenafil 1 mg TID
Sildenafil 5 mg TID
Sildenafil 20 mg TID

*$P=0.005$ and †$P=0.009$, sildenafil 20 vs 1 mg TID.

Mean Change (95% CI) From Baseline in BNP, pg/mL

n=38 n=39 n=42　n=29 n=33 n=34

Week 12　　　Week 24

B

Mean Change (95% CI) From Baseline in Pro-BNP, pg/mL

n=39 n=40 n=43　n=30 n=33 n=34

Week 12　　　Week 24

Fig. 6 Changes from baseline in BNP (**a**) and pro-BNP (**b**) during double-blind (week 12) and open-label (week 24) phases of the study. All patients received sildenafil 20 mg TID in the open-label phase of the study (weeks 13–24). BNP = B-type natriuretic peptide; TID = 3 times daily

EC_{50} and approaching EC_{90}, and the observed exposure with sildenafil 20 mg TID was mainly above EC_{90}.

The pharmacokinetic data justify the different clinical responses between sildenafil 1 and 20 mg TID and explain the small difference observed between sildenafil 20 and 5 mg TID because most of the patients on 5 mg TID had a sildenafil plasma level between 3 and 20 ng/mL.

A significant correlation among mean sildenafil plasma concentration and 6MWD could be observed, although the relationship between average sildenafil plasma concentration and PVR appeared to show only a shallow trend. Whether this was due to the missing placebo group or was a consequence of the smaller sample size and larger variability on PVR cannot be concluded but should be interpreted on the basis of the complex interplay between pharmacokinetics and pharmacodynamics. The vasodilator effect is the result of the interplay of several factors: tissue penetration of the drug, density and activity of PDE5 enzyme, and severity of vascular lesions.

Smaller improvement in 6MWD at week 12 with sildenafil 20 mg TID was observed in this study (38 m) compared with SUPER-1 (45 m); however, patient populations differed. Both studies had similar baseline 6MWD, but a greater proportion of patients in this study had baseline functional class II status compared with those in SUPER-1 (57% vs 39%, respectively); therefore, patients in this study had lower-than-expected 6MWD at baseline. Patients in our study were also younger (45 vs 49 years), with a shorter time since diagnosis (median, 0.17 vs 0.85 years) and an increased percentage of Asian patients (67% vs 7%). Geographic variation in 6MWD has been described for

Table 5 Adverse Event Summary

All-Cause (Treatment-Related) AEs, n	Sildenafil Dose, TID					
	Double-Blind Phase (Week 12)			Open-Label Phase[a] (Week 24)		
	1 mg ($n = 41$)	5 mg ($n = 43$)	20 mg ($n = 45$)	1 mg ($n = 41$)	5 mg ($n = 43$)	20 mg ($n = 45$)
Patients with AEs	17 (9)	17 (10)	19 (14)	23 (11)	22 (12)	22 (15)
Patients with serious AEs	4 (0)	2 (0)	3 (1)	6 (0)	3 (0)	5 (2)
Discontinuations due to AEs	1 (1)	1 (0)	3 (2)	1 (1)	1 (0)	3 (2)
Deaths	1 (0)	1 (0)	0	0	0	0
Number of AEs	46 (12)	41 (17)	47 (24)	90 (19)	69 (27)	74 (31)
AEs occurring in ≥3 patients						
Anemia	1 (0)	0 (0)	3 (1)	1 (0)	1 (0)	3 (1)
Fatigue	2 (1)	1 (0)	0 (0)	3 (1)	1 (0)	0 (0)
Nasopharyngitis	2 (0)	1 (0)	1 (0)	2 (0)	1 (0)	3 (0)
Dizziness	2 (1)	1 (0)	1 (1)	3 (1)	2 (1)	2 (2)
Dyspnea	2 (0)	3 (0)	3 (0)	2 (0)	4 (1)	3 (0)
Headache	1 (1)	1 (1)	3 (3)	2 (2)	3 (2)	3 (3)
Epistaxis	0 (0)	2 (2)	0 (0)	1 (0)	3 (3)	0 (0)
Back pain	0 (0)	1 (0)	2 (1)	1 (0)	1 (0)	3 (2)

AE adverse event, *TID* 3 times daily
[a]Includes AEs from the double-blind and open-label portions of the study

patients with PAH and was reported to be independent of anthropometric factors [9]. Although few non-Asian patients enrolled in this study, 6MWD did not appear to differ between groups, with the exception of sildenafil 1 mg TID (Fig. 5).

Interestingly, results from the open-label phase suggest the possibility of further improvement in 6MWD after the first 3 months of therapy with sildenafil 20 mg TID. The mean increase in 6MWD from baseline at the end of the double-blind phase (41 m) was maintained in the sildenafil 5-mg group uptitrated to sildenafil 20 mg TID in the extension study (50 m), yet larger increases were observed from the end of the double-blind study to the end of the open-label study in the sildenafil 1- and 20-mg groups (from 14–47 m and from 38–70 m, respectively). Thus, sildenafil 20 mg TID maintains treatment effects regardless of prior low-dose treatment. However, 6MWD did not increase to the same degree in patients previously treated with lower doses as in patients who continuously received 20 mg TID, suggesting that a longer duration of an adequate dose may confer a larger improvement in 6MWD. Interestingly, the total improvement observed after 24 weeks in the 20-mg group (70 m) was larger than in the SUPER-1 study at 12 weeks (48 m) or 1 year (51 m) for all sildenafil doses combined. It may be possible that in a population of young and mainly incident cases, as in our study, further improvements in 6MWD may be observed with continued sildenafil treatment.

Decreases for BNP and pro-BNP versus baseline were significantly higher with sildenafil 20 mg versus 1 mg TID at week 12, paralleling findings with 6MWD. BNP levels similarly paralleled improvements (BNP levels decreased) or worsening (BNP levels increased) in pulmonary hemodynamics and functional parameters, including 6MWD, in patients with PAH in a previous study [10]. Elevated plasma BNP levels are associated with increased mortality in patients with PAH, and a decrease in BNP levels after therapy is associated with improved survival [11, 12]. Pro-BNP levels have recently been shown to identify poor outcome in patients with PAH [13, 14]. Longer-term follow-up of patients from our study is not ongoing, which prevents any correlation with mortality.

The main limitation of the present study is its premature termination. The study was designed to assess the relative efficacy of sildenafil 20 mg TID and lower doses and powered for the primary endpoint but the sample size was not reached because of premature termination [4, 6]. Looking at the results, this does not seem a major issue, as the difference in the primary and secondary endpoints between 1 mgTID and 20 mg TID is statistically significant and coherent. Regarding the comparison between the 5-mg and 20-mg groups, the differences were small enough that, even with the completion of the

study, similar results may have been observed. A noninferiority study comparing sildenafil 5 mg TID versus 20 mg TID would require an unrealistically large sample size for a rare disease like PAH. Estimating from the results of the current study, 382 patients would be required for a study with a noninferiority margin of 15 m at 90% power and a 1-sided significance level of 0.05, assuming a true difference (5 vs 20 mg TID) of 0 m and a standard deviation of 50 m. The required sample size would increase if patient dropout was considered or if a smaller noninferiority margin was desired.

Conclusion

Despite this study having the limitation of premature termination, sildenafil 1 mg TID, but not 5 mg TID, was shown to be inferior to 20 mg TID for improvement in 6MWD in patients with PAH. Sildenafil 5 mg TID appeared to have similar clinical and hemodynamic effects as 20 mg TID. Interestingly, 6MWD results from the open-label phase of the study suggest that patients on the approved sildenafil dose (20 mg TID) continued to show clinical improvement after the first 12 weeks of treatment. Hence, the question remains whether doses lower than 20 mg TID have therapeutic value and needs to be seen in light of the current therapeutic approach in PAH.

Abbreviations

6MWD: 6-minute walk distance; AE: Adverse event; ANCOVA: Analysis of covariance; BLQ: Below the limit of quantification; BNP: B-type natriuretic peptide; CYP: Cytochrome P450; DMC: Data monitoring committee; ETRA: Endothelin-receptor antagonists; FDA: US Food and Drug Administration; ITT: Intent to treat; LOCF: Last observation carried forward; mPAP: Mean pulmonary arterial pressure; OR: Odds ratio; PAH: Pulmonary arterial hypertension; PDE5: Phosphodiesterase type 5; PVR: Pulmonary vascular resistance; PVRI: Pulmonary vascular resistance index; RHC: Right heart catheterization; TAPSE: Tricuspid annular plane systolic excursion; TID: 3 times daily; TTCW: Time to clinical worsening

Acknowledgements

The authors would like to thank Susan Raber for assistance with the analyses presented in the manuscript. Editorial support was provided by Tiffany Brake, PhD, Candace Lundin, DVM, MS, and Janet E. Matsuura, PhD, from Complete Healthcare Communications, LLC, and was funded by Pfizer Inc.

Funding

This study was funded by Pfizer Inc.

Authors' contributions

CDV, BKSS, ZS, LH, XG and Z-CJ participated in the acquisition of data, analysis and interpretation of data, and drafted the manuscript or revised it critically for intellectual content; MZ performed the statistical analysis, analyzed and interpreted the data, and drafted the manuscript or revised it critically for intellectual content; ML analyzed and interpreted the data and drafted the manuscript or revised it critically for intellectual content. All authors read and approved the final manuscript.

Competing interests

C.D.V. has received fees for serving as a speaker, consultant, and advisory board member from Actelion, Dompè, GlaxoSmithKline, Italfarmaco, Lilly,

Pfizer, and United Therapeutics. B.K.S.S. has received research funding from
Pfizer and Actelion. Z.S. has been a consultant and served as a speaker and
advisory board member for United Therapeutics, Gilead, and Actelion. L.H.,
M.L., and M.Z. are Pfizer employees. X.G. is a former Pfizer employee. Z.-C.J.
has received fees for serving as a speaker, consultant, and advisory board
member from Actelion, Bayer, GlaxoSmithKline, Lilly, Pfizer, and United
Therapeutics.

Author details
[1]Department of Cardiovascular and Respiratory Disease, University of Rome
La Sapienza, Viale del Policlinico 155, 00161 Rome, Italy. [2]CARE Hospitals,
Gandhi Bhavan Road Nampally, Hyderabad, India. [3]Baylor College of
Medicine, 1 Baylor Plaza, Houston, TX 77030, USA. [4]Pfizer Ltd, Ramsgate
Road, Sandwich Kent CT13 9NJ, UK. [5]Pfizer Inc, 558 Eastern Point Rd, Groton,
CT 06340, USA. [6]Pfizer Inc, 10646 Science Center Dr, La Jolla Campus, San
Diego, CA 92121, USA. [7]Shanghai Pulmonary Hospital, Tongji University
School of Medicine, 507, Zhengmin Road, Shanghai, China.

References
1. McLaughlin W, Archer SL, Badesch DB, Barst RJ, Farber HW, Lindner JR, et al. ACCF/AHA 2009 expert consensus document on pulmonary hypertension: a report of the American College of Cardiology Foundation Task Force on Expert Consensus Documents and the American Heart Association developed in collaboration with the American College of Chest Physicians; American Thoracic Society, Inc.; and the Pulmonary Hypertension Association. J Am Coll Cardiol. 2009;53:1573–619.
2. Galie N, Corris PA, Frost A, Girgis RE, Granton J, Jing ZC, et al. Updated treatment algorithm of pulmonary arterial hypertension. J Am Coll Cardiol. 2013;62:D60–72.
3. Galie N, Ghofrani HA, Torbicki A, Barst RJ, Rubin LJ, Badesch D, et al. Sildenafil citrate therapy for pulmonary arterial hypertension. N Engl J Med. 2005;353:2148–57.
4. Harnisch L, Hayashi N. Population pharmacokinetic (PK) of sildenafil in paediatric and adult pulmonary arterial hypertension (PAH) patients. Eur Respir J 2009;34(Suppl. 53):3916.
5. Revatio® (sildenafil citrate). Full Prescribing Information. New York: Pfizer Inc; 2014.
6. Simonneau G, Rubin LJ, Galie N, Barst RJ, Fleming TR, Frost AE, et al. Addition of sildenafil to long-term intravenous epoprostenol therapy in patients with pulmonary arterial hypertension: a randomized trial. Ann Intern Med. 2008;149:521–30.
7. Gabler NB, French B, Strom BL, Palevsky HI, Taichman DB, Kawut SM, et al. Validation of 6-minute walk distance as a surrogate end point in pulmonary arterial hypertension trials. Circulation. 2012;126:349–56.
8. Mathai SC, Puhan MA, Lam D, Wise RA. The minimal important difference in the 6-minute walk test for patients with pulmonary arterial hypertension. Am J Respir Crit Care Med. 2012;186:428–33.
9. Casanova C, Celli BR, Barria P, Casas A, Cote C, de Torres JP, et al. The 6-min walk distance in healthy subjects: reference standards from seven countries. Eur Respir J. 2011;37:150–6.
10. Leuchte HH, Holzapfel M, Baumgartner RA, Neurohr C, Vogeser M, Behr J. Characterization of brain natriuretic peptide in long-term follow-up of pulmonary arterial hypertension. Chest. 2005;128:2368–74.
11. Casserly B, Klinger JR. Brain natriuretic peptide in pulmonary arterial hypertension: biomarker and potential therapeutic agent. Drug Des Devel Ther. 2009;3:269–87.
12. Nagaya N, Nishikimi T, Uematsu M, Satoh T, Kyotani S, Sakamaki F, et al. Plasma brain natriuretic peptide as a prognostic indicator in patients with primary pulmonary hypertension. Circulation. 2000;102:865–70.
13. Mauritz GJ, Rizopoulos D, Groepenhoff H, Tiede H, Felix J, Eilers P, et al. Usefulness of serial N-terminal pro-B-type natriuretic peptide measurements for determining prognosis in patients with pulmonary arterial hypertension. Am J Cardiol. 2011;108:1645–50.
14. Fijalkowska A, Kurzyna M, Torbicki A, Szewczyk G, Florczyk M, Pruszczyk P, et al. Serum N-terminal brain natriuretic peptide as a prognostic parameter in patients with pulmonary hypertension. Chest. 2006;129:1313–21.

Effects of treadmill exercise versus Flutter® on respiratory flow and sputum properties in adults with cystic fibrosis

Tiffany J. Dwyer[1,2,3]*, Rahizan Zainuldin[1,4,5], Evangelia Daviskas[2], Peter T. P. Bye[2,3] and Jennifer A. Alison[1,6]

Abstract

Background: Treadmill exercise and airway clearance with the Flutter® device have previously been shown to improve mucus clearance mechanisms in people with cystic fibrosis (CF) but have not been compared. It is therefore not known if treadmill exercise is an adequate form of airway clearance that could replace established airway clearance techniques, such as the Flutter®. The aim of this study was to evaluate respiratory flow, sputum properties and subjective responses of treadmill exercise and Flutter® therapy, compared to resting breathing (control).

Methods: Twenty-four adults with mild to severe CF lung disease (FEV_1 28–86% predicted) completed a three-day randomised, controlled, cross-over study. Interventions consisted of 20 min of resting breathing (control), treadmill exercise at 60% of the participant's peak oxygen consumption and Flutter® therapy. Respiratory flow was measured during the interventions. Sputum properties (solids content and mechanical impedance) and subjective responses (ease of expectoration and sense of chest congestion) were measured before, immediately after the interventions and after 20 min of recovery.

Results: Treadmill exercise and Flutter® resulted in similar significant increases in peak expiratory flow, but only Flutter® created an expiratory airflow bias (i.e. peak expiratory flow was at least 10% higher than peak inspiratory flow). Treadmill exercise and Flutter® therapy resulted in similar significant reductions in sputum mechanical impedance, but only treadmill exercise caused a transient increase in sputum hydration. Treadmill exercise improved ease of expectoration and Flutter® therapy improved subjective sense of chest congestion.

Conclusions: A single bout of treadmill exercise and Flutter® therapy were equally effective in augmenting mucus clearance mechanisms in adults with CF. Only longer term studies, however, will determine if exercise alone is an adequate form of airway clearance therapy that could replace other airway clearance techniques.

Keywords: Cystic fibrosis, Exercise, Oscillating PEP, Flutter®, Airway clearance, Physiotherapy, Sputum

* Correspondence: tiffany.dwyer@sydney.edu.au
[1]Discipline of Physiotherapy, Faculty of Health Sciences, University of Sydney, Sydney, Australia
[2]Department of Respiratory Medicine, Royal Prince Alfred Hospital, Sydney, Australia
Full list of author information is available at the end of the article

Background

Cystic fibrosis (CF) lung disease is characterised by reduced hydration at the airway surface and dehydrated mucus, [1] resulting in impaired mucus clearance that leads to a cascade of inflammation and progressive lung damage [2]. Interventions to improve mucus clearance are integral to the respiratory management of CF [3].

Most therapies are required daily and adults with CF report spending an average of 108 min on treatment activities each day, the majority of that time performing airway clearance and exercise [4]. Strategies to combine effective interventions to minimise treatment time are needed. Exercise improves physical fitness and may also improve lung function and quality of life in people with CF [5]. If exercise also aids mucus clearance, it would reduce treatment time, as exercise could substitute airway clearance interventions, while gaining the other known benefits of exercise.

Airway clearance or physiotherapy techniques aim to improve mucus clearance by the following mechanisms: altering airflow (increasing the peak expiratory flow and creating an expiratory airflow bias, with the ratio of peak expiratory to peak inspiratory flow, PEF:PIF > 1.10); [6, 7] improving the physical properties of the mucus; [8] potentially increasing airway surface hydration; [9–13] and coughing [14].

Treadmill exercise improves mucus clearance mechanisms in CF by increasing PEF and reducing sputum mechanical impedance [15]. Physiotherapy with a device creating oscillating positive expiratory pressure, the Flutter®, is an established form of airway clearance in CF and is equally effective to other airway clearance techniques [16]. The Flutter® improves mucus clearance

mechanisms in CF by increasing PEF and creating an expiratory airflow bias, [17] as well as reducing sputum mechanical impedance [18]. Exercise and Flutter®, however, have not been compared. Therefore, the aim of this study was to determine the effects of treadmill exercise and Flutter® therapy, compared to resting breathing (control), on respiratory flow (including airflow bias), sputum properties and subjective responses in adults with CF.

Methods

Participants

Participants were recruited from the Adult CF Clinic at Royal Prince Alfred Hospital, Sydney, Australia. Patients were eligible for inclusion if they were at least 17 years old, had a confirmed diagnosis of CF (genetic testing and/or previous positive sweat test results) and their treating physician deemed them to be clinically stable [19]. Patients were excluded if they had received a lung transplant, were infected with *Burkholderia cepacia* complex or were pregnant. Potential participants were volunteers or personally approached by one of the researchers (TJD) at either a routine clinic visit or at the end of a hospital admission. Research procedures were approved by the Sydney South West Area Health Service Ethics Committee (Protocol X08-0175) and participants provided written informed consent prior to trial enrolment.

Study design

The trial was a randomised, cross-over design, registered with the Australian and New Zealand Clinical Trials Registry (#ACTRN12609000168257). The study involved four visits (Fig. 1). On Visit 1, participants' spirometry

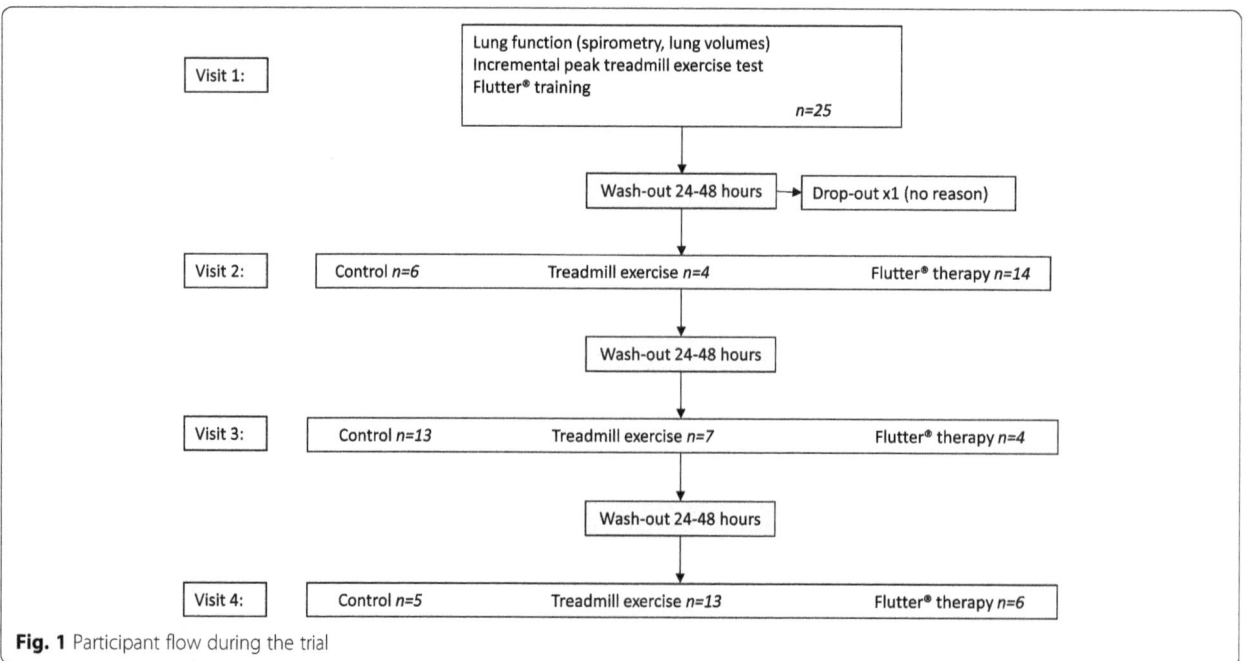

Fig. 1 Participant flow during the trial

and lung volumes (via body plethysmography) (VMax229, SensorMedics, Yorba Linda, USA) were measured according to the American Thoracic Society/European Respiratory Society guidelines [20, 21]. Participants then completed an incremental peak treadmill exercise test, according to a modified Balke protocol, [22] with breath-by-breath measurement of ventilatory and metabolic variables (VMax229 system) and pulse oximetry (Radical^{TM}, Masimo, Irvine, USA). All exercise tests were classified as maximal effort according to the criteria outlined in the CF exercise testing guidelines [23]. Participants were taught to use the Flutter® device (Flutter VRP1 valve®; Axcan Scandipharm Inc., Birmingham, USA) by a senior physiotherapist. If participants were using the Flutter® on a regular basis, any corrections to their technique were made if necessary. After completion of all study procedures on Visit 1, participants were randomised to the order of interventions for the following three sessions (Visits 2, 3 and 4). Intervention order was determined by computer-generated randomisation (with a random integer generator on www.random.org). Randomisation was performed by a person not involved in the interventions on Visits 2, 3 and 4 and stored in sealed, sequentially numbered, opaque envelopes.

On Visits 2, 3 and 4, participants completed the three-day, randomised, cross-over study, according to the data collection procedures in Fig. 2. Visits 2, 3 and 4 were scheduled at the same time in the morning within a one-week period (during which medication, airway clearance and exercise regimens were unchanged). Participants were also asked to withhold routine mucolytic therapy, airway clearance and exercise on the morning of a trial visit. On each Visit 2, 3 and 4, sputum samples were collected immediately before (pre) and after (post + 0) a 20-min intervention, and after a further 20 min of resting breathing/recovery (post + 20). If participants spontaneously expectorated a sputum sample in the five minutes following the intervention (i.e. they were not requested to do so), this was also collected (post + 5). The three interventions were resting breathing (control), constant-load treadmill exercise and Flutter® plus the forced expiratory technique (FET), [24] from now on referred to as "Flutter® therapy".

Treatment interventions

For the control intervention, participants sat quietly for 20 min. For the exercise intervention, participants exercised on the treadmill for 20 min at a constant work rate equivalent to 60% of the peak oxygen consumption (VO$_2$) achieved in the incremental peak treadmill test on Visit 1. This intensity and duration were chosen to replicate a typical prescription used for exercise training [25]. The Flutter® therapy intervention consisted of breathing through the Flutter® for 15 breaths, followed by relaxed and deep breathing, huffing and coughing, according to the FET [24]. This cycle was repeated six times. The Flutter® angle/inclination was chosen for each participant that maximised the sensation of vibrations within the lungs [26] and held in a constant position with a clamp during the intervention. The Flutter® angle was measured with an inclinometer.

Measurements
Respiratory flow

During each 20-min intervention, respiratory flow was measured with a heated pneumotachograph (Hans Rudolf model 3813, Hans Rudolf Inc., Kansas City, USA), calibrated on each occasion, where scaling factors were pre-determined by a rotameter (Model 2000 Fisher Controls, Croydon, England). The Flutter® was attached to the expiratory port of a two-way non-rebreathing valve (2700 series, Hans Rudolf Inc.) in order to collect inspiratory and expiratory flow (i.e. the participant inspired through the pneumotachograph and expired through the pneumotachograph and Flutter®). Data were collected at 125 Hz and flow signals were later analysed by a blinded assessor using custom-made software (PhysioDAQxs v3.0 and Breathalyser v1.0, University of Sydney, Australia) to determine PEF and airflow bias (PEF:PIF) for all interventions, and oscillation frequency during the Flutter® intervention. For the Flutter® intervention, respiratory flow was measured only whilst participants breathed in and out through the Flutter® (i.e. not during the FET component of the intervention).

Sputum properties

Sputum samples were manually separated from saliva and stored in 1.2 mL tubes in a –80 °C freezer. The

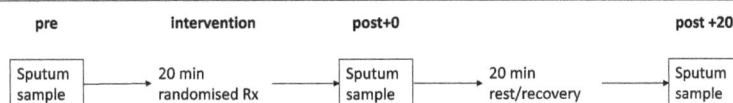

---

	pre	intervention	post+0		post +20
	Sputum sample	→ 20 min randomised Rx →	Sputum sample	→ 20 min rest/recovery →	Sputum sample

Fig. 2 Data collection procedures on Visits 2, 3 and 4. Participants completed visual analogue scores for subjective sense of chest congestion and ease of sputum expectoration with each sputum sample. A sputum sample was also collected five minutes after the intervention (post + 5) if spontaneously expectorated (i.e. it was not requested from participants). Respiratory flow data were collected during the 20 min treatment and coughs were counted during the 20 min treatment and rest/recovery periods

storage tubes were coded, to ensure de-identification at later analysis when measured by a blinded assessor. Sputum analysis procedures were followed as reported previously [15, 27, 28]. The sputum solids content percentage, from which inferences of airway hydration are made, was estimated by measuring the weight of a 50 μL aliquot of sputum before and after lyophilisation to dryness for 24 h using a freeze dryer (Kinetics, Stone Ridge, USA). Sputum elasticity (dynamic G') and viscosity (dynamic G'') were measured using a 20 μL aliquot of sputum and a controlled stress rheometer with geometry 20 mm, 0.5° aluminium cone and plate over the frequency of 1–100 rad/s (AR2000, TA Instruments, New Castle, USA). The results were reported as sputum mechanical impedance (G*), also known as rigidity factor, which is the vector sum of viscosity and elasticity. Sputum mechanical impedance values at 1 rad/s represent sputum properties during resting breathing and mucociliary clearance, values at 100 rad/s represent those during cough and cough clearance.

Cough

All coughs (spontaneous and those directed, according to the FET) were manually counted during each 20-min intervention and recovery period.

Subjective responses

For each requested sputum sample, participants recorded on a 10 cm visual analogue scale the subjective sense of chest congestion (0 = very congested, 10 = very clear) and ease of expectoration (0 = very difficult to expectorate, 10 = very easy to expectorate). The visual analogue scales were later measured by an assessor blinded to the intervention.

Statistical analyses

Repeated measures ANOVA were performed to compare differences between the interventions in subjective responses and sputum properties data. Paired t-tests were used to compare respiratory flow between the interventions. Wilcoxon signed rank tests were used to determine differences between the interventions in the number of coughs, as these data were not normally distributed. Statistical significance was set at $p < 0.05$.

The difference in sputum mechanical impedance between interventions was the primary outcome measure. Data from our previous study showed that 20 participants would be required to provide 80% power to detect the anticipated between group differences as significant for three of the four measures of sputum mechanical impedance (alpha 0.05) [15]. We sought to recruit 25 participants to allow for a 20% dropout and increase precision around our estimates.

Results

Twenty-five adults with mild to severe CF lung disease were recruited and 24 completed the study (one participant withdrew after Visit 1 without giving a reason). Participant baseline characteristics are presented in Tables 1 and 2 [29–32]. Routine mucolytic therapy was: hypertonic saline only for 6 participants; rhDNase only for 9 participants; both hypertonic saline and rhDNase for 7 participants. No participant used mannitol and 2 participants did not use any mucolytic medication. Twenty-one of the 24 participants exercised regularly when well and 22 performed some form of airway clearance routinely (3 only exercised; 1 performed established airway clearance only and 18 performed a combination of exercise and established airway clearance techniques, including 2 who performed Flutter® therapy on a regular basis (see Additional file 1 for full details).

All participants were able to spontaneously expectorate a sputum sample at each requested time point. There were no significant differences in pre-intervention sputum properties or subjective sense of chest congestion and ease of expectoration on Visits 2, 3 and 4, and no carry-over or order effect between interventions was detected (Additional file 1).

Treatment descriptors

Pulse rate, oxygen saturation and treatment descriptors (work rate and perceived intensity during treadmill exercise; [33, 34] Flutter® angle, oscillation frequency and average expiratory pressure) for the 20-min interventions are presented in Table 3. Treadmill exercise was moderate intensity for breathlessness and perceived exertion. All treatments were well-tolerated with no adverse events.

Table 1 Participant characteristics

	Mean ± SD	Range
Age (yr)	30 ± 8	19–48
Sex (F : M)	9 : 15	
BMI (kg/m²)	21.0 ± 2.2	17.1–26.2
FEV₁ (L)	1.81 ± 0.72	0.90–3.40
FEV₁ (predicted %)	51 ± 18	28–86
FVC (predicted %)	71 ± 14	46–98
RV/TLC (%)	40 ± 10	24–57
Treadmill peak VO₂ (mL/kg/min)	30.6 ± 7.8	18.9–50.5
Treadmill peak VO₂ (predicted %)	82 ± 19	48–127

Mean ± standard deviation and range of participant baseline characteristics for the 24 participants who completed the study. Forced expiratory volume in 1 s (FEV₁), forced vital capacity (FVC) [30] and treadmill peak VO₂ [31, 32] expressed as a percentage of predicted values. Residual volume (RV) divided by total lung capacity (TLC) reflects the degree of air trapping

Table 2 Baseline sputum properties and subjective reports

	Mean ± SD	Range
Sputum solids content (%)	6.4 ± 2.6	1.6–13.3
Sputum mechanical impedance (G*) at 1 rad/s (Pa)	21.0 ± 15.9	5.7–59.1
Sputum mechanical impedance (G*) at 100 rad/s (Pa)	174.8 ± 76.7	84.1–396.7
Sense of chest congestion (cm)	5.5 ± 2.4	0.5–9.8
Ease of expectoration (cm)	4.9 ± 2.5	0.1–10.0

Mean ± standard deviation and range of sputum properties and subjective reports for the first sputum sample collected from the 24 participants who completed the study. Sputum mechanical impedance (G*, the vector sum of sputum viscosity and elasticity). Subjective sense of chest congestion (0 = very congested, 10 = very clear) and ease of expectoration (0 = very difficult to expectorate, 10 = very easy to expectorate) scored by participant on a 10 cm visual analogue scale

Mucus clearance mechanisms

Respiratory flow

Peak expiratory flow (PEF) was significantly higher during treadmill exercise and Flutter® compared to control (Table 4). Only Flutter® resulted in an expiratory airflow bias (PEF:PIF > 1.10).

Sputum properties

There were no significant differences in sputum water content, measured by sputum percent solids, between any interventions immediately after (post + 0) or after 20-min recovery (post + 20) (Fig. 3). However, for those who spontaneously expectorated a sputum sample in the five minutes following an intervention (post + 5; $n = 12/15/16$ for control/exercise/Flutter® therapy respectively), treadmill exercise resulted in significantly lower sputum percent solids than control (pre-post + 5 mean difference 1.2%, 95% CI 0.4 to 1.9) and a trend for lower sputum percent solids compared to Flutter® therapy (pre-post + 5 mean difference 1.1%, 95% CI –0.1 to 2.3).

Treadmill exercise resulted in significant reductions in sputum mechanical impedance compared to control both

Table 3 Treatment descriptors

	PR (bpm)	SpO₂ (%)	Treatment descriptors
Control	81 ± 14	96 ± 3	resting breathing
Treadmill	129 ± 18	96 ± 3	5.4 km/h ± 0.7 at 3% incline ± 3, dyspnoea 3 ± 1, RPE 3 ± 2
Flutter®	84 ± 10	97 ± 2	7.3° ± 3.6 at 17.5 Hz ± 1.7, 31 cmH₂O ± 10

Data are presented as mean ± standard deviation for group values of the pulse rate (PR) and oxygen saturation (SpO₂), and treatment descriptors (treadmill speed and incline, modified Borg dyspnoea [34] and modified 0-to-10-point rate of perceived exertion (RPE) [33]; Flutter® angle and oscillation frequency, average expiratory pressure). Treadmill work rate was set at the speed and incline equivalent to 60% of the participant's peak VO₂ achieved on Visit 1 of the study. Flutter® angle (positive numbers represent an inclination above the horizontal at 0°) was set at the inclination determined to be the most effective by the senior physiotherapist on Visit 1 of the study (i.e. that maximised the sensation of vibrations within the lungs)

Table 4 Respiratory flow during the interventions

	PEF (L/s)	PEF:PIF
Control	0.68 ± 0.28	0.85 ± 0.14
Treadmill	1.68* ± 0.51	0.90 ± 0.10
Flutter®	1.53* ± 0.25	1.13* ± 0.37

Data are presented as mean ± standard deviation for group values of peak expiratory flow (PEF) and ratio of peak expiratory to peak inspiratory flow (PEF:PIF). Mean difference and (95% CI): Treadmill v control PEF 1.00 L/s (0.82 to 1.18); Flutter® v control PEF 0.85 L/s (0.69 to 1.01); Flutter® v control PEF:PIF: 0.28 (0.11 to 0.45)
*$p < 0.01$ compared to control

immediately following the intervention (pre-post + 0 mean difference at 1 rad/s 7.1 Pa, 95% CI 1.9 to 12.3; at 100 rad/s 32.5 Pa, 95% CI 5.5 to 59.6) and after 20-min recovery (pre-post + 20 mean difference at 1 rad/s 11.5 Pa, 95% CI 4.0 to 19.1) (Fig. 4). Flutter® therapy resulted in significant reductions in sputum mechanical impedance both immediately following the intervention (pre-post + 0 mean difference 6.4 Pa, 95% CI 0.7 to 12.2) and after 20-min recovery (pre-post + 20 mean difference at 1 rad/s 7.3 Pa, 95% CI 3.3 to 11.2; at 100 rad/s 29.9 Pa, 95% CI 29.9 Pa, 9.0 to 50.9). There were no significant differences in sputum mechanical impedance following treadmill exercise compared to Flutter® therapy.

Cough

There were significantly more coughs during treadmill exercise and Flutter® therapy compared to control, and during Flutter® therapy compared to treadmill exercise (Table 5). Note that participants were instructed to cough 18 times during the FET in the Flutter® therapy intervention. There were no differences between interventions in the number of spontaneous coughs during the 20-min recovery.

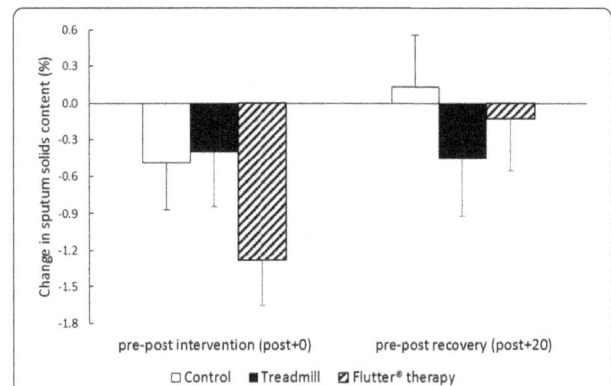

Fig. 3 Change in sputum hydration. Measured by sputum solids content, from pre to post intervention (post + 0) and pre to post recovery (post + 20). A negative change represents an improvement in sputum hydration. Results are group mean and SE for the control (*white*), treadmill exercise (*black*) and Flutter® therapy (diagonal lines) interventions

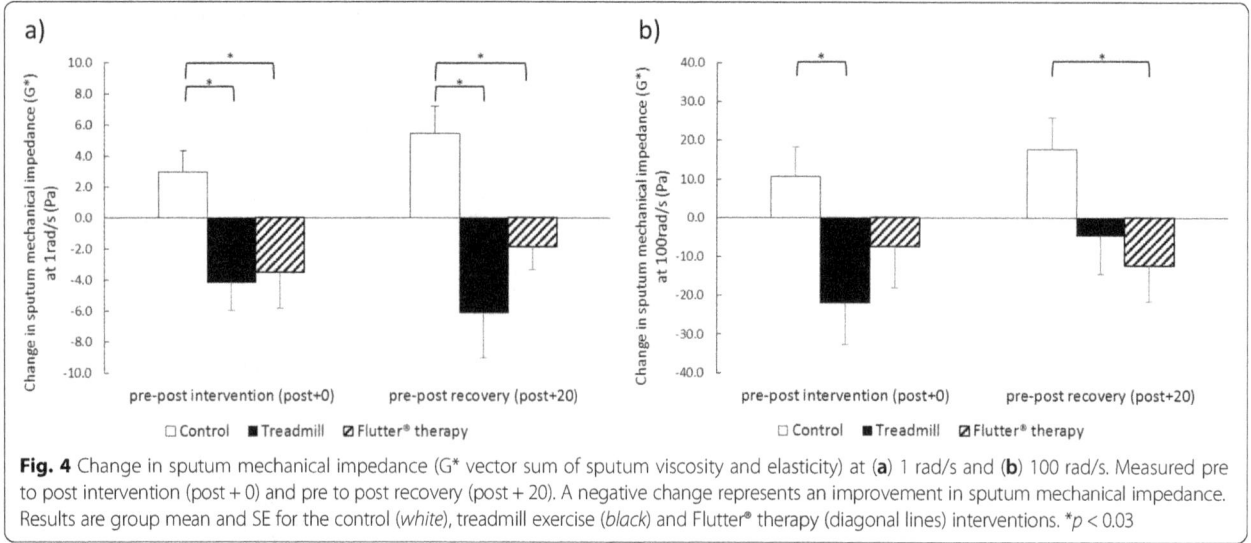

Fig. 4 Change in sputum mechanical impedance (G* vector sum of sputum viscosity and elasticity) at (**a**) 1 rad/s and (**b**) 100 rad/s. Measured pre to post intervention (post + 0) and pre to post recovery (post + 20). A negative change represents an improvement in sputum mechanical impedance. Results are group mean and SE for the control (*white*), treadmill exercise (*black*) and Flutter® therapy (diagonal lines) interventions. *$p < 0.03$

Subjective responses

Treadmill exercise significantly improved subjective ease of expectoration compared to control after 20-min recovery (pre-post + 20 mean difference 1.3 cm, 95% CI 0.3 to 2.3) (Fig. 5a). There were no significant differences in ease of expectoration following Flutter® therapy compared to control or Flutter® therapy compared to treadmill exercise.

There were no significant differences in subjective sense of chest congestion following treadmill exercise compared to control or treadmill exercise compared to Flutter® therapy (Fig. 5b). Flutter® therapy significantly improved subjective sense of chest congestion compared to control both immediately post intervention (pre-post + 0 mean difference 0.8 cm, 95% CI 0.1 to 1.4) and after 20-min recovery (pre-post + 20 mean difference 0.9 cm, 95% CI 0.2 to 1.7).

Discussion

The primary purpose of this study was to compare treadmill exercise and Flutter® therapy on mucus clearance mechanisms in CF. The main findings were that both treadmill exercise and Flutter® resulted in similar significant increases in PEF, but only Flutter® created an expiratory airflow bias. In addition both treadmill

Table 5 Coughs during and following the interventions

	Coughs during intervention	Coughs during recovery
Control	2 (0–5)	1 (0–3)
Treadmill	4* (1–9)	2 (1–5)
Flutter® therapy	24* (18–34)	2 (1–4)

Data are presented as median (interquartile range) for group values of the number of coughs during the 20-min intervention and 20-min resting breathing/recovery period. NB. Participants were instructed to cough 18 times during the Flutter® therapy intervention
*$p < 0.01$ compared to control

exercise and Flutter® therapy resulted in similar significant reductions in sputum mechanical impedance, but only treadmill exercise caused a transient increase in sputum hydration.

The PEF and airflow bias measured during treadmill exercise was similar to that reported by our group previously [15]. The PEF and oscillation frequency measured during Flutter were higher than previously reported by our group (1.53 L/s v 1.13 L/s and 17.5 Hz v 11.3 Hz respectively), yet the airflow bias was similar (1.13 v 1.15), [17] and above the 1.10 threshold proposed to augment annular flow of mucus towards the oropharynx [6]. The higher PEF and oscillation frequency with Flutter® in this study compared to our earlier work may be explained by the Flutter® position. In the earlier study the Flutter® was used in the horizontal position for all participants, [17] however in the current study the Flutter® inclination was individually determined (with an average angle 7.3° above the horizontal). Holding the Flutter® at higher inclinations results in higher oscillations [35, 36].

The reductions in sputum mechanical impedance following treadmill exercise were similar to those reported previously by our group [15]. Different techniques to measure sputum viscosity and elasticity prevented comparing the changes following Flutter® therapy in this study to those reported by other researchers [18]. Our study found no significant difference between treadmill exercise and Flutter® therapy in the reductions in sputum mechanical impedance, suggesting that the combined effects of shearing forces and airway oscillations with the two interventions were similar.

There was no change in sputum hydration immediately following treadmill exercise or after 20 min of recovery, similar to our previous study [15]. However, we found a significant reduction in sputum solids content in the five minutes following treadmill exercise but

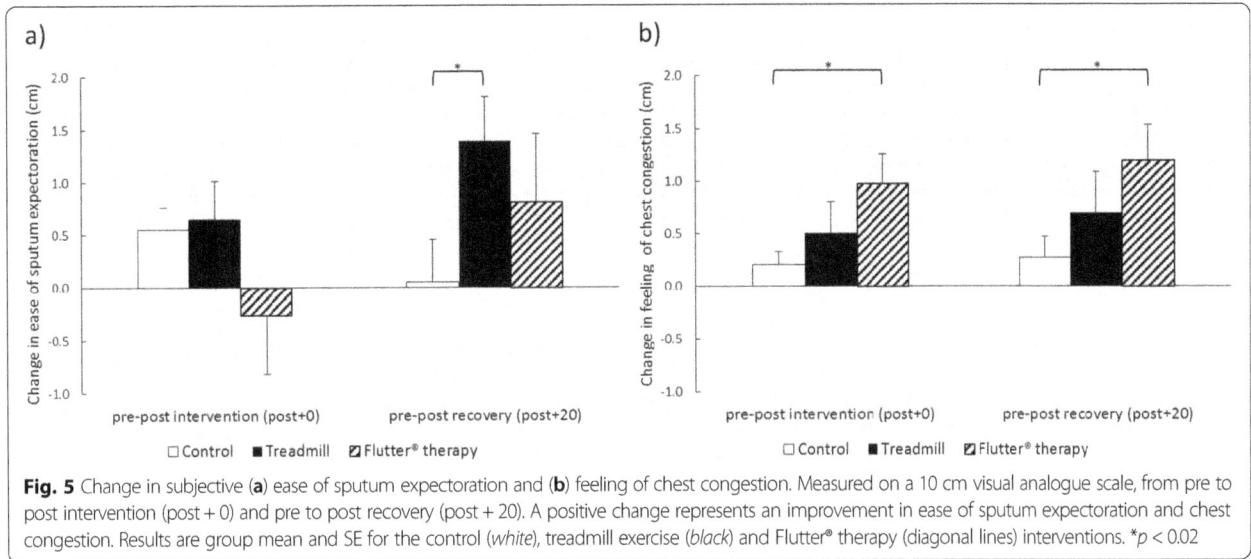

Fig. 5 Change in subjective (**a**) ease of sputum expectoration and (**b**) feeling of chest congestion. Measured on a 10 cm visual analogue scale, from pre to post intervention (post + 0) and pre to post recovery (post + 20). A positive change represents an improvement in ease of sputum expectoration and chest congestion. Results are group mean and SE for the control (*white*), treadmill exercise (*black*) and Flutter® therapy (diagonal lines) interventions. *$p < 0.02$

not after Flutter® therapy. Previously researchers have shown an inhibition of sodium conductance channels [11, 12, 37] and altered ion regulation with submaximal cycle exercise in adults with CF [13], suggesting improved airway hydration or airway surface liquid, however these changes only lasted for four minutes after ceasing exercise [37]. Our study provides some evidence to support the proposed increase in mucus water content with exercise in CF [10–12]. The 1.2% reduction in sputum solids content that we observed is likely to be clinically significant as it is similar to that achieved with mannitol in people with CF, [28] which results in significant improvements in mucus clearance [38] and lung function in the long term [39].

Consistent with the improved changes in sputum properties, participants reported significant improvements in ease of expectoration following treadmill exercise but not following Flutter® therapy. Alternately, participants reported significant improvements in subjective sense of chest congestion following Flutter® therapy but not following treadmill exercise. We did not measure the amount of sputum expectorated, as this would have interfered with sputum rheology and solids content measurements. Perhaps treadmill exercise facilitated sputum expectoration (due to increased PEF and reduced sputum mechanical impedance), but participants did not spontaneously expectorate sufficient sputum to feel less chest congestion. Also, potentially the format of the FET during Flutter® treatment (18 directed coughs in 20 min) increased the amount of sputum expectorated (and hence sensation of less chest congestion), but it was a taxing treatment and so participants did not consider it easier to expectorate.

Conclusions

A single bout of moderate-intensity treadmill exercise and Flutter® therapy improved mucus clearance mechanisms in adults with CF. Both treatments increased PEF, but only Flutter® created an expiratory airflow bias. Both treatments resulted in similar significant reductions in sputum mechanical impedance, however only treadmill exercise created a significant transient reduction in sputum solids content. It would therefore appear that treadmill exercise and Flutter® therapy are equally effective in augmenting mucus clearance mechanisms in adults with CF. Physiological or mechanistic findings on their own, however, are insufficient to implement changes to clinical practice. Studies that directly measure mucus and mucociliary clearance or longer term studies with clinically important outcomes (such as exacerbation frequency, antibiotic use, quality of life and lung function) are required to ascertain the relative merit of these interventions and to determine if people with CF can use exercise alone as an adequate form of airway clearance therapy.

Abbreviations
CF: cystic fibrosis; FET: forced expiratory technique; FEV$_1$: forced expiratory volume in 1 s; G*: sputum mechanical impedance; PEF: peak expiratory flow; PIF: peak inspiratory flow; RPE: rate of perceived exertion; RV: residual volume; Rx: treatment; TLC: total lung capacity; VO$_2$: oxygen consumption

Acknowledgements
Thank you to John Eisenhuth (Faculty of Health Sciences, University of Sydney, Sydney, Australia) for developing the PhysioDAQxs v3.0 and Breathalyser v1.0.

Funding
The Australian Respiratory Council funded the study. The Australian Respiratory Council had no input or contribution to the design of the study and collection, analysis, and interpretation of data and in writing the manuscript.

Authors' contributions

TJD, PTPB and JAA were involved in the conception and design of the study. TJD and RZ were responsible for data acquisition. TJD and ED were responsible for the sputum analyses and interpretation. TJD was responsible for data and statistical analyses. TJD and JAA were responsible for interpretation of findings. TJD was responsible for drafting the manuscript. All authors were involved in revising, critically appraising and providing final approval of the published version and agree to be accountable for all aspects of the work.

Competing interests

The authors declare that they have no competing interests.

Author details

[1]Discipline of Physiotherapy, Faculty of Health Sciences, University of Sydney, Sydney, Australia. [2]Department of Respiratory Medicine, Royal Prince Alfred Hospital, Sydney, Australia. [3]Central Clinical School, Sydney Medical School, University of Sydney, Sydney, Australia. [4]Rehabilitation Department, Ng Teng Fong General Hospital, Jurong Health Services, Jurong East, Singapore. [5]Health and Social Sciences, Academic Programme, Singapore Institute of Technology, Jurong East, Singapore. [6]Department of Physiotherapy, Royal Prince Alfred Hospital, Sydney, Australia.

References

1. Matsui H, et al. Evidence for periciliary liquid layer depletion, not abnormal ion composition, in the pathogenesis of cystic fibrosis airways disease. Cell. 1998;95(7):1005–15.
2. Robinson M, Bye PTB. Mucociliary clearance in cystic fibrosis. Pediatr Pulmonol. 2002;33(4):293–306.
3. Dodd ME, Prasad SA. Physiotherapy management of cystic fibrosis. Chron Respir Dis. 2005;2(3):139–49.
4. Sawicki GS, Sellers DE, Robinson WM. High treatment burden in adults with cystic fibrosis: challenges to disease self-management. J Cyst Fibros. 2009;8(2):91–6.
5. Radtke T, et al. Physical exercise training for cystic fibrosis. Cochrane Database Syst Rev. 2015;6, CD002768.
6. Kim CS, Iglesias AJ, Sackner MA. Mucus clearance by two-phase gas–liquid flow mechanism: Asymmetric periodic flow model. J Appl Physiol. 1987;62(3):959–71.
7. Olseni L, Lannefors L, van der Schans CP. Airway-clearance techniques individually tailored to each patient, in Therapy for mucus-clearance disorders. Rubin BK and van der Schans CP, Editors. Therapy for mucus-clearance disorders. New York: Marcel Dekker, Inc; 2004. p. 413–431.
8. King M. Role of mucus viscoelasticity in clearance by cough. Eur J Respir Dis Suppl. 1987;153:165–72.
9. Button B, Boucher RC, University of North Carolina Virtual Lung Group. Role of mechanical stress in regulating airway surface hydration and mucus clearance rates. Respir Physiol Neurobiol. 2008;163(1–3):189–201.
10. Button B, Picher M, Boucher RC. Differential effects of cyclic and constant stress on ATP release and mucociliary transport by human airway epithelia. J Physiol. 2007;580(2):577–92.
11. Hebestreit A, et al. Exercise inhibits epithelial sodium channels in patients with cystic fibrosis. Am J Respir Crit Care Med. 2001;164(3):443–6.
12. Schmitt L, et al. Exercise reduces airway sodium ion reabsorption in cystic fibrosis but not in exercise asthma. Eur Respir J. 2011;37(2):342–8.
13. Wheatley CM, et al. Moderate intensity exercise mediates comparable increases in exhaled chloride as albuterol in individuals with cystic fibrosis. Respir Med. 2015;109(8):1001–11.
14. Mellins RB. Pulmonary physiotherapy in the pediatric age group. Am Rev Respir Dis. 1974;110(6 Pt 2):137–42.
15. Dwyer TJ, et al. Effects of exercise on respiratory flow and sputum properties in cystic fibrosis. Chest. 2011;139(4):870–7.
16. Morrison L, Agnew J. Oscillating devices for airway clearance in people with cystic fibrosis. Cochrane Database Syst Rev. 2014;7, CD006842.
17. McCarren B, Alison JA. Physiological effects of vibration in subjects with cystic fibrosis. Eur Respir J. 2006;27(6):1204–9.
18. App EM, et al. Sputum rheology changes in cystic fibrosis lung disease following two different types of physiotherapy: flutter vs autogenic drainage. Chest. 1998;114(1):171–7.
19. Fuchs HJ, et al. Effect of aerosolized recombinant human DNase on exacerbations of respiratory symptoms and on pulmonary function in patients with cystic fibrosis. N Engl J Med. 1994;331(10):637–42.
20. Miller MR, et al. Standardisation of spirometry. Eur Respir J. 2005;26(2):319–38.
21. Wanger J, et al. Standardisation of the measurement of lung volumes. Eur Respir J. 2005;26(3):511–22.
22. Balke B, Ware RW. An experimental study of physical fitness of Air Force personnel. U S Armed Forces Med J. 1959;10(6):675–88.
23. Hebestreit H, et al. Statement on Exercise Testing in Cystic Fibrosis. Respiration. 2015;90(4):332–51.
24. Pryor J. The forced expiration technique, in Respiratory Care. Pryor J, Editor. Respiratory care. Edinburgh: Churchill Livingstone; 1991. p. 79–100.
25. American College of Sports Medicine. ACSM's guidelines for exercise testing and prescription. 9th ed. Philadelphia: Wolters Kluwer/Lippincott Williams & Wilkins Health; 2014.
26. Konstan MW, Stern RC, Doershuk CF. Efficacy of the Flutter device for airway mucus clearance in patients with cystic fibrosis. J Pediatr. 1994;124(5 Pt 1):689–93.
27. Daviskas E, Anderson SD, Young IH. Inhaled mannitol changes the sputum properties in asthmatics with mucus hypersecretion. Respirology. 2007;12(5):683–91.
28. Daviskas E, et al. Inhaled mannitol improves the hydration and surface properties of sputum in patients with cystic fibrosis. Chest. 2010;137(4):861–8.
29. Goldman HI, Becklake MR. Respiratory function tests; normal values at median altitudes and the prediction of normal results. Am Rev Tuberc. 1959;79(4):457–67.
30. Morris JF, Koski A, Johnson LC. Spirometric standards for healthy nonsmoking adults. Am Rev Respir Dis. 1971;103(1):57–67.
31. Drinkwater BL, Horvath SM, Wells CL. Aerobic power of females, ages 10 to 68. J Gerontol. 1975;30(4):385–94.
32. Froelicher Jr VF, Allen M, Lancaster MC. Maximal treadmill testing of normal USAF aircrewmen. Aerosp Med. 1974;45(3):310–5.
33. Borg GA. Psychophysical bases of perceived exertion. Med Sci Sports Exerc. 1982;14(5):377–81.
34. Mahler DA, et al. Continuous measurement of breathlessness during exercise: validity, reliability, and responsiveness. J Appl Physiol. 2001;90(6):2188–96.
35. Alves LA, Pitta F, Brunetto AF. Performance analysis of the Flutter VRP1 under different flows and angles. Respir Care. 2008;53(3):316–23.
36. Brooks D, et al. The flutter device and expiratory pressures. J Cardiopulm Rehabil. 2002;22(1):53–7.
37. Alsuwaidan S, et al. Effect of exercise on the nasal transmucosal potential difference in patients with cystic fibrosis and normal subjects. Thorax. 1994;49(12):1249–50.
38. Robinson M, et al. The effect of inhaled mannitol on bronchial mucus clearance in cystic fibrosis patients: a pilot study. Eur Respir J. 1999;14(3):678–85.
39. Nolan SJ, et al. Inhaled mannitol for cystic fibrosis. Cochrane Database Syst Rev. 2015;10, CD008649.

Successful treatment of severe *Pneumocystis* pneumonia in an immunosuppressed patient using caspofungin combined with clindamycin

Hongjuan Li[1*], Haoming Huang[2] and Hangyong He[3*]

Abstract

Background: *Pneumocystis jirovecii* is responsible for *Pneumocystis* pneumonia (PCP), which occurs almost exclusively in immunocompromised individuals. Trimethoprim-sulfamethoxazole (TMP-SMZ) is regarded as the first-line treatment and prophylaxis for *P. jirovecii* infection, but the frequency of adverse reactions and newly emerged antibiotic resistance limit its use.

Case presentation: Ulcerations and hemorrhages involving the tongue were noted secondary to TMP-SMZ desensitization against PCP in a 46-year-old male who had previously been diagnosed with IgA nephropathy and sustained prolonged corticosteroid therapy. There was an urgent need for an alternative regimen due to the severe response to TMP-SMZ. The patient was successfully treated with a combination therapy of caspofungin and clindamycin.

Conclusion: Caspofungin combined with clindamycin is an optional treatment for PCP when treatment with TMP-SMZ fails or in patients who cannot tolerate TMP-SMZ.

Keywords: *Pneumocystis* pneumonia, Caspofungin, Clindamycin

Background

Pneumocystis pneumonia (PCP) is an opportunistic infection caused by *Pneumocystis jirovecii*, which mainly occurs when cellular immunity is depressed because of AIDS, malignancies, prolonged corticosteroid therapy, or organ transplantation. Recent research has indicated that underlying renal dysfunction and chronic renal pathology are risk factors for PCP in patients with IgA nephropathy [1]. The PCP mortality rate is high among patients with delayed diagnosis and treatment, and death is due to severe respiratory failure [2, 3].

The first-line medication of treatment and prophylaxis for *P. jirovecii* infection is trimethoprim-sulfamethoxazole (TMP-SMZ) [4]; however, use of TMP-SMZ could be problematic in patients with adverse reactions and drug resistance. Caspofungin-based therapy has been shown to be effective against *Pneumocystis* in animal models of PCP [5–7]; however, the clinical experience with caspofungin in human PCP are limited and controversial. Herein, we report a case involving salvage therapy with caspofungin and clindamycin in the successful management of an immunosuppressed PCP patient who was allergic to TMP-SMZ.

Case presentation

A 46-year-old male had been diagnosed with IgA nephropathy based on renal biopsy 3 months before admission. A concurrent diagnosis of chronic kidney dysfunction was

* Correspondence: lihon-002@163.com; yonghang2004@sina.com
[1]Department of Emergency, Guangdong Hospital of Traditional Chinese Medicine, Guangzhou, Guangdong 510105, China
[3]Department of Respiratory and Critical Care Medicine, Beijing Chao-Yang Hospital, Capital Medical University, Beijing 100020, China
Full list of author information is available at the end of the article

established. He was treated with cyclophosphamide and high-dose methylprednisolone, followed by methylprednisolone (40 mg orally per day) for maintenance. He also had hypertension, diabetes mellitus, gout, and leukoderma. He was shown to be allergic to TMP-SMZ when treated for a respiratory infection some years before. The allergic reaction manifested as ulcerations involving the tongue and genitalia, which resolved gradually with discontinuation of TMP-SMZ.

The patient had a fever of 38 °C and sought medical care at a local clinic with complaints of fever, chills, wheezing, and a productive cough. No significant findings were noted on chest X-ray (Fig. 1), and the patient was offered symptomatic treatment and discharged. He returned to the local clinic one week later because of worsening symptoms. Arterial blood gas analysis showed type I respiratory failure. A thoracic computed tomography (CT) scan reported bilateral lung infiltrates with ground-glass attenuation (Fig. 2a). The temperature climbed to 40 °C and the patient was then transferred to the respiratory intensive care unit (RICU).

After transfer to the RICU (day 1), the patient received non-invasive positive pressure ventilation (NIPPV) for respiratory support with continuous positive airway pressure at 4 cmH$_2$O (FiO$_2$ 50 %), and high-flow nasal cannula oxygen supplement (FiO$_2$ 50 %) between gaps. Chest auscultation demonstrated bibasilar crepitation.

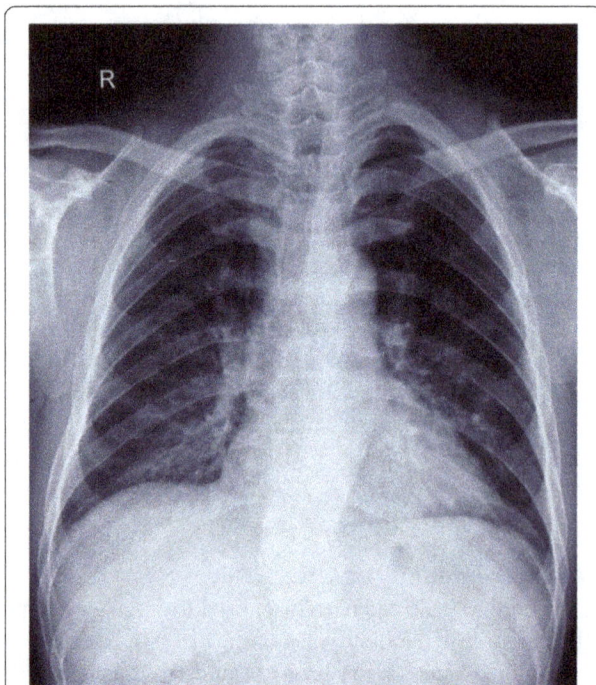

Fig. 1 Posteroanterior chest X-ray image one week before the patient's transfer to the respiratory intensive care unit (RICU). No significant finding was observed on the X-ray image at this date (December 2015)

An arterial blood sample was acquired under NIPPV support (FiO$_2$ 50 %), and blood gas analysis showed the following: pH, 7.39; PaCO$_2$, 36 mmHg; PaO$_2$, 88 mmHg; and A-a O$_2$ gradient, 68 mmHg. The leukocyte count was 12.2×10^9/L. The procalcitonin level was 22.09 ng/ml. Other laboratory findings included the following: serum urea nitrogen, 30.83 mmol/L; serum creatinine, 478.50 umol/L; potassium, 5.3 mmol/L; and lactic acid dehydrogenase, 729 U/L. The serum 1,3-β-D-glucan level was > 1000 pg/ml (beyond the testing range). The CD4$^+$ T-cell count was 46 cells/mm^3. HIV was excluded by real-time polymerase chain reaction (PCR) analysis. *Pneumocystis jirovecii* was visualized under light microscopy in both induced sputum and bronchoalveolar lavage fluid (BALF) with Gomori methenamine silver staining. Cytomegalovirus (CMV)-pp65 antigen and CMV-DNA were positive in blood samples. Induced sputum and BALF were collected for real-time PCR analysis, yielding positive *P. jirovecii* DNA and CMV-DNA. A high-resolution CT (HRCT) scan on day 14 demonstrated aggravation of the bilateral lower lobe consolidation (Fig. 2b).

Because of the low oxygen index (PaO$_2$/FiO$_2$ = 166 mmHg) and infiltrates, the patient was thought to have developed moderate acute respiratory distress syndrome (ARDS), and a 21-day adjunctive corticosteroid therapy was initiated on day 1. Methylprednisolone (80 mg IVggt qd) was administered for the first 5 days, then tapered to 40 mg IVggt qd for another 5 days, and 20 mg po qd for 11 days more. Because the patient was allergic to TMP-SMZ which is a first-line choice for PCP, a TMP-SMZ desensitization protocol (0.12 g po q6h for 2 days, 0.48 g q6h for 2 days, and 0.96 g q6h for 2 days) was instituted on day 2. Ulcers and hemorrhages were observed on the left side of the tongue on day 7, which was believed to be an adverse reaction to TMP-SMZ. Therefore, TMP-SMZ therapy was abandoned on day 7, and was subsequently replaced by a 21-day combination therapy of caspofungin (50 mg IVggt qd) and clindamycin (0.3 g IVggt q6h) from days 8 to 28. Ganciclovir was added to cover CMV infection. Other pathogens, such as bacteria, could not be excluded in this case, thus cefoperazone-sulbactam and moxifloxacin were added empirically.

The patient's condition gradually remitted and the oxygen index improved. The patient was transferred back to the general ward on day 33. The 1,3-β-D-glucan levels and absolute cell counts of T-cell subsets were carefully monitored. The CD4$^+$ T-cell count decreased when TMP-SMZ was discontinued, but gradually normalized, which was accompanied by a decreasing 1,3-β-D-glucan level (Fig. 3). *Pneumocystis jirovecii* was undetectable microscopically in induced sputum on day 9. The PCR became negative for

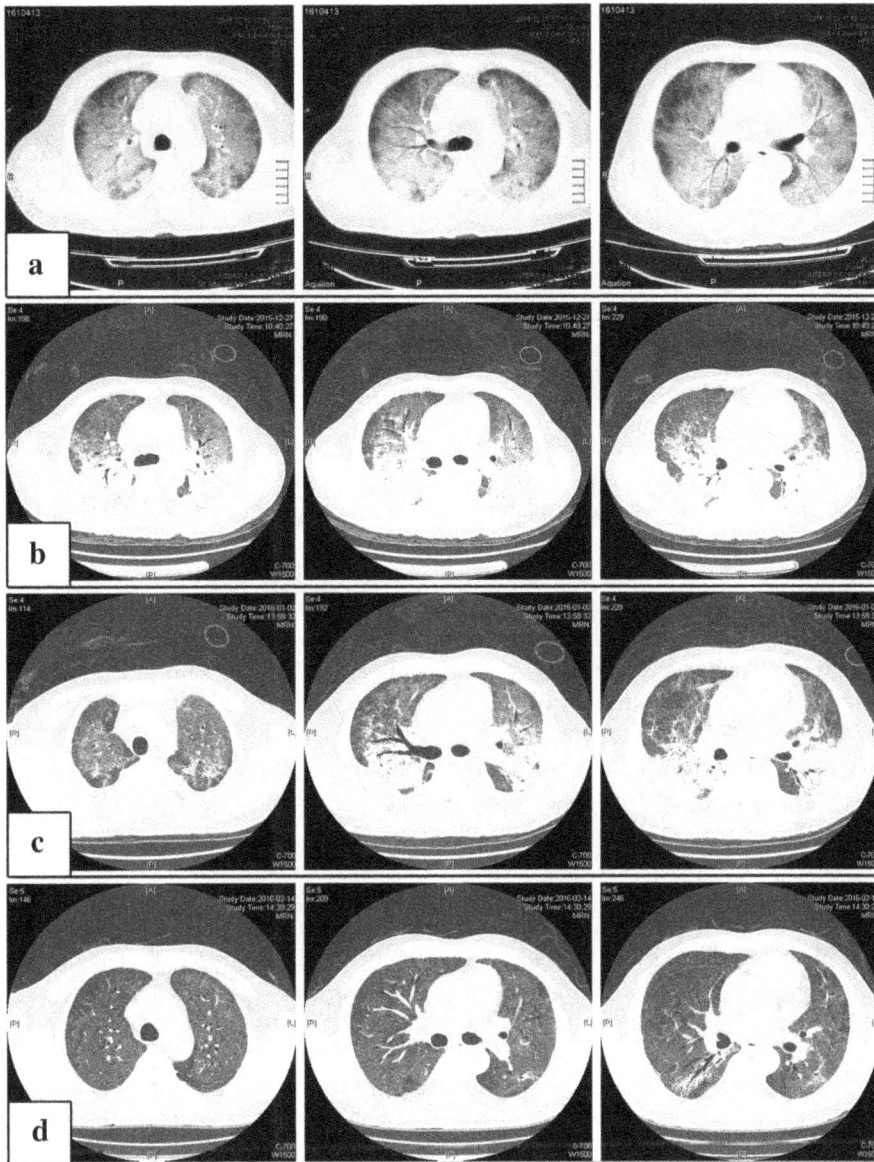

Fig. 2 High resolution CT scans of the chest at the levels of aortic arch, root of ascending aorta and pulmonary arteries from left to right, performed from top to down on days 1 (**a**: December 2015), 14 (**b**: December 2015), 20 (**c**: January 2016) and 90 (**d**: February 2016). Bilateral lung infiltrates with ground-glass attenuation (**a**). Bilateral infiltrates and dense consolidations aggravated (**b**). Minimal absorption compared to day 14 (**c**). Dense consolidations were significantly absorbed (**d**)

sputum *P. jirovecii* and CMV-DNA on days 13 and 29, respectively. On day 20, HRCT revealed that the upper lobe infiltrates and dense consolidations in the lower lobes were absorbed compared to the last scan (Fig. 2c). A follow-up HRCT was arranged on day 90, which showed significant absorption of the dense consolidations (Fig. 2d). The symptoms were nearly relieved by the time he was discharged, with the exception of occasional coughing. Because the patient restored his normal CD4$^+$ T-cell count, secondary prophylaxis for PCP was not needed.

Discussion

Pneumocystis jirovecii (formerly *Pneumocystis carinii*) was initially classified as a protozoan parasite, and molecular and genetic evidence categorized *P. jirovecii* among the fungi. Although *Pneumocystis* cannot be cultivated on standard artificial media and the lifecycle of the organism is unclear, *Pneumocystis* does share some biological characteristics with protozoa. Indeed, two apparently distinctive forms can be observed under microscope (trophic and cystic forms) [8]. Although trophic forms are predominant in infected tissues, glucans are only found in cystic forms [9].

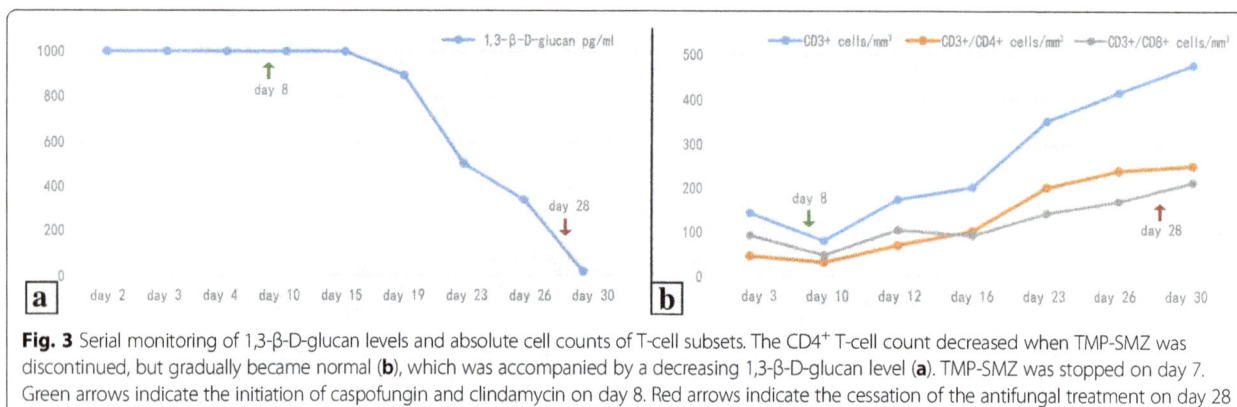

Fig. 3 Serial monitoring of 1,3-β-D-glucan levels and absolute cell counts of T-cell subsets. The CD4+ T-cell count decreased when TMP-SMZ was discontinued, but gradually became normal (**b**), which was accompanied by a decreasing 1,3-β-D-glucan level (**a**). TMP-SMZ was stopped on day 7. Green arrows indicate the initiation of caspofungin and clindamycin on day 8. Red arrows indicate the cessation of the antifungal treatment on day 28

Clinical manifestations, and laboratory and imaging studies are not pathognomonic in PCP, thus a heightened clinical suspicion should be maintained in patients known to be HIV-infected and immunosuppressed. HRCT may be valuable in assessing lung injury and the severity of PCP [10, 11]. A definitive diagnosis of PCP requires the detection of trophic and/or cystic forms of *P. jirovecii* at direct microscopic examination of lower respiratory tract samples, such as induced sputum, BALF and lung biopsy specimens [4]. With the development of PCR technology, especially real-time PCR assays, the detection of *P. jirovecii* DNA in respiratory samples has become an essential part of the laboratory diagnosis of PCP [4, 12]. Nevertheless, due to its high sensitivity, PCR may allow detection of *P. jirovecii* in latent infections without PCP, which decreases its specificity [13].

All polysaccharides of the fungal cell wall are different from those produced by mammalian cells. Among them, 1,3-β-D-glucan is a reliable adjunctive diagnostic marker for PCP, but not a prognosis predictor [14]; negative results are useful to rule out PCP in HIV patients [15]. Nevertheless, Kamada et al. [16] reported an HIV-infected patient with PCP and normal 1,3-β-D-glucan levels throughout the course of infection, which might reflect an early phase infection with limited lung injury. Interpreting 1,3-β-D-glucan results among non-HIV individuals should be done with care and in parallel with other clinical findings [15]. Furthermore, 1,3-β-D-glucan could be elevated in other invasive fungal diseases and may obscure the diagnosis.

In HIV-infected patients, PCP rarely occurs when the CD4+ T-cell count is > 200 cells/mm^3 [17]. Moreover, CD4+ T-cell counts are of concern when initiating and discontinuing PCP prophylaxis in HIV-infected individuals [4]. Yet, consensus about CD4+ T-cell counts has not been well-established towards PCP unrelated to HIV. Nevertheless, non-HIV patients with CD4+ T-cell counts < 200 cells/mm^3 appear to be at increased risk for developing PCP [18], thus it is reasonable to monitor CD4+ T-cell counts in such patients.

TMP-SMZ, an antibiotic used to treat a variety of infections, is the first-line drug for PCP prophylaxis and treatment, but treatment failure may occur because of dihydropteroate synthase and dihydrofolate reductase mutations during the course of the treatment [19, 20]. Adverse effects of TMP-SMZ are also common, such as fever, rash, nausea, vomiting, transaminase elevation, and more serious toxicities, including neutropenia, thrombocytopenia, Stevens-Johnson syndrome, and toxic epidermal necrolysis [21]. With mild adverse reactions, TMP-SMZ should be continued with a gradual dose increment (desensitization) or at a reduced dose or frequency. TMP-SMZ therapy should be aborted in patients with possible or definite life-threatening reactions [4].

Echinocandins are antifungal agents that noncompetitively inhibit 1,3-β-D-glucan synthase [22]. Thus, echinocandins are toxic to fungi in which the glucans play an important role in maintaining the integrity of the fungal cell wall [22] and partly contribute to the host inflammatory response in the lung [23]. Caspofungin used alone or with low-dose TMP-SMZ has been shown to be efficient in treating PCP on experimental animal PCP models [5, 6]. Unlike TMP-SMZ, which primarily eliminates trophic forms of *Pneumocystis*, caspofungin clears cystic forms which might play a key role in transmission [7]. Nevertheless, the clinical use of echinocandins, such as caspofungin, against *P. jirovecii* infection is still controversial. Utili et al. [24] reported 4 cases of solid organ transplant recipients infected by PCP who were treated by caspofungin and TMP-SMZ with favorable outcomes. While Utili et al. [24] summarized 8 reported cases involving echinocandin-containing regimens for PCP before 2007, two lymphoblastic leukemia patients died in spite of prolonged echinocandin treatment in addition to other anti-*Pneumocystis* therapies. In a retrospective analysis among 80 HIV-PCP patients, 10 of whom had confirmed PCP microbiologically, received caspofungin-based salvage therapies, and showed satisfactory outcomes, one patient died with bilateral pneumothoraces [25].

Clindamycin combined with primaquine has activity against *P. jirovecii*, although the mechanism is still unclear. In protozoa, clindamycin targets protein synthesis in a parasite-specific organelle (the apicoplast) [26], which is related to mitochondrial function and the lifecycle of the organism. In addition, reduction of protein and nucleic acid synthesis has been observed in *Plasmodium falciparum* when exposed to clindamycin [27]. Primaquine could interfere with the microbial electron transport system by generating quinone metabolites and superoxides in vivo [28], which may prevent the proliferation of *P. jirovecii*. A previous study by Queener et al. [29] demonstrated a higher efficacy of clindamycin combined with primaquine compared to the use of each drug alone for treatment and prophylaxis of PCP in rat models. Clindamycin/primaquine regimens, the clinical efficacy of which have been proven by clinical trial [30], appear to have the highest efficacy among alternative therapies for PCP [31] and are now used as second-line therapy in PCP management [4].

A moderate-to-severe PCP infection is defined as a PaO_2 < 70 mmHg at room air or an A-a O_2 gradient $\geq$ 35 mmHg [4]. Because our patient's blood gas analysis was tested under NIPPV, the severity of PCP had to be evaluated with all of the clinical findings. In the current case, this middle-aged man, who had undergone prolonged corticosteroid therapy for an underlying IgA nephropathy, was diagnosed with PCP and developed ARDS. The adjunctive corticosteroid dose needed to be individualized to balance anti-inflammatory against immunosuppressed effects. Thus, we began high-dose methylprednisolone tapering. The patient failed desensitization to TMP-SMZ. Given that primaquine is not routinely available in our hospital, alternative therapy with caspofungin plus clindamycin was initiated. The only report of concomitant use of caspofungin with clindamycin for PCP involves a patient who did not respond to combination therapy and the infection was eventually controlled following TMP-SMZ desensitization [32]. Our patient showed an impressive response to the treatment and ultimately recovered.

Because the microscopic images of respiratory tract specimens were not attached to the patient's documents, we have no way to determine how the trophic and cystic forms changed during the course of treatment, but elevated 1,3-β-D-glucan levels implied that cysts had been producing glucans on which caspofungin might have an effect. The efficacy of clindamycin could not be determined clearly in our case. Given that clindamycin improves the outcome together with primaquine, the efficacy with caspofungin may warrant further investigation. Our patient showed a concomitant CMV infection and received ganciclovir for the treatment, while clinical study suggested that concomitant CMV infection in non-HIV related PCP did not affect prognosis and antiviral drugs might be unnecessary [33].

Conclusion
In summary, this new combination therapy of caspofungin plus clindamycin in managing PCP may be considered in patients who fail standard treatment. Monitoring 1,3-β-D-glucan is of more convenience than other forms of testing, such as BALF, and may provide early diagnostic clues. Based on our case and a review of the literature, we suggest that highly elevated 1,3-β-D-glucan levels may be a predictor of a satisfactory caspofungin response to PCP.

Abbreviations
ARDS: Acute respiratory distress syndrome; BALF: Bronchoalveolar lavage fluid; CMV: Cytomegalovirus; CT: Computed tomography; HRCT: High-resolution computed tomography; NIPPV: Non-invasive positive pressure ventilation; PCP: *Pneumocystis* pneumonia; PCR: Polymerase chain reaction; RICU: Respiratory intensive care unit; TMP-SMZ: Trimethoprim-sulfamethoxazole

Acknowledgments
We are grateful to Prof. Junling Zuo from Guangzhou University of Traditional Chinese Medicine for his instructions and inspiring guidance.

Funding
No funding has been received for this project.

Authors' contributions
HL and HYH were the physicians involved in the follow-up of the patient. HMH and HL were responsible for the initial manuscript writing. HYH revised the manuscript. All authors read and approved the final manuscript.

Competing interests
The authors declare that they have no competing interests.

Author details
[1]Department of Emergency, Guangdong Hospital of Traditional Chinese Medicine, Guangzhou, Guangdong 510105, China. [2]Department of Emergency, Guangzhou University of Traditional Chinese Medicine First Affiliated Hospital, Guangzhou, Guangdong 510405, China. [3]Department of Respiratory and Critical Care Medicine, Beijing Chao-Yang Hospital, Capital Medical University, Beijing 100020, China.

References
1. Ye W-L, Tang N, Wen Y-B, Li H, Li M-X, Bin D, Li X-M. Underlying renal insufficiency: the pivotal risk factor for *Pneumocystis jirovecii* pneumonia in immunosuppressed patients with non-transplant glomerular disease. Int Urol Nephrol. 2016. doi:10.1007/s11255-016-1324-x.
2. Boonsarngsuk V, Sirilak S, Kiatboonsri S. Acute respiratory failure due to *Pneumocystis* pneumonia: outcome and prognostic factors. Int J Infect Dis. 2008;13:59–66.
3. Li M-C, Lee N-Y, Lee C-C, Lee H-C, Chang C-M, Ko W-C. *Pneumocystis jiroveci* pneumonia in immunocompromised patients: delayed diagnosis and poor outcomes in non-HIV-infected individuals. J Microbiol Immunol Infect. 2012;47:42–7.
4. Kaplan JE, Benson C, Holmes KK, Brooks JT, Pau A, Masur H. Guidelines for prevention and treatment of opportunistic infections in HIV-infected adults and adolescents: recommendations from CDC, the National Institutes of

Health, and the HIV Medicine Association of the Infectious Diseases Society of America. MMWR Recomm Rep. 2009;58:1–198.

5. Sun P, Tong Z. Efficacy of caspofungin, a 1,3-β-D-glucan synthase inhibitor, on *Pneumocystis carinii* pneumonia in rats. Med Mycol. 2014;52:798–803.

6. Lobo ML, Esteves F, de Sousa B, Cardoso F, Cushion MT, Antunes F, Matos O. Therapeutic potential of caspofungin combined with trimethoprim-sulfamethoxazole for *Pneumocystis* pneumonia: a pilot study in mice. PLoS ONE. 2013;8:e70619.

7. Cushion MT, Linke MJ, Ashbaugh A, Sesterhenn T, Collins MS, Lynch K, Brubaker R, Walzer PD. Echinocandin treatment of *pneumocystis* pneumonia in rodent models depletes cysts leaving trophic burdens that cannot transmit the infection. PLoS ONE. 2010;5:e8524.

8. Wyder MA, Rasch EM, Kaneshiro ES. Quantitation of absolute *Pneumocystis carinii* nuclear DNA content. Trophic and cystic forms isolated from infected rat lungs are haploid organisms. J Eukaryot Microbiol. 1998;45:233–9.

9. Nollstadt KH, Powles MA, Fujioka H, Aikawa M, Schmatz DM. Use of beta-1,3-glucan-specific antibody to study the cyst wall of *Pneumocystis carinii* and effects of pneumocandin B0 analog L-733,560. Antimicrob Agents Chemother. 1994;38:2258–65.

10. Chou C-W, Chao H-S, Lin F-C, Tsai H-C, Yuan W-H, Chang S-C. Clinical usefulness of HRCT in assessing the severity of *Pneumocystis jirovecii* Pneumonia: a cross-sectional study. Medicine. 2015;94:e768.

11. Vogel MN, Vatlach M, Weissgerber P, Goeppert B, Claussen CD, Hetzel J, Horger M. HRCT-features of *Pneumocystis jiroveci* pneumonia and their evolution before and after treatment in non-HIV immunocompromised patients. Eur J Radiol. 2011;81:1315–20.

12. Sasso M, Chastang-Dumas E, Bastide S, Alonso S, Lechiche C, Bourgeois N, Lachaud L. Performances of four real-time PCR assays for diagnosis of *Pneumocystis jirovecii* pneumonia. J Clin Microbiol. 2015;54:625–30.

13. Hauser PM, Bille J, Lass-Flörl C, Geltner C, Feldmesser M, Levi M, Patel H, Muggia V, Alexander B, Hughes M, Follett SA, Cui X, Leung F, Morgan G, Moody A, Perlin DS, Denning DW. Multicenter, prospective clinical evaluation of respiratory samples from subjects at risk for *Pneumocystis jirovecii* infection by use of a commercial real-time PCR assay. J Clin Microbiol. 2011;49:1872–8.

14. Held J, Koch MS, Reischl U, Danner T, Serr A. Serum (1 → 3)-β-D-glucan measurement as an early indicator of *Pneumocystis jirovecii* pneumonia and evaluation of its prognostic value. Clin Microbiol Infect. 2010;17:595–602.

15. Li W-J, Guo Y-L, Liu T-J, Wang K, Kong J-L. Diagnosis of *pneumocystis* pneumonia using serum (1–3)-β-D-Glucan: a bivariate meta-analysis and systematic review. J Thorac Dis. 2015;7:2214–25.

16. Kamada T, Furuta K, Tomioka H. *Pneumocystis* pneumonia associated with human immunodeficiency virus infection without elevated (1 → 3)-β-D glucan: A case report. Respir Med Case Rep. 2016;18:73–5.

17. Phair J, Muñoz A, Detels R, Kaslow R, Rinaldo C, Saah A. The risk of *Pneumocystis carinii* pneumonia among men infected with human immunodeficiency virus type 1. Multicenter AIDS Cohort Study Group. N Engl J Med. 1990;322:161–5.

18. Avino LJ, Naylor SM, Roecker AM. *Pneumocystis jirovecii* pneumonia in the non-HIV-infected population. Ann Pharmacother. 2016;50:673–9.

19. Moukhlis R, Boyer J, Lacube P, Bolognini J, Roux P, Hennequin C. Linking *Pneumocystis jiroveci* sulfamethoxazole resistance to the alleles of the DHPS gene using functional complementation in *Saccharomyces cerevisiae*. Clin Microbiol Infect. 2009;16:501–7.

20. Queener SF, Cody V, Pace J, Torkelson P, Gangjee A. Trimethoprim resistance of dihydrofolate reductase variants from clinical isolates of *Pneumocystis jirovecii*. Antimicrob Agents Chemother. 2013;57:4990–8.

21. Xinqiang L. An analysis of adverse reactions induced by compound sulfamethoxazole tablets in 267 cases. Chin J Pharmaco Epidemiol. 2004;13:139–40.

22. Borchani C, Fonteyn F, Jamin G, Destain J, Willems L, Paquot M, Blecker C, Thonart P. Structural characterization, technological functionality, and physiological aspects of fungal β-D-glucans: a review. Crit Rev Food Sci Nutr. 2015;56:1746–52.

23. Vassallo R, Standing JE, Limper AH. Isolated *Pneumocystis carinii* cell wall glucan provokes lower respiratory tract inflammatory responses. J Immunol. 2000;164:3755–63.

24. Utili R, Durante-Mangoni E, Basilico C, Mattei A, Ragone E, Grossi P. Efficacy of caspofungin addition to trimethoprim-sulfamethoxazole treatment for severe Pneumocystis pneumonia in solid organ transplant recipients. Transplantation. 2007;84:685–8.

25. Armstrong-James D, Stebbing J, John L, Murungi A, Bower M, Gazzard B, Nelson M. A trial of caspofungin salvage treatment in PCP pneumonia. Thorax. 2011;66:537–8.

26. Fichera M, Roos D. A plastid organelle as a drug target in apicomplexan parasites. Nature. 1997;390:407–9.

27. Seaberg LS, Parquette AR, Gluzman IY, Phillips GW, Brodasky TF, Krogstad DJ. Clindamycin activity against chloroquine-resistant *Plasmodium falciparum*. J Infect Dis. 1984;150:904–11.

28. Vale N, Moreira R, Gomes P. Primaquine revisited six decades after its discovery. Eur J Med Chem. 2009;44:937–53.

29. Queener SF, Bartlett MS, Richardson JD, Durkin MM, Jay MA, Smith JW. Activity of clindamycin with primaquine against *Pneumocystis carinii in vitro* and *in vivo*. Antimicrob Agents Chemother. 1988;32:807–13.

30. Toma E, Thorne A, Singer J, Raboud J, Lemieux C, Trottier S, Bergeron MG, Tsoukas C, Falutz J, Lalonde R, Gaudreau C, Therrien R. Clindamycin with primaquine vs. Trimethoprim-sulfamethoxazole therapy for mild and moderately severe *Pneumocystis carinii* pneumonia in patients with AIDS: a multicenter, double-blind, randomized trial (CTN 004). CTN-PCP Study Group. Clin Infect Dis. 1998;27:524–30.

31. Smego J, Nagar S, Maloba B, Popara M. A meta-analysis of salvage therapy for *Pneumocystis carinii* pneumonia. Arch Intern Med. 2001;161:1529–33.

32. Zhang Y, Zhang H, Xu J, Wu C, Ma X. Lack of response in severe *pneumocystis* pneumonia to combined caspofungin and clindamycin treatment: a case report. Chin Med Sci J. 2011;26:246–8.

33. Chou C-W, Lin F-C, Tsai H-C, Chang S-C. The impact of concomitant pulmonary infection on immune dysregulation in *Pneumocystis jirovecii* pneumonia. BMC Pulm Med. 2014;14:182.

Efficacy of concurrent treatments in idiopathic pulmonary fibrosis patients with a rapid progression of respiratory failure: an analysis of a national administrative database in Japan

Keishi Oda[1], Kazuhiro Yatera[1*], Yoshihisa Fujino[2], Hiroshi Ishimoto[1,5], Hiroyuki Nakao[3], Tetsuya Hanaka[1], Takaaki Ogoshi[1], Takashi Kido[1], Kiyohide Fushimi[4], Shinya Matsuda[2] and Hiroshi Mukae[1,5]

Abstract

Background: Some IPF patients show a rapid progression of respiratory failure. Most patients are treated with high-dose corticosteroids. However, no large clinical studies have investigated the prognosis or efficacy of combined treatments including high-dose corticosteroids in IPF patients with a rapid progression of respiratory failure.

Methods: We enrolled IPF patients who received mechanical ventilation and high-dose corticosteroids between April 2010 and March 2013. Records were extracted from a Japanese nationwide inpatient database. We conducted a retrospective epidemiologic and prognostic analysis.

Results: Two hundred nine patients receiving an average of 12.8 days of ventilatory support were enrolled. There were 138 (66 %) fatal cases; the median survival was 21 days. The short-term (within 30 days) and long-term (within 90 days) survival rates were 44.6 and 24.6 %, respectively. The average monthly admission rate among the IPF patients with the rapid progression of respiratory failure in the winter was significantly higher than that in spring ($p = 0.018$). Survival did not differ to a statistically significant extent in the different geographic areas of Japan. Survivors were significantly younger ($p = 0.002$) with higher rates of mild dyspnea on admission ($p = 0.012$), they more frequently underwent bronchoscopy ($p < 0.001$), and received anticoagulants ($p = 0.027$), co-trimoxazole ($p < 0.001$) and macrolide ($p = 0.02$) more frequently than non-survivors. A multivariate logistic analysis demonstrated that two factors were significantly associated with a poor prognosis: >80 years of age (OR = 2.94, 95 % CI 1.044–8.303; $p = 0.041$) and the intravenous administration of high-dose cyclophosphamide (OR = 3.17, 95 % CI 1.101–9.148; $p = 0.033$). Undergoing bronchoscopy during intubation (OR = 0.25, 95 % CI 0.079–0.798; $p = 0.019$) and the administration of co-trimoxazole (OR = 0.28, 95 % CI 0.132–0.607; $p = 0.001$) and macrolides (OR = 0.37, 95 % CI 0.155–0.867; $p = 0.033$) were significantly associated with a good prognosis. The dosage of co-trimoxazole significantly correlated with survival.

Conclusions: Co-trimoxazole and macrolides may be a good addition to high-dose corticosteroids in the treatment of IPF patients with a rapid progression of respiratory failure.

Keywords: Acute exacerbation of idiopathic pulmonary fibrosis, Mechanical ventilation, Corticosteroid, Co-trimoxazole, Macrolide, Nationwide database, Acute respiratory failure

* Correspondence: yatera@med.uoeh-u.ac.jp
[1]Department of Respiratory Medicine, University of Occupational and Environmental Health, Japan, 1-1, Iseigaoka, Yahatanishiku, Kitakyushu City, Fukuoka 807-8555, Japan
Full list of author information is available at the end of the article

Background

Idiopathic pulmonary fibrosis (IPF) is a progressive parenchymal lung disease with an estimated median survival of 3–5 years from the time of diagnosis [1, 2]. The disease behavior in patients with IPF is usually diverse, with some IPF patients showing the rapid progression of respiratory failure [3, 4]. The mortality rate in IPF patients with severe respiratory failure who require a ventilator is around 90 % [5].

Most of the severe IPF patients who show rapid progression of respiratory failure receive high-dose corticosteroids [3, 6]. The 2011 international evidence-based guideline indicates that it as weak positive recommendation [2] in patients with definite or suspected [7] acute exacerbation of IPF (AE-IPF). Thus far, however, there have been no large clinical data sets to investigate the prognosis of patients with AE-IPF who receive ventilator treatment and high-dose corticosteroids. In addition, patients with AE-IPF are pathologically heterogeneous [8], and the appropriate treatment strategy for AE-IPF patients is not fully understood. Recent treatments for patients with AE-IPF include new agents, such as thrombomodulin [9, 10] and new ventilator setting strategies that aim to avoid valotrauma [11, 12]. Such treatments show some promise in their potential to improve the survival rate.

The aim of the present study was to evaluate the epidemiology and prognosis of IPF patients with severe rapid progression of respiratory failure who required ventilator support in Japan, using a large, contemporary, and comprehensive Japanese clinical database, and to explore effective combined treatment options that include the administration of high-dose corticosteroids.

Methods

Data source

We used the Japanese Diagnosis Procedure Combination (DPC) database, a nationwide inpatient database, to collect patient data. The details of the DPC inpatient database have been described previously [13]. Briefly, the DPC is a case-mix patient classification system which includes the clinical data and information on the date of admission, the charges, and the quantity of medical care items. The database is linked with a lump-sum per-diem payment system. Data from hospitals including all 82 university hospitals in Japan are gathered and merged into a standardized electronic format by the Japanese Ministry of Health, Labour, and Welfare. The database covers more than 1,500 acute care hospitals located throughout Japan and about 50,000 hospital beds. It represents approximately 50 % of all of the acute care hospitalizations during the same period in Japan. The database includes the main diagnoses, comorbidities present at admission and in-hospital complications as

defined in the International Classification of Diseases and Related Health Problems, 10th Revision (ICD-10) codes and text data (in Japanese). The database also includes the following data: patient age and sex; height; body weight; Fletcher, Hugh-Jones (F, H-J) classification; Brinkman Index; drug use; diagnostic and therapeutic procedures; date of admission; length of stay; status at discharge; and the unique identifiers of the hospitals. Attending physicians are obliged to record the diagnoses for each patient at discharge with reference to medical charts to optimize the accuracy of the recorded diagnoses. All of the data were anonymously collected in the database, thus the requirements for informed consent were waived. This study was approved by the Ethics Committee of Tokyo Medical and Dental University, Tokyo, Japan (approval number 788).

Patient selection and data retrieval

From the total of 39,504 patients who were admitted to the hospitals with a principal diagnosis of other interstitial pulmonary diseases with fibrosis (ICD-10 code J841) and who were discharged between April 2010 and March 2013 patients, we excluded 35,900 patients who did not receive invasive mechanical ventilation within one week after admission because we intended to only evaluate IPF patients with the rapid progression of respiratory failure. Next, non-IPF patients ($n = 1,655$) were excluded based on the text data, followed by patients who were not treated with high-dose corticosteroids (methylprednisolone: ≥ 500 mg, daily) within one week after admission ($n = 1,740$). The final study population included 209 patients (Fig. 1). These patients did not include any patients with viral, fungal or infectious bacterial pulmonary diseases as the main diagnosis or as comorbidities at the time of admission.

Definition of variables

Subjective respiratory symptoms, such as cough and dyspnea, were measured using the F, H-J classification [14]. The institution criteria authorized by The Japanese Respiratory Society were used for defining a respiratory specialized hospital. The seasons on admission were defined as follows: "spring," from March to May; "summer," from June to August; "fall," from September to November; and "winter" from December to February.

Statistical analyses

A poisson multivariable regression analysis was used to evaluate the differences in the admission rates between the seasons to adjust for the effect of the fiscal year. The chi-squared test or Fisher's exact test were used as appropriate to analyze the differences in the clinical features between survivors and non-survivors. To analyze the prognostic factors for overall survival, a univariate

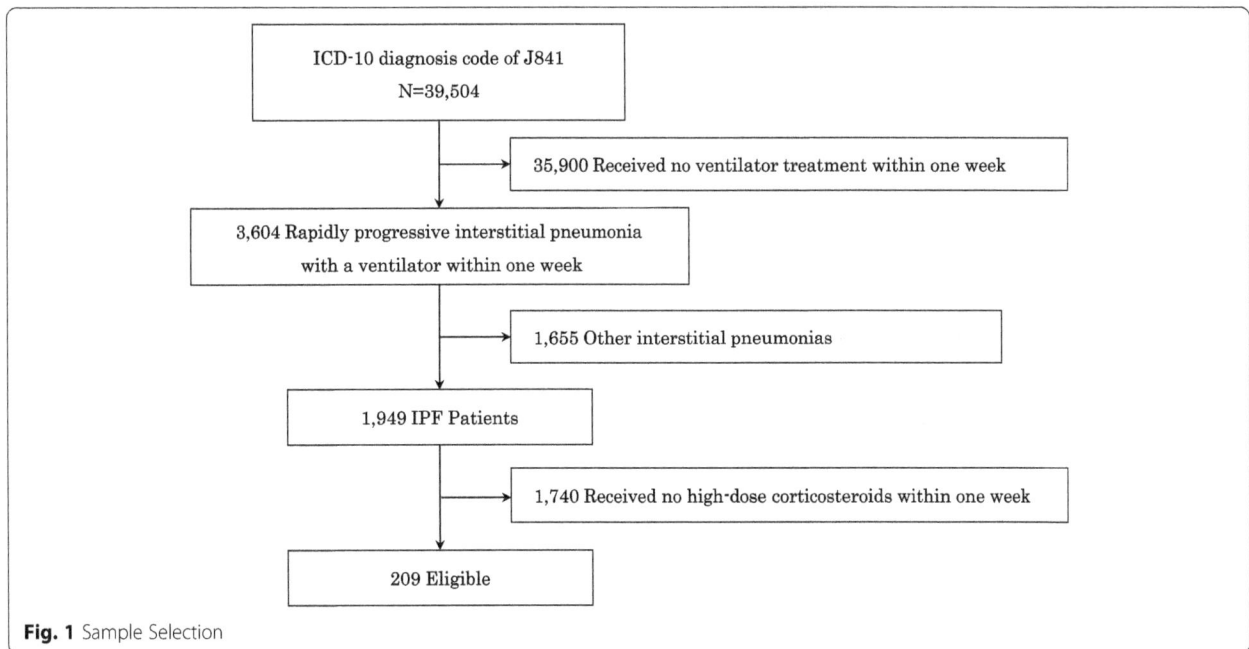

Fig. 1 Sample Selection

logistic regression were initially used to select statistically significant clinical characteristics (sex, age, performing bronchoscopy and an F, H-J classification) and to evaluate each treatment effect (the variables included treatments were applicable at least 10 % of all patients). The final multivariate logistic regression models with backward elimination were also used including the predictors (sex, age, significant clinical characteristics and the treatment). Odds ratios (OR) and 95 % confidence intervals (CI) were calculated. P values of <0.05 were considered to be statistically significant. All calculations were performed using the STATA 13 software program (Stata, College Station, TX).

Results
Patient characteristics
The clinical characteristics of the patients are shown in Table 1. The mean (standard deviation; SD) age was 72.3 (9.6) years and 82.3 % of the patients were men. The average monthly admission rate among the IPF patients with the rapid progression of respiratory failure in the winter was significantly higher than that in spring ($p = 0.018$), but was not significantly different to the rates in summer ($p = 0.065$) and fall ($p = 0.379$). The rate of emergent transfer was 48.3, and 82.8 % of the patients were admitted to specialty hospitals. Ventilatory support was provided for an average of 12.8 days.

Outcome
The number of patients with fatal outcomes was 138 of 209 (66 %) during the observation period. The

median survival period was approximately 21 days after admission. The short-term (within 30 days) and long-term (within 90 days) survival rates were 44.6 and 24.6 %, respectively (Fig. 2). The Hokuriku area had the highest rate of short-term survival (60 %), however, this rate was not significantly different from other areas (Fig. 3). Bronchoscopy and tracheostomy was performed in 20 (9.6 %) and 16 (7.7 %) patients during hospitalization, respectively. The patient characteristics of the survivors (patients who discharged alive) and the non-survivor (patients who died in the hospital) are summarized in Table 2. The survivors were younger ($p = 0.002$), with mild symptoms of dyspnea on admission ($p = 0.012$), higher rates of bronchoscopy during intubation ($p < 0.001$), anticoagulant (unfractionated and low-molecular-weight heparin) use ($p = 0.027$), co-trimoxazole use ($p < 0.001$) and macrolide use ($p = 0.020$) in comparison to non-survivors. Twenty-seven of 71 (38 %) survivors who were discharged from the hospitals received home oxygen therapy.

Prognostic factors
A univariate logistic analysis indicated two significant risk factors for in-hospital mortality: ≥80 years of age ($p = 0.033$) and an F, H-J classification scale of 5 ($p = 0.012$), whereas the performance bronchoscopy, and the use of anticoagulants, co-trimoxazole and macrolides were correlated with a good prognosis (Table 3). The multivariate logistic analysis demonstrated that two variables were significantly correlated with in-hospital mortality: ≥80 years of age ($p = 0.041$) and

Table 1 The clinical characteristics of the participants

	N (%)	Mean ± SD
Patients	209	
Age, years	209	72.3 ± 9.6
<60	17 (8.1)	
60–69	52 (24.9)	
70–79	98 (46.9)	
≥80	42 (20.1)	
Male	172 (82.3)	
BMI, kg/m²	178	22.3 ± 3.8
<18.5	27 (15.2)	
18.5–25	114 (64.0)	
>25	37 (20.8)	
Brinkman Index	184	599.5 ± 675.7
0	68 (37.0)	
1–800	45 (24.5)	
>800	71 (33.6)	
F, H-J Classification scale	166	
1	2 (1.2)	
2	4 (2.4)	
3	7 (4.2)	
4	28 (16.9)	
5	125 (75.3)	
Season		
Spring	48 (23.0)	
Summer	34 (16.2)	
Fall	56 (26.8)	
Winter	71 (34.0)*	
Specialty hospital		
Yes/No	173 (82.8)/36 (17.2)	
Arrival by ambulance		
Yes/No	101 (48.3)/108 (51.7)	

Abbreviations: BMI body mass index, *F, H-J* Fletcher, Hugh-Jones. Values are given as mean ± SD or n (%). The total dose was not equal to 209 because there were missing values in the data file. *Significantly different in comparison to spring (*p* = 0.018, poisson regression)

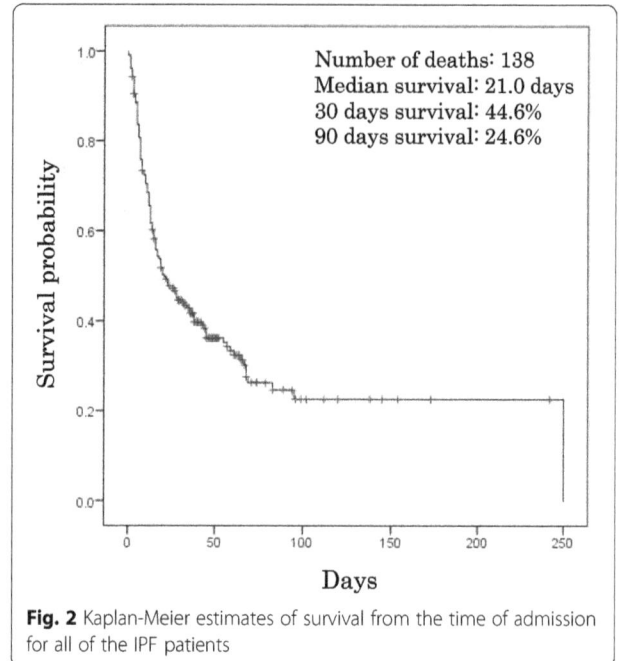

Fig. 2 Kaplan-Meier estimates of survival from the time of admission for all of the IPF patients

Number of deaths: 138
Median survival: 21.0 days
30 days survival: 44.6%
90 days survival: 24.6%

the intravenous administration of high-dose cyclophosphamide (≥100 mg, daily) (*p* = 0.033). In contrast, the following variables were significantly correlated with a good prognosis: the performance of bronchoscopy during intubation (OR = 0.25, 95 % Cl 0.079–0.798; *p* = 0.019), and the administration of co-trimoxazole (OR = 0.28, 95 % Cl 0.132–0.607; *p* = 0.001) and macrolides (OR = 0.37, 95 % Cl 0.155–0.867; *p* = 0.022). The mortality rates of the patients who were treated in specialty and non-specialty hospitals did not differ to a statistically significant extent.

The relationship between survival and co-trimoxazole dosage

We examined the difference in the survival rates of patients who were treated with by co-trimoxazole tablets (sulfamethoxazole [400 mg] and trimethoprim [80 mg]) or the equivalent dose of co-trimoxazole granules and injections. Figure 4 represents the relationship between the survival rates of three groups of patients who were treated with different doses of co-trimoxazole. The doses were defined as follows: high dose (solid line; ≥6 tablets daily, *n* = 74), low dose (broken line; 1–5 tablets daily, *n* = 41) and no co-trimoxazole (dotted line; *n* = 94). Co-trimoxazole treatment in the low-dose and high-dose groups was initiated an average of 7.9 and 8.3 days after admission, respectively. The survival of the patients in the high-dose group was significantly longer than that in the low-dose and no co-trimoxazole groups (log rank *p* < 0.001). The survival of the patients in the low-dose group was also significantly longer than that in the no co-trimoxazole group (log rank *p* = 0.009) (Fig. 4).

Discussion

Thus far, there have been no large data sets on the prognosis and prognostic factors in IPF patients with rapid progression of respiratory failure. The data of the present study, which were extracted from a nation-wide Japanese epidemiological database show, for the first time, the current prognosis of IPF patients with rapid progression of respiratory failure who receive treatment with high-dose corticosteroids. Treatments with co-trimoxazole and macrolides were significantly associated

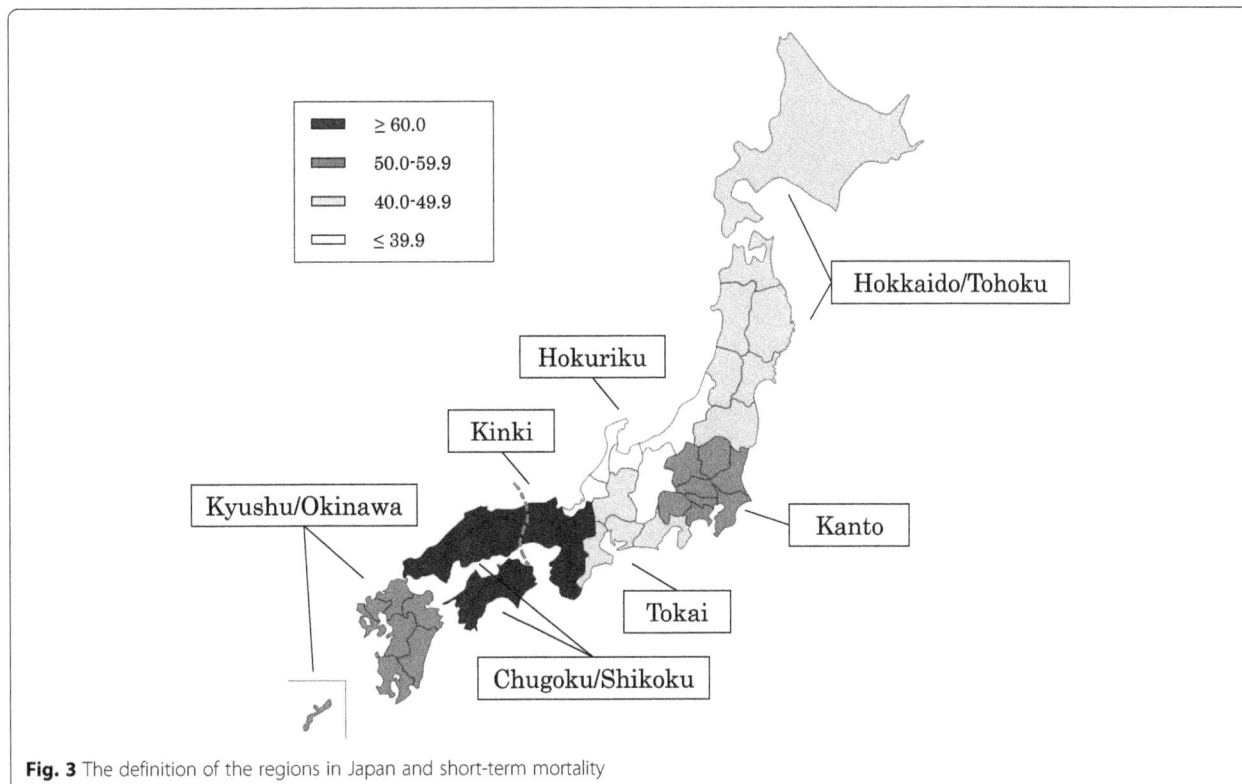

Fig. 3 The definition of the regions in Japan and short-term mortality

with a good prognosis and are considered to be effective when administered in combination with high-dose corticosteroids. The performance of bronchoscopy during ventilatory support was also correlated with a good prognosis. Conversely, the intravenous administration of high-dose cyclophosphamide was significantly associated with a poor prognosis. Our findings suggest that these managements may improve the morbidities associated with severe rapidly progressive of IPF.

Using a large, nationally representative Japanese database allowed us to investigate the prognostic factors for in-hospital mortality in IPF patients with rapid progression of respiratory failure. The application of mechanical ventilation in IPF patients with respiratory failure is considered to be a "weak" recommendation [2]. The 90-day mortality rate of patients with severe rapidly progressive IPF who received mechanical ventilation (75.4 %) was lower than the previously reported rate (approximately 90 %) [5, 15]. Our results indicate that in such patients, the provision of mechanical ventilation may still be controversial. Similarly to stable patients with IPF [16], IPF patients who were older than 80 years of age showed a very poor prognosis in the present study. According to our data, ventilatory support may not be recommended in these patients. Similar to a previous report [17], a significantly higher number of patients were admitted due to IPF with rapid progression of respiratory failure in

winter than in spring; however, there were no location-based differences in Japan. In contrast with stable patients with IPF [18], no differences of mortality were observed according to whether or patients were admitted to specialty or non-specialty hospitals.

Although there have only been limited data on the role of bacterial infection in IPF patients, recent reports suggest the high importance of infectious causes and the importance of the progression of IPF [19, 20] in the development of AE-IPF [21]. In cases where the exclusion of infectious causes was insufficient (e.g. when they were diagnosed by the analysis of endotracheal aspirate or bronchoalveolar lavage fluid), they were considered as cases of suspected AE-IPF. It has been reported that the prognosis of patients with suspected AE-IPF is not significantly different to that of patients with definite AE-IPF [7]. The data in the present study showed that the performance of bronchoscopy might be related to a better prognosis (Table 3). The majority of AE-IPF patients received empiric antimicrobial treatments, which targeted common respiratory pathogens (although there has been no data to support their use in AE-IPF patients) [22]. The infectious causes of respiratory failure can easily missed, even when several microbiological tests are performed for clinical reasons: in the treatment of such patients it is not usually possible to wait for microbiological results, and antimicrobial treatments are

Table 2 The comparison of the clinical features of survivors and the non-survivors

	Survivors	Non-survivors	p-value
Patients	71	138	
Age, years	69.3 ± 10.2	73.8 ± 8.8	0.002
Male	56 (78.9)	116 (84.1)	0.352
BMI, kg/m^2	22.2 ± 3.9	22.3 ± 3.8	0.795
Brinkman Index			
0/1–800/>800	26/14/25	42/31/46	0.719
F, H-J Classification scale			
1/2/3/4/5	1/3/3/16/42	1/1/4/12/83	0.012
Specialty hospital care	60 (84.5)	113 (81.9)	0.634
Ambulance transfer	32 (45.1)	69 (50.0)	0.499
Performing bronchoscopy	14 (19.7)	6 (4.4)	<0.001
Treatment regimen use			
Sivelestat	37 (52.1)	67 (48.9)	0.626
Diuretic drug	37 (52.1)	65 (47.1)	0.492
Anticoagulant therapy	37 (52.1)	50 (36.2)	0.027
Immunosuppressive therapy	30 (42.3)	45 (32.6)	0.169
Intravenous high-dose cyclophosphamide	9 (12.7)	23 (16.7)	0.448
PMX	4 (5.6)	9 (6.5)	0.801
Recombinant human soluble thrombomodulin	3 (4.2)	6 (4.4)	0.967
Antibiotic therapy	71 (100)	135 (97.8)	0.211
β-Lactams	60 (84.5)	116 (84.1)	0.933
Co-trimoxazole	56 (78.9)	59 (42.8)	<0.001
Quinolones	38 (53.5)	65 (47.1)	0.379
Macrolides	23 (32.4)	25 (18.1)	0.020
Tetracycline	6 (8.5)	12 (8.7)	0.952
Anti-MRSA antibiotics	6 (8.5)	11 (7.8)	0.904
Clindamycin	3 (4.2)	2 (1.5)	0.214
Aminoglycoside	2 (2.8)	1 (0.7)	0.228
Others	5 (7.0)	7 (5.1)	0.562

Data are presented as mean ± SD or n (%), unless otherwise indicated. Definition of abbreviations: BMI = Body Mass Index, F, H-J = Fletcher, Hugh-Jones, PMX = Direct hemoperfusion with polymyxin B-immobilized fiber, MRSA = Methicillin-resistant *Staphylococcus aureus*. The total dose was not equal to 209 because there were missing values in the data file

considered to be low risk. The results of the present study suggest that antibiotic treatments (other than co-trimoxazole and macrolides) may not contribute to the survival of AE-IPF patients with respiratory failure. This study also showed a trend towards poor survival in patients who were treated with immunosuppressants, especially intravenous high-dose cyclophosphamide. Currently, there is no strong evidence to support the use of immunosuppressants in AE-IPF patients with respiratory failure, and further studies will be needed to evaluate the role of immunosuppressants when they are administered in combination with high-dose corticosteroids.

Several reports have described the relationship between the prognosis of IPF patients and the administration of co-trimoxazole or macrolides. Shimizu et al. hypothesized that the specific role of co-trimoxazole was linked to a high prevalence of *Pneumocystis jiroveci* colonization among patients with stable IPF [23]. Shulgina et al. also reported that the addition of co-trimoxazole therapy to the standard treatment for stable patients with fibrotic idiopathic interstitial pneumonia resulted in improved quality of life and a reduction in mortality [24]. Huie et al. investigated the potential role of infection in the exacerbation of acute respiratory symptoms in patients with IPF [25] and showed *P. jiroveci* may be associated with the onset of AE-IPF. Our data indicated that the administration of co-trimoxazole mortality in IPF patients with rapid progression of respiratory failure, not only at the treatment

Table 3 Prognostic factors for survival

Variable	N (%)	Univariate logistic analysis			Multivariate logistic analysis		
		OR	95 % CI	p-value	OR	95 % CI	p-value
Age, years	209						
<60	17 (8.1)	ref			ref		
60–69	52 (24.9)	1.12	0.374–3.362	0.839			
70–79	98 (46.9)	1.83	0.647–5.196	0.254			
≥80	42 (20.1)	3.78	1.110–12.858	0.033	2.94	1.044–8.303	0.041
Male	172 (82.3)	1.41	0.681–2.930	0.354			
BMI, kg/m^2	178						
<18.5	27 (15.2)	ref					
18.5–25	114 (64.0)	1.43	0.604–3.388	0.415			
>25	37 (20.8)	1.13	0.409–3.117	0.814			
Brinkman Index	184						
0	68 (37.0)	ref					
1–800	45 (24.5)	1.37	0.617–3.046	0.439			
>800	71 (33.6)	1.14	0.571–2.271	0.712			
F, H-J Classification scale	166						
1–4	41 (24.7)	ref			ref		
5	125 (75.3)	2.53	1.229–5.187	0.012	2.13	0.931–4.856	0.073
Specialty hospital care	173 (82.8)	0.83	0.382–1.799	0.635			
Ambulance transfer	101 (48.3)	1.22	0.686–2.164				
Performing bronchoscopy	20 (9.6)	0.19	0.068–0.506	0.001	0.25	0.079–0.798	0.019
Sivelestat	104 (49.8)	0.87	0.489–1.538	0.626			
Diuretic drug	102 (48.8)	0.82	0.461–1.451	0.493			
Anticoagulant therapy	87 (41.6)	0.52	0.292–0.933	0.028			
Immunosuppressive therapy	75 (35.9)	0.66	0.366–1.193	0.17			
Intravenous high-dose cyclophosphamide	32 (15.3)	1.38	0.601–3.160	0.449	3.17	1.101–9.148	0.033
PMX	13 (6.2)	1.17	0.347–3.935	0.801			
Recombinant human soluble thrombomodulin	9 (4.3)	1.03	0.250–4.247	0.967			
Antibiotic therapy	206 (98.6)	–	–				
β-Lactams	176 (84.2)	0.97	0.440–2.126	0.933			
Co-trimoxazole	115 (55.0)	0.20	0.103–0.388	<0.001		0.28	0.132–0.607
Quinolones	103 (49.3)	0.77	0.436–1.372	0.38			
Macrolides	48 (23.0)	0.46	0.239–0.893	0.022		0.37	0.155–0.867
Tetracycline	18 (8.6)	1.03	0.370–2.875	0.952			
Anti-MRSA antibiotics	17 (8.1)	0.94	0.332–2.651	0.904			
Clindamycin	5 (2.4)	0.33	0.054–2.042	0.235			
Aminoglycoside	3 (1.4)	0.25	0.022–2.826	0.264			
Others	12 (5.7)	0.71	0.216–2.307	0.564			

Data are presented as n (%), unless otherwise indicated. Definition of abbreviations: *BMI* body mass index, *F, H-J* Fletcher, Hugh-Jones, *PMX* Direct hemoperfusion with polymyxin B-immobilized fiber, *MRSA* Methicillin-resistant *Staphylococcus aureus*

dose for *P. jiroveci* but also at lower doses. This favorable effect of co-trimoxazole might, in addition to its antimicrobial activity against *P. jiroveci*, may be due to its anti-inflammatory effect: co-trimoxazole might have reduced the neutrophil-derived oxidative stress [26]. Macrolides have also been reported to have anti-inflammatory effects [27, 28]. Kawamura et al. reported that azithromycin was associated with improved outcomes in patients with acute exacerbation of chronic fibrosing interstitial pneumonia [29]. The administration of macrolides and co-trimoxazol

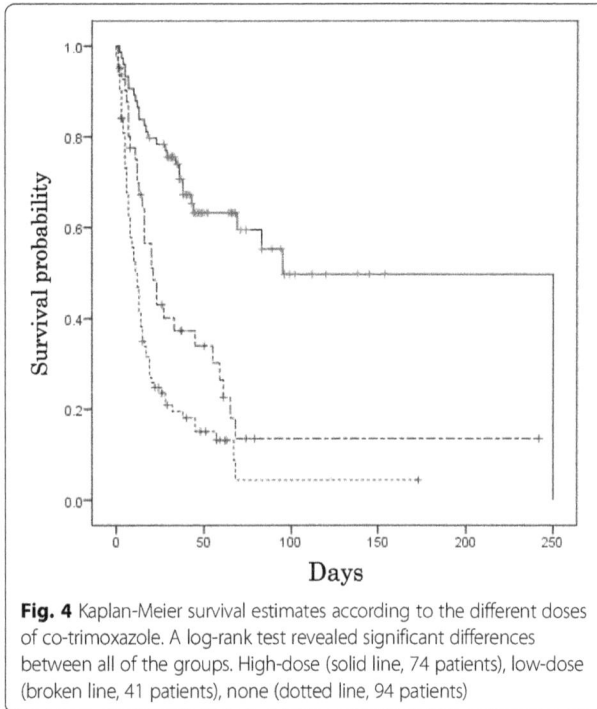

Fig. 4 Kaplan-Meier survival estimates according to the different doses of co-trimoxazole. A log-rank test revealed significant differences between all of the groups. High-dose (solid line, 74 patients), low-dose (broken line, 41 patients), none (dotted line, 94 patients)

may therefore increase the survival rate in patients with AE-IPF.

The present study is associated with several limitations. First, this study was a retrospective observational study. However, the analysis of the large data set of the DPC database system allowed us to perform our study in a large patient population. Tzilas et al. reported the weakness of the ICD coding system [30]; however, in addition to the ICD data our study also used the text data that were recorded in the DPC database system to clarify the physicians' diagnoses. Second, several clinical variables were not obtained, including the medication data and the patients' respiratory function before admission, and the results of bacteriological tests. However, we only enrolled IPF patients with rapid progression of respiratory failure in whom a ventilator was used on admission to ensure that the severity of IPF in our study population was uniform at the start of the observation period. Third, the DPC database system can only record in-hospital data, thus the data of the patients who were discharged from the DPC hospitals was not available and the contribution of their medications to survival may be underestimated. Finally, it is uncertain whether the regional clinical pathway would work the same way in other countries where health systems and policies differ from those in Japan. The effectiveness of the clinical pathway has been shown to be inconsistent in different areas and further studies are necessary to examine the applicability of this system to other countries.

Conclusion

We herein showed the epidemiology and prognosis of IPF patients with rapid progression of respiratory failure in recent years using a national administrative database in Japan. The performance of bronchoscopy during intubation, and the administration of co-trimoxazole and macrolides were significantly good prognostic factors. The concomitant use of co-trimoxazole in addition to high-dose corticosteroids may improve survival in IPF patients with rapid exacerbation of respiratory failure. Further clinical trials are necessary to verify the findings of the present study.

Key messages

- Rapid progression of respiratory failure in IPF patients was frequently seen in the winter. Older age and a higher grade of dyspnea on admission were poor prognostic factors. In addition, the prognosis of the patients did not differ in relation to the geographic area of Japan or in patients who were treated in a specialized hospital.

- The results of this study indicate that the prognosis of patients who underwent a bronchoscopic examination was better prognosis than those who did not; however, the performance of bronchoscopy in AE-IPF patients might be controversial.

- Regarding the treatment of IPF patients with rapid progression of respiratory failure, the use of high-dose corticosteroids in combination with macrolides and co-trimoxazole may lead to a better prognosis. However, prospective randomized controlled trials are necessary to elucidate the clinical effects of these agents.

Abbreviations
AE-IPF, Acute exacerbation of IPF; CI, Confidence Intervals; DPC, Diagnosis Procedure Combination; F, H-J, Fletcher, Hugh-Jones; ICD-10, International Classification of Diseases and Related Health Problems, 10th Revision; IPF, Idiopathic Pulmonary Fibrosis; OR, Odds ratios

Acknowledgements
This research was partly supported by a grant to the Diffuse Lung Diseases Research Group from the Ministry of Health, Labour and Welfare, Japan and was a Ministry of Education, Science, Sports and Culture Grant-in-Aid for Scientific Research (B), 2013–2015 (25860665, Keishi Oda).

Funding
None.

Authors' contributions
KO and KY had full access to all the data in the study and takes responsibility for the integrity of the data and the accuracy of the data analysis. YF, KF, SM contributed to the data collection. KY and HM contributed to preparing the manuscript. T.H, T.O and T.K contributed to the design of the protocol. YF

and HN contributed to the statistical data analysis. All authors read and approved the final manuscript.

Competing interests

The authors declare that they have no competing interests.

Author details

[1]Department of Respiratory Medicine, University of Occupational and Environmental Health, Japan, 1-1, Iseigaoka, Yahatanishiku, Kitakyushu City, Fukuoka 807-8555, Japan. [2]Department of Preventive Medicine and Community Health, University of Occupational and Environmental Health, Japan, 1-1, Iseigaoka, Yahatanishiku, Kitakyushu City, Fukuoka 807-8555, Japan. [3]Miyazaki Prefectural Nursing University, 3-5-1 Manabino, Miyazaki city, Miyazaki 880-0929, Japan. [4]Department of Health Care Informatics, Tokyo Medical and Dental University Graduate School, 1-5-45 Yushima, Bunkyoku, Tokyo 113-8510, Japan. [5]Second Department of Internal Medicine, Nagasaki University School of Medicine, 1-7-1 Sakamoto, Nagasaki 852-8501, Japan.

References

1. Natsuizaka M, Chiba H, Kuronuma K, Otsuka M, Kudo K, Mori M, Bando M, Sugiyama Y, Takahashi H. Epidemiologic survey of Japanese patients with idiopathic pulmonary fibrosis and investigation of ethnic differences. Am J Respir Crit Care Med. 2014;190(7):773–9.
2. Raghu G, Collard HR, Egan JJ, Martinez FJ, Behr J, Brown KK, Colby TV, Cordier JF, Flaherty KR, Lasky JA, et al. An official ATS/ERS/JRS/ALAT statement: idiopathic pulmonary fibrosis: evidence-based guidelines for diagnosis and management. Am J Respir Crit Care Med. 2011;183(6):788–824.
3. Kondoh Y, Taniguchi H, Kawabata Y, Yokoi T, Suzuki K, Takagi K. Acute exacerbation in idiopathic pulmonary fibrosis. Analysis of clinical and pathologic findings in three cases. Chest. 1993;103(6):1808–12.
4. Collard HR, Moore BB, Flaherty KR, Brown KK, Kaner RJ, King TE, Lasky JA, Loyd JE, Noth I, Olman MA, et al. Acute exacerbations of idiopathic pulmonary fibrosis. Am J Respir Crit Care Med. 2007;176(7):636–43.
5. Mallick S. Outcome of patients with idiopathic pulmonary fibrosis (IPF) ventilated in intensive care unit. Respir Med. 2008;102(10):1355–9.
6. Song JW, Hong SB, Lim CM, Koh Y, Kim DS. Acute exacerbation of idiopathic pulmonary fibrosis: incidence, risk factors and outcome. Eur Respir J. 2011;37(2):356–63.
7. Collard HR, Yow E, Richeldi L, Anstrom KJ, Glazer C, investigators I. Suspected acute exacerbation of idiopathic pulmonary fibrosis as an outcome measure in clinical trials. Respir Res. 2013;14:73.
8. Oda K, Ishimoto H, Yamada S, Kushima H, Ishii H, Imanaga T, Harada T, Ishimatsu Y, Matsumoto N, Naito K, et al. Autopsy analyses in acute exacerbation of idiopathic pulmonary fibrosis. Respir Res. 2014;15(1):109.
9. Juarez MM, Chan AL, Norris AG, Morrissey BM, Albertson TE. Acute exacerbation of idiopathic pulmonary fibrosis-a review of current and novel pharmacotherapies. J Thorac Dis. 2015;7(3):499–519.
10. Kataoka K, Taniguchi H, Kondoh Y, Nishiyama O, Kimura T, Matsuda T, Yokoyama T, Sakamoto K, Ando M. Recombinant human thrombomodulin in acute exacerbation of idiopathic pulmonary fibrosis. Chest 2015;148(2):436–43.
11. Bhatti H, Girdhar A, Usman F, Cury J, Bajwa A. Approach to acute exacerbation of idiopathic pulmonary fibrosis. Ann Thorac Med. 2013;8(2):71–7.
12. Antoniou KM, Wells AU. Acute exacerbations of idiopathic pulmonary fibrosis. Respiration. 2013;86(4):265–74.
13. Kuwabara K, Matsuda S, Fushimi K, Ishikawa KB, Horiguchi H, Hayashida K, Fujimori K. Contribution of case-mix classification to profiling hospital characteristics and productivity. Int J Health Plann Manage. 2011;26(3):e138–50.
14. FLETCHER CM. The clinical diagnosis of pulmonary emphysema; an experimental study. Proc R Soc Med. 1952;45(9):577–84.
15. Gaudry S, Vincent F, Rabbat A, Nunes H, Crestani B, Naccache JM, Wolff M, Thabut G, Valeyre D, Cohen Y, et al. Invasive mechanical ventilation in patients with fibrosing interstitial pneumonia. J Thorac Cardiovasc Surg. 2014;147(1):47–53.
16. Raghu G, Chen SY, Yeh WS, Maroni B, Li Q, Lee YC, Collard HR. Idiopathic pulmonary fibrosis in US Medicare beneficiaries aged 65 years and older: incidence, prevalence, and survival, 2001–11. Lancet Respir Med. 2014;2(7):566–72.
17. Olson AL, Swigris JJ, Raghu G, Brown KK. Seasonal variation: mortality from pulmonary fibrosis is greatest in the winter. Chest. 2009;136(1):16–22.
18. Lamas DJ, Kawut SM, Bagiella E, Philip N, Arcasoy SM, Lederer DJ. Delayed access and survival in idiopathic pulmonary fibrosis: a cohort study. Am J Respir Crit Care Med. 2011;184(7):842–7.
19. Molyneaux PL, Cox MJ, Willis-Owen SA, Mallia P, Russell KE, Russell AM, Murphy E, Johnston SL, Schwartz DA, Wells AU, et al. The role of bacteria in the pathogenesis and progression of idiopathic pulmonary fibrosis. Am J Respir Crit Care Med. 2014;190(8):906–13.
20. Han MK, Zhou Y, Murray S, Tayob N, Noth I, Lama VN, Moore BB, White ES, Flaherty KR, Huffnagle GB, et al. Lung microbiome and disease progression in idiopathic pulmonary fibrosis: an analysis of the COMET study. Lancet Respir Med. 2014;2(7):548–56.
21. Kim DS, Park JH, Park BK, Lee JS, Nicholson AG, Colby T. Acute exacerbation of idiopathic pulmonary fibrosis: frequency and clinical features. Eur Respir J. 2006;27(1):143–50.
22. Collard HR, Loyd JE, King TE, Lancaster LH. Current diagnosis and management of idiopathic pulmonary fibrosis: a survey of academic physicians. Respir Med. 2007;101(9):2011–6.
23. Shimizu Y, Sunaga N, Dobashi K, Fueki M, Fueki N, Makino S, Mori M. Serum markers in interstitial pneumonia with and without Pneumocystis jirovecii colonization: a prospective study. BMC Infect Dis. 2009;9:47.
24. Shulgina L, Cahn AP, Chilvers ER, Parfrey H, Clark AB, Wilson EC, Twentyman OP, Davison AG, Curtin JJ, Crawford MB, et al. Treating idiopathic pulmonary fibrosis with the addition of co-trimoxazole: a randomised controlled trial. Thorax. 2013;68(2):155–62.
25. Huie TJ, Olson AL, Cosgrove GP, Janssen WJ, Lara AR, Lynch DA, Groshong SD, Moss M, Schwarz MI, Brown KK, et al. A detailed evaluation of acute respiratory decline in patients with fibrotic lung disease: aetiology and outcomes. Respirology. 2010;15(6):909–17.
26. Anderson R, Grabow G, Oosthuizen R, Theron A, Van Rensburg AJ. Effects of sulfamethoxazole and trimethoprim on human neutrophil and lymphocyte functions in vitro: in vivo effects of co-trimoxazole. Antimicrob Agents Chemother. 1980;17(3):322–6.
27. Kanoh S, Rubin BK. Mechanisms of action and clinical application of macrolides as immunomodulatory medications. Clin Microbiol Rev. 2010;23(3):590–615.
28. Ishimoto H, Mukae H, Sakamoto N, Amenomori M, Kitazaki T, Imamura Y, Fujita H, Ishii H, Nakayama S, Yanagihara K, et al. Different effects of telithromycin on MUC5AC production induced by human neutrophil peptide-1 or lipopolysaccharide in NCI-H292 cells compared with azithromycin and clarithromycin. J Antimicrob Chemother. 2009;63(1):109–14.
29. Kawamura K, Ichikado K, Suga M, Yoshioka M. Efficacy of azithromycin for treatment of acute exacerbation of chronic fibrosing interstitial pneumonia: a prospective, open-label study with historical controls. Respiration. 2014;87(6):478–84.
30. Tzilas V, Bouros D. Inherent weaknesses of the current ICD coding system regarding idiopathic pulmonary fibrosis. Eur Respir J. 2015;45(4):1194–6.

Permissions

The contributors of this book come from diverse backgrounds, making this book a truly international effort. This book will bring forth new frontiers with its revolutionizing research information and detailed analysis of the nascent developments around the world.

We would like to thank all the contributing authors for lending their expertise to make the book truly unique. They have played a crucial role in the development of this book. Without their invaluable contributions this book wouldn't have been possible. They have made vital efforts to compile up to date information on the varied aspects of this subject to make this book a valuable addition to the collection of many professionals and students.

This book was conceptualized with the vision of imparting up-to-date information and advanced data in this field. To ensure the same, a matchless editorial board was set up. Every individual on the board went through rigorous rounds of assessment to prove their worth. After which they invested a large part of their time researching and compiling the most relevant data for our readers.

The editorial board has been involved in producing this book since its inception. They have spent rigorous hours researching and exploring the diverse topics which have resulted in the successful publishing of this book. They have passed on their knowledge of decades through this book. To expedite this challenging task, the publisher supported the team at every step. A small team of assistant editors was also appointed to further simplify the editing procedure and attain best results for the readers.

Apart from the editorial board, the designing team has also invested a significant amount of their time in understanding the subject and creating the most relevant covers. They scrutinized every image to scout for the most suitable representation of the subject and create an appropriate cover for the book.

The publishing team has been an ardent support to the editorial, designing and production team. Their endless efforts to recruit the best for this project, has resulted in the accomplishment of this book. They are a veteran in the field of academics and their pool of knowledge is as vast as their experience in printing. Their expertise and guidance has proved useful at every step. Their uncompromising quality standards have made this book an exceptional effort. Their encouragement from time to time has been an inspiration for everyone.

The publisher and the editorial board hope that this book will prove to be a valuable piece of knowledge for researchers, students, practitioners and scholars across the globe.

List of Contributors

Philip J. Langridge, Reyenna L. Sheehan and David W. Denning
The National Aspergillosis Centre, ERC, 2nd floor, University Hospital South Manchester, Southmoor Road, Manchester M23 9LT, UK

David W. Denning
The University of Manchester; Manchester Academic Health Science Centre, Manchester, UK

Elaine Nguyen, Craig I. Coleman and Erin R. Weeda
University of Connecticut School of Pharmacy, 69 North Eagleville Road, Unit 3092, Storrs, CT 06269, USA

W. Frank Peacock
Department of Emergency Medicine, Baylor College of Medicine, 1504 Taub Loop, Houston, TX, USA

Philip S. Wells
Department of Medicine, University of Ottawa, Ottawa Hospital Research Institute, 501 Smyth Road, Ottawa, ON, Canada

Concetta Crivera, Peter Wildgoose, Jeff R. Schein and Veronica Ashton
Janssen Scientific Affairs, LLC, 1000 Route 202, Raritan, NJ, USA

Thomas J. Bunz
New England Health Analytics, LLC, Granby, CT, USA

Gregory J. Fermann
Department of Emergency Medicine, University of Cincinnati, 231 Albert Sabin Way, Cincinnati, OH, USA

Joshua J. Mooney
Stanford University, Stanford, CA, USA

Karina Raimundo
Genentech, Inc, South San Francisco, CA, USA

Eunice Chang and Michael S. Broder
Partnership for Health Analytic Research, LLC, Beverly Hills, CA, USA

Shenglan Pu, Daoxin Wang, Yan Zhao, Di Qi, Jing He and Guoqi Zhou
Department of Respiratory Medicine, Second Affiliated Hospital of Chongqing Medical University, Chongqing 400010, China

Daishun Liu
Department of Respiratory and Critical Care Medicine, The First People's Hospital of Zunyi, Zunyi, China

Nicole Ezer, Kevin Schwartzman and Anne V. Gonzalez
Respiratory Epidemiology and Clinical Research Unit, Montreal Chest Institute, McGill University Health Centre, Montreal, QC, Canada

Linda Ofiara, Nicole Ezer, Kevin Schwartzman and Anne V. Gonzalez
Respiratory Division, McGill University Health Centre, Montreal, QC, Canada

Asma Navasakulpong
Respiratory and Respiratory Critical Care Medicine, Faculty of Medicine, Prince of Songkla University, Songkhla, Thailand

Youfeng Zhu, Haiyan Yin and Rui Zhang
Department of Intensive Care Unit, Guangzhou Red Cross Hospital, Medical College, Jinan University, Tongfuzhong Road No. 396, Guangzhou, Guangdong province 510220, China

Jianrui Wei
Department of Cardiology, Guangzhou Red Cross Hospital, Medical College, Jinan University, Guangzhou, Guangdong province 510220, China

Jong Sik Lee, Sung Koo Han and Jae-Joon Yim
Division of Pulmonary and Critical Care Medicine, Department of Internal Medicine, Seoul National University College of Medicine, 101, Daehak-ro, Jongno-gu, Seoul 03080, Republic of Korea

Jong Hyuk Lee and Soon Ho Yoon
Department of Radiology, Seoul National University College of Medicine, 101, Daehak-ro, Jongno-gu, Seoul 03080, Republic of Korea

Taek Soo Kim and Moon-Woo Seong
Department of Laboratory Medicine, Seoul National University Hospital, 101, Daehak-ro, Jongno-gu, Seoul 03080, Republic of Korea

Ruth L. Dentice
Physiotherapy Department, Royal Prince Alfred Hospital, Sydney, Australia

Peter T. P. Bye and Mark R. Elkins
Sydney Medical School, University of Sydney, Sydney, Australia

Mark R. Elkins
Centre for Education and Workforce Development, Sydney Local Health District, Sydney, Australia

Genevieve M. Dwyer
Physiotherapy Program, Western Sydney University, Sydney, Australia

Peter T. P. Bye
Department of Respiratory and Sleep Medicine, Royal Prince Alfred Hospital, Sydney, Australia

Takashi Kido, Takaaki Ogoshi, Keishi Oda, Hiroshi Mukae and Kazuhiro Yatera
Department of Respiratory Medicine, University of Occupational and Environmental Health, 1-1 Iseigaoka, Yahatanishi-ku, Kitakyushu, Japan

Toshihiko Mayumi, Hiroki Otsubo and Takashi Kido
Department of Emergency Medicine, University of Occupational and Environmental Health, Kitakyushu, Japan

Yoshihisa Fujino, Shinya Matsuda, Tatsuhiko Kubo and Keiji Muramatsu
Department of Preventive Medicine and Community Health, University of Occupational and Environmental Health, Kitakyushu, Japan

Takeshi Asakawa
Department of Information Systems Center, University of Occupational and Environmental Health, Kitakyushu, Japan

Hiroshi Mukae
Second Department of Internal Medicine, Nagasaki University Hospital, Nagasaki, Japan

Mario Boehm, Changwu Lu, Tatyana Novoyatleva, Friedrich Grimminger, Hossein A. Ghofrani, Norbert Weissmann, Werner Seeger, Ralph T. Schermuly and Baktybek Kojonazarov
Universities of Giessen and Marburg Lung Center (UGMLC), Excellence Cluster Cardio-Pulmonary System (ECCPS), Member of the German Center for Lung Research (DZL), Aulweg 130, 35392, Giessen, Germany

Allan Lawrie, Nadine Arnold, Adam Braithwaite and Josephine Pickworth
Department of Infection, Immunity and Cardiovascular Disease, University of Sheffield, Sheffield, UK

David G. Kiely
Sheffield Pulmonary Vascular Disease Unit, Royal Hallamshire Hospital, Sheffield, UK

Giorgio Conti, Giorgia Spinazzola, Giuliano Ferrone, Olimpia Festa, Marco Piastra, Luca Tortorolo and Roberta Costa
Intensive Care and Anaesthesia Department and Ventilab, Catholic University of Rome, Policlinico A. Gemelli, Largo Agostino Gemelli 8, 00168 Rome, Italy

Cesare Gregoretti and Andrea Cortegiani
Department of Biopathology and Medical Biotechnologies (DIBIMED), Section of Anesthesia, Analgesia, Intensive Care and Emergency. Policlinico Paolo Giaccone, University of Palermo, Via del vespro 129, 90127 Palermo, Italy

M. Molina-Molina, V. Vicens-Zygmunt, J. Dorca and A. Montes-Worboys
Department of Pneumology, Bellvitge University Hospital, Barcelona, Spain

C. Machahua-Huamani, J. Dorca, V. Vicens-Zygmunt, M. Molina-Molina and A. Montes-Worboys
Pneumology Research Group, IDIBELL, University of Barcelona, Barcelona, Spain

E. Sala-Llinas, J. Dorca, M. Molina-Molina and A. Montes-Worboys
Research Network in Respiratory Diseases (CIBERES), ISCIII, Madrid, Spain

R. Llatjós
Department of Pathology, Bellvitge University Hospital, Barcelona, Spain

I. Escobar
Department of Thoracic Surgery, Bellvitge University Hospital, Barcelona, Spain

P. Luburich-Hernaiz
Servei de Diagnostic per la Imatge El Prat (SDPI El Prat) Department of Radiology, Bellvitge University Hospital, Barcelona, Spain

E. Sala-Llinas
Department of Penumology, Son Espases University Hospital, Palma de Mallorca, Spain

A. Montes-Worboys
Laboratori de Pneumologia Experimental (Lab. 4126). IDIBELL, Pavelló de Govern. Campus de Bellvitge, Universitat de Barcelona, Hospital de Bellvitge, Carrer de la Feixa Llarga, 08907 L'Hospitalet de Llobregat, Barcelona, Spain

Paola Faverio, Federica De Giacomi, Luca Sardella, Grazia Messinesi and Alberto Pesci
Dipartimento Cardio-Toraco-Vascolare, University of Milan Bicocca, Respiratory Unit, San Gerardo Hospital, ASST di Monza, Via Pergolesi 33, 20900 Monza, Italy

Giuseppe Fiorentino
UOC di Fisiopatologia e Riabilitazione Respiratoria, AO Ospedali dei Colli Monaldi, Naples, Italy

Francesco Salerno and Mauro Carone
UOC Pulmonology and Pulmonary Rehabilitation, Istituti Clinici Scientifici Maugeri, IRCCS di Cassano Murge (BA), Cassano delle Murge, Italy

Jousel Ora and Paola Rogliani
Division of Respiratory Medicine, University Hospital Tor Vergata, Rome, Italy

Giulia Pellegrino and Giuseppe Francesco Sferrazza Papa
Dipartimento di Scienze Neuroriabilitative, Casa di Cura del Policlinico, Milan, Italy

Francesco Bini
Department of Internal Medicine, UOC Pulmonology, Ospedale ASST-Rhodense, Garbagnate Milanese, Italy

Bruno Dino Bodini
Pulmonology Unit, Ospedale Maggiore della Carità, University of Piemonte Orientale, Novara, Italy

Antonio Esquinas
Internsive Care Unit, Hospital Morales Meseguer, Múrcia, Spain

Andrzej Labyk, Dominik Wretowski, Sabina Zybińska-Oksiutowicz, Aleksandra Furdyna, Katarzyna Ciesielska, Olga Dzikowska –Diduch, Barbara Lichodziejewska, Piotr Pruszczyk and Marek Roik
Center for Diagnostics and Treatment of Venous Thromboembolism, Department of Internal Medicine and Cardiology, Warsaw Medical University, Infant Jesus Hospital, Lindleya Street 4, 02-005 Warsaw, Poland

Dorota Piotrowska-Kownacka
Department of Radiology, Infant Jesus Hospital, Lindleya Street 4, 02-005 Warsaw, Poland

Andrzej Biederman
Cardiac Surgery Department Medicover Hospital, Rzeczypospolitej 5 Avenue, 02-972 Warsaw, Poland

Camilla Koch Ryrsø, Peter Lange and Ulrik Winning Iepsen
The Centre of Inflammation and Metabolism and the Centre for Physical Activity Research, Rigshospitalet, University of Copenhagen, Blegdamsvej 9, DK-2100 Copenhagen, Denmark

Henriette Edemann Callesen, Britta Tendal and Camilla Koch Ryrsø
Danish Health Authority, Copenhagen, Denmark

Nina Skavlan Godtfredsen
Department of Respiratory Medicine, Copenhagen University Hospital, Hvidovre, Denmark
Department of Clinical Medicine, University of Copenhagen, Copenhagen, Denmark

Linette Marie Kofod
Department of Physiotherapy, Copenhagen University Hospital, Hvidovre, Denmark

Marie Lavesen
Department of Pulmonary and Infectious Diseases, Copenhagen University Hospital, Nordsjælland, Hillerød, Denmark

Line Mogensen
The Department of the Elderly and Disabled, Odense Municipality, Odense, Denmark

Randi Tobberup
Department of Gastroenterology, Center for Nutrition and Bowel Disease, Aalborg University Hospital, Aalborg, Denmark

Ingeborg Farver-Vestergaard
Unit for Psychooncology and Health Psychology, Aarhus University Hospital and Aarhus University, Aarhus, Denmark

Peter Lange
Department of Public Health, Section of Social Medicine, University of Copenhagen, Copenhagen, Denmark
Medical Department O, Respiratory Section, Herlev and Gentofte Hospital, Herlev, Denmark

Kamran Khan Sumalani and Nadeem Ahmed Rizvi
Department of Chest Medicine, Jinnah Postgraduate Medical Centre, Karachi 75400, Pakistan

Asif Asghar
Department of Thoracic Surgery, Combined Military Hospital, Peshawar, Pakistan

Adolfo Baloira
Hospital de Montecelo, Mourente, s/n, 36071 Pontevedra, Spain

José Miguel Rodriguez Gonzalez-Moro
Hospital Universitario Príncipe de Asturias, Alcalá de Henares, Madrid, Spain

Estefanía Sanjuán
CAP María Bernades, Viladecans, Barcelona, Spain

Juan Antonio Trigueros
Centro de Salud Menasalbas, Toledo, Spain

Ricard Casamor
Novartis Farmacéutica S.A, Barcelona, Spain

Luca Valko, Szabolcs Baglyas, Janos Gal and Andras Lorx
Department of Anesthesiology and Intensive Therapy, Semmelweis University, 1082 Üllői út 78B, Budapest, Hungary

Carmine Dario Vizza
Department of Cardiovascular and Respiratory Disease, University of Rome La Sapienza, Viale del Policlinico 155, 00161 Rome, Italy

B. K. S. Sastry
CARE Hospitals, Gandhi Bhavan Road Nampally, Hyderabad, India

Zeenat Safdar
Baylor College of Medicine, 1 Baylor Plaza, Houston, TX 77030, USA

Lutz Harnisch
Pfizer Ltd, Ramsgate Road, Sandwich Kent CT13 9NJ, UK

Xiang Gao and Manisha Lamba
Pfizer Inc, 558 Eastern Point Rd, Groton, CT 06340, USA

Min Zhang
Pfizer Inc, 10646 Science Center Dr, La Jolla Campus, San Diego, CA 92121, USA

Zhi-Cheng Jing
Shanghai Pulmonary Hospital, Tongji University School of Medicine, 507, Zhengmin Road, Shanghai, China

Tiffany J. Dwyer, Rahizan Zainuldin and Jennifer A. Alison
Discipline of Physiotherapy, Faculty of Health Sciences, University of Sydney, Sydney, Australia

Evangelia Daviskas, Peter T. P. Bye and Tiffany J. Dwyer
Department of Respiratory Medicine, Royal Prince Alfred Hospital, Sydney, Australia

Peter T. P. Bye and Tiffany J. Dwyer
Central Clinical School, Sydney Medical School, University of Sydney, Sydney, Australia

Rahizan Zainuldin
Rehabilitation Department, Ng Teng Fong General Hospital, Jurong Health Services, Jurong East, Singapore
Health and Social Sciences, Academic Programme, Singapore Institute of Technology, Jurong East, Singapore

Jennifer A. Alison
Department of Physiotherapy, Royal Prince Alfred Hospital, Sydney, Australia

Hongjuan Li
Department of Emergency, Guangdong Hospital of Traditional Chinese Medicine, Guangzhou, Guangdong 510105, China

Haoming Huang
Department of Emergency, Guangzhou University of Traditional Chinese Medicine First Affiliated Hospital, Guangzhou, Guangdong 510405, China

Hangyong He
Department of Respiratory and Critical Care Medicine, Beijing Chao-Yang Hospital, Capital Medical University, Beijing 100020, China

Keishi Oda, Kazuhiro Yatera, Hiroshi Ishimoto, Tetsuya Hanaka, Takaaki Ogoshi, Takashi Kido and Hiroshi Mukae
Department of Respiratory Medicine, University of Occupational and Environmental Health, Japan, 1-1, Iseigaoka, Yahatanishiku, Kitakyushu City, Fukuoka 807-8555, Japan

Shinya Matsuda and Yoshihisa Fujino
Department of Preventive Medicine and Community Health, University of Occupational and Environmental Health, Japan, 1-1, Iseigaoka, Yahatanishiku, Kitakyushu City, Fukuoka 807-8555, Japan

Hiroyuki Nakao
Miyazaki Prefectural Nursing University, 3-5-1 Manabino, Miyazaki city, Miyazaki 880-0929, Japan

Kiyohide Fushimi
Department of Health Care Informatics, Tokyo Medical and Dental University Graduate School, 1-5-45 Yushima, Bunkyoku, Tokyo 113-8510, Japan

Hiroshi Ishimoto and Hiroshi Mukae
Second Department of Internal Medicine, Nagasaki University School of Medicine, 1-7-1 Sakamoto, Nagasaki 852-8501, Japan

Index

A

Acute Eosinophilic Pneumonia, 102, 106, 109

Acute Interstitial Pneumonia, 102, 106, 108

Acute Respiratory Distress Syndrome, 22-23, 28-30, 47, 62-63, 67-68, 78, 83, 102, 106, 176, 179

Acute Respiratory Failure, 20, 39-42, 47-48, 77, 83-84, 98-103, 106, 109-110, 179, 181

Aldosterone, 69-76

Allergic Bronchopulmonary Aspergillosis, 2, 7-8

Arterial Blood Pressure Regulation, 69

Arterial Oxygen Partial Pressure, 22-23, 27-29

Aspergillus, 1-8

Aspergillus Bronchitis, 2, 6, 8

Aspergillus Fumigatus, 1, 6-8

B

Balloon Pulmonary Angioplasty, 111-112, 114-115

Bronchoalveolar Lavage, 5, 8, 98, 100-102, 106, 108-109, 176, 179, 185

Burkholderia Cepacia Complex, 58, 168

C

Chronic Hypersensitivity Pneumonitis, 101, 106, 108

Chronic Obstructive Pulmonary Disease, 14, 17, 20, 40, 103, 106, 116-117, 130, 132-133, 140, 142, 144, 146-147, 149-150, 153-154

Chronic Pulmonary Aspergillosis, 2, 7-8

Chronic Thromboembolic Pulmonary Hypertension, 111, 114-115

Clarithromycin Resistance, 49

Continuous Positive Airway Pressure, 40, 47, 81, 84, 103, 106, 153, 176

Conventional Oxygen Therapy, 39-42, 47-48, 98, 104, 109

Corticosteroid, 62-67, 102, 175-176, 179, 181

Cryptogenic Organizing Pneumonia, 102, 106

Cystic Fibrosis, 4, 7-8, 56-61, 167-168, 173-174

E

Endobronchial Ultrasound-guided Needle Aspiration (ebus), 31

Endotracheal Intubation, 43, 48, 104, 106

Endotracheal Tube, 77-79, 81-83

Enzyme-linked Immunosorbent Assay, 96

Eplerenone, 69-76

Extracorporeal Membrane Oxygenation, 98, 103, 105-106, 109-110

F

Forced Expiratory Volume, 58-60, 132, 141-143, 146, 170, 173

Forced Vital Capacity, 59-60, 96, 100, 141-142, 146, 170

H

High-flow Nasal Cannula, 39-40, 47-48, 84, 98, 100, 103, 106, 109, 176

High-flow Nasal Cannula Oxygen Therapy, 39, 48, 109

I

Idiopathic Pulmonary Fibrosis, 13, 20-21, 85, 96-100, 107-110, 158, 181-182, 188-189

Inhalation Therapy, 42, 56, 59

Inhaled Tobramycin, 57, 60

Intensive Care Unit, 20, 22-23, 29, 47-48, 77-78, 83-84, 100, 107-109, 150, 152, 176, 179, 189

Interstitial Lung Diseases, 68, 98-100, 105, 107-109

L

Lymphangioleiomiomatosis, 86, 96

M

Mechanical Ventilation, 13, 15, 18-20, 22, 27, 30, 40, 47, 63-67, 77, 81, 84, 98, 100-101, 104, 107-109, 148-154, 181-182, 185, 189

Methicillin Resistant Staphylococcus Aureus, 6-7

Multiloculated Empyema, 134

Mycobacterium Abscessus Subspecies Abscessus, 49, 55

Mycobacterium Avium Complex, 49, 55

Myocardial Infarction, 10-11, 14, 17-20, 76, 135

N

Nebullsation, 56-58

Non-invasive Ventilation, 13-16, 18, 47-48, 77, 81, 83-84, 98, 100, 103-105, 107, 109

Non-small Cell Lung Cancer, 32, 37-38

Noninvasive Ventilation, 13, 20, 30, 40, 47, 83-84, 105, 109-110, 148-154

Nontuberculous Mycobacteria, 49, 51-52, 54-55

P

Pirfenidone, 20-21, 85-97, 107

Pneumocystis Pneumonia, 1, 7-8, 175, 179-180

Positive End Expiratory Pressure, 78, 83, 105

Pressure Support Ventilation, 77, 83-84

Pseudomonas Aeruginosa, 1, 3, 6

Pulmonary Angiography, 10, 111-114

Pulmonary Arterial Hypertension, 69, 75-76, 155, 165-166

Pulmonary Artery Endothelial Cells, 70, 73, 75

Pulmonary Artery Wedge Pressure, 112, 114, 156

Pulmonary Embolism, 9-12, 98, 101, 106, 111

Pulmonary Fibrosis, 13, 20-21, 85-86, 88, 94-100, 107-110, 158, 181-182, 188-189

Pulmonary Hypertension, 14, 17, 69, 75-76, 100, 111, 114-115, 155, 157, 166

Pulmonary Pressure Ratio, 113-114

Pulmonary Tuberculosis, 2, 61

Pulmonary Vascular Resistance, 69, 112, 114, 155, 159, 163, 165

R

Radio Immunoprecipitation Assay, 96

Rapamycin, 75, 85-97

Reperfusion Pulmonary Injury, 113-115

S

Sarcoidosis, 33, 99-100, 107-108, 110-115

Simplified Pulmonary Embolism Severity Index, 11

Sivelestat Sodium, 22, 30

Small Cell Lung Cancer, 32-33, 37-38

Sputum, 1-8, 50-51, 55, 109, 167-174, 176-178

Streptococcus Pneumoniae, 1, 6

T

Total Pulmonary Resistance Index, 71-72

Transthoracic Needle Aspiration, 32, 37

V

Vascular Endothelial Growth Factor Receptor, 72

Video-assisted Thoracoscopic Surgery, 134-135

www.ingramcontent.com/pod-product-compliance
Lightning Source LLC
Chambersburg PA
CBHW082015190326
41458CB00010B/3197